The Pharmacy Practice
Handbook of Medication Facts

The Pharmacy Practice Handbook of Medication Facts

Harold L. Kirschenbaum, M.S., Pharm.D.
Associate Professor of Pharmacy Practice
Assistant Dean for Experiential Education
Arnold & Marie Schwartz College of Pharmacy and Health Sciences
Long Island University, 75 Dekalb Avenue, Brooklyn, New York

Michelle M. Kalis, Ph.D., R.Ph.
Associate Professor of Pharmacology
Arnold & Marie Schwartz College of Pharmacy and Health Sciences
Long Island University, 75 Dekalb Avenue, Brooklyn, New York

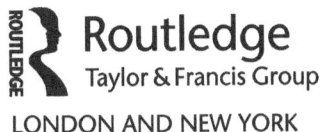

Routledge
Taylor & Francis Group

LONDON AND NEW YORK

The Pharmacy Practice Handbook of Medication Facts

First published 2000 by Technomic Publishing Company, Inc.

Published 2019 by Routledge
2 Park Square, Milton Park, Abingdon, Oxon OX14 4RN
52 Vanderbilt Avenue, New York, NY 10017

Routledge is an imprint of the Taylor & Francis Group, an informa business

Copyright © 2000 Taylor & Francis

All rights reserved. No part of this book may be reprinted or reproduced or utilised in any form or by any electronic, mechanical, or other means, now known or hereafter invented, including photocopying and recording, or in any information storage or retrieval system, without permission in writing from the publishers.

Notice:
Product or corporate names may be trademarks or registered trademarks, and are used only for identification and explanation without intent to infringe.

Main entry under title:
 The Pharmacy Practice Handbook of Medication Facts

Bibliography: p.
Includes index p. 761

Library of Congress Catalog Card No. 99-67719

ISBN 13: 978-1-56676-762-0 (pbk)

Contents

Preface   ix

Cardiovascular Agents. 1
    Calcium Channel Blockers   3
    Alpha-1 Blockers   16
    Alpha-2 Agonists   21
    Angiotensin II Receptor Antagonists   25
    Miscellaneous Antihypertensive Agents   29
    Angiotensin Converting Enzyme (ACE) Inhibitors   38
    Beta Adrenergic Blocking Agents   55
    Nitrates   78
    Antihypertensive Agents   88
    Antiarrhythmic Agents   89
    Digitalis Glycosides   107
    Diuretics—Thiazides and Related Agents   111
    Diuretics—Loop   122
    Diuretics—Potassium Sparing   129

Lipid Lowering Agents 135
    Antilipemics   137

Blood Modifiers. 149
    Anticoagulants   151
    Antiplatelet Agents   159

Respiratory Agents 163
    Antiinflammatory Agents for the Respiratory Tract   165
    Bronchodilators   180

Antihistamines 193
    Antihistamines (H_1 Receptors)   195

Antiinfectives 211
    Tetracyclines   213
    Macrolide Antibiotics   218
    Penicillins   225

vi   *Contents*

    Cephalosporins and Other Beta-lactam Antibiotics   230
    Quinolone Antibiotics and Related Agents   237
    Sulfonamides   245
    Urinary Antiinfectives   251
    Aminoglycosides   256
    Antituberculosis Agents   261
    Antifungal Agents   277
    AIDS Chemotherapeutic Agents   288
    Antimalarial Agents   301
    Miscellaneous Antiinfectives   310

Antineoplastic Agents 319
    Selected Antineoplastic Agents   321

Antiarthritic/Antigout Agents. 357
    Antiarthritic Agents   359
    Agents for Gouty Arthritis   371

Analgesics. 377
    Opioid Analgesics   379
    Non-Steroidal Antiinflammatory Agents and
        Related Agents   394

Psychotherapeutic Agents. 415
    Antianxiety Agents   428
    Antidepressants and Agents for Obsessive
        Compulsive Disorder   428
    Anti-Manic and Anti-Panic Agents   454
    Antipsychotics   460
    Sedative Hypnotics   480

Antiparkinsonian Agents 491
    Antiparkinsonian Agents   493

Antiepileptics 509
    Antiepileptics   511

Migraine Preparations. 529
    Migraine Preparations   531

Hormones 545
    Androgens   547
    Estrogens and Select Estrogen Combinations   554
    Selected Oral Contraceptives   562
    Thyroid Hormones   565
    Glucocorticoids (systemic)   569
    Miscellaneous Hormones   576

Fertility Agents 583
    Fertility Agents   585

Osteoporosis Treatments 595
    Medications for Osteoporosis   597

Antidiabetic Agents 603
    Oral Hypoglycemics and Related Agents   605
    Insulin   618

Gastrointestinal Agents 627
    Antidiarrheals   629
    Antiemetics   639
    Antispasmodics   652
    Agents for Peptic Ulcer Disease, Gastroesophageal
        Reflux Disease (GERD), and Related Conditions   661

Topical Corticosteroids 675
    Topical Corticosteroids   677

Alzheimers's Disease Agents 685
    Alzheimer's Disease Agents   687

Agents for Glaucoma 691
    Selected Glaucoma Agents   693

Agent for Erectile Dysfunction 703
    Agent for Erectile Dysfunction   705

Appendices 707
    Appendix A: Common Medical Abbreviations   709
    Appendix B: Common Pharmaceutical Abbreviations   715
    Appendix C: Common Drug Name/Category
        Abbreviations and Acronyms   718
    Appendix D: Key Laboratory Tests and
        Reference Intervals   722
    Appendix E: FDA Pregnancy Categories   726
    Appendix F: Selected Nonprescription (OTC)
        Agents Frequently Found in Combination Products   727
    Appendix G: An English-Spanish Guide for Pharmacists   733
    Appendix H: Metered Dose Inhalers   737
    Appendix I: Spacers/Holding Chambers   740
    Appendix J: Nose Drops   742
    Appendix K: Nasal Sprays, Pumps, and Inhalers   744
    Appendix L: Eye Drops   746
    Appendix M: Eye Ointments and Gels   748

Appendix N: Ear Drops 750
Appendix O: Guidelines for Administering Subcutaneous Injections 752
Appendix P: Nomograms to Determine Body Surface Area of Adults, Children, and Infants 753
Appendix Q: Conversions Among Systems Used in Pharmaceutical Calculations 756
Appendix R: Calculating Milliequivalents 758
Appendix S: Temperature Conversions 759

Index 761

Preface

With the rapidly increasing number of marketed pharmacologic agents, pharmacists, physicians, physician assistants, nurses, other health care professionals, and students in the health care field are finding it increasingly difficult to provide colleagues and patients with the types of patient-oriented information they need. The overall goal of this book is to provide this essential data in an easy-to-use, readily available, concise, and easily portable format. Chapters are arranged by therapeutic class and, in many cases, are subdivided into separate tables for the reader's convenience. The tables follow a specific format throughout the text.

Following these chapters are appendices of useful information for the health care professional and student, such as medical and pharmaceutical abbreviations as well as reference intervals for common laboratory tests. Appended as well are diagrams and text suitable for patient counseling sessions that illustrate and/or describe the proper technique for administering medications via various routes. Also, given the widespread use of the Spanish language within the United States, one appendix provides English to Spanish translations for commonly used medical/pharmaceutical words and phrases.

To use this handbook the reader should first consult the index, which indicates a specific page/table in the text where the medication is listed. In situations where a product has more than one indication, complete details about the product usually are provided in only one chapter or table, but are cross-referenced. The tables were designed to provide the reader with the opportunity to read about a specific agent or to examine a group of products used for the same or a similar condition.

In the individual tables, the most common prescription medications available in the United States are listed alphabetically by generic name. The tables also provide many of the most common trade or brand names for these products, the usual adult dosages (for FDA-approved indications as delineated in the Prescribing Information [PI]), contraindications, most common adverse effects, and other considerations such as warnings and precautions that need to be placed into perspective when evaluating an individual patient, and essential information that should be discussed with a patient during counseling sessions.

The last point highlights one of the major goals of this handbook—to provide the health care professional and student with key information that should be conveyed to patients in order to improve compliance and other outcomes. Consistent with the goals of this text as well, and to minimize duplication, material is not described twice. Thus, the reader should review at least the section on contraindications/considerations/adverse effects as well as the section on counseling before speaking with a patient. As this handbook provides the factual information or the "what" to discuss with patients, the reader may wish to review other sources that review "how" to communicate with patients. Clearly, the only way to enhance a patient's understanding and proper use of a medication is to provide accurate information in a manner that is acceptable and tailored to the individual patient's needs.

The text was developed as a "pocket handbook." Consistent with the handbook nature of this publication, there was no attempt to make the text all inclusive; similarly, it is not intended to replace standard drug information sources. The information provided concerning common trade names, adult dosages, warnings, adverse effects, etc. should be used only as a general guideline and should not be considered an official or complete source. One should also note that the majority of the medications included in this text are those used in an ambulatory setting and thus are administered orally, via inhalation/nebulizer, or topically—only select parenteral medications are included. In addition, with the exception of some of the most common combination products (eg, sulfamethoxazole/trimethoprim and carbidopa + levodopa), multiple ingredient medications are not included—the reader should review the individual components of combination products to obtain required information. If a discrepancy exists between the information found in this handbook and an official source such as the product labeling, the reader is urged to use the official source.

Due to the volume of information and the complex nature of interpreting drug-drug, drug-food, and drug-laboratory test interactions, this type of information is not included in this handbook. The reader should refer to the appropriate prescribing information (PI), tertiary sources, computer programs, and primary literature devoted to drug interactions to obtain this information. Also, due to the fact that virtually all medications are "contraindicated" in persons allergic to it or similar products, this general warning has not been listed for each medication. Nevertheless, it is essential that a patient's medication history, medication allergies, food allergies, concomitant prescription/non-prescription therapies, social history (eg, smoking and alcohol use), and other pertinent items are assessed prior to prescribing/dispensing/administering a medication.

When counseling a patient, several other key points should be conveyed:

- Use child-resistant containers whenever possible

- Medications should be kept out of the reach of children
- Medications should be stored away from heat and direct sunlight
- Do not store medications in the bathroom or in any other damp area
- Do not store medications in the refrigerator or freezer unless specifically directed to do so
- For medications available in canisters or aerosol containers, do not puncture, break, or burn them, even after they are empty
- Discard outdated medications promptly and safely
- For medications being refilled, if the medication looks different than the one used previously check with the pharmacist
- If anyone accidentally takes an overdose of the medication, seek immediate medical attention by contacting a Poison Control Center or going to a hospital's emergency department

This handbook has, for the most part, been compiled from the product labeling, the tertiary literature, and the authors' experience/opinion as to the most important information that should be conveyed to a patient. Tertiary reference sources used to prepare this text include the following:

- Anon. American Hospital Formulary Service: Drug Information. Bethesda, MD: American Society of Health System Pharmacists, Inc; 1998.
- Anon. Physicians' Desk Reference. 52nd ed. Montvale, NJ: Medical Economics Company, Inc; 1998.
- Anon. USP Dispensing Information Volume I: Drug Information for the Health Care Professional. 18th ed. Rockville, MD: The United States Pharmacopeial Convention Inc; 1998.
- Anon. USP Dispensing Information Volume II: Advice for the Patient. 18th ed, 1998. Rockville, MD: The United States Pharmacopeial Convention Inc; 1997.
- Olin BR, ed. Facts and Comparisons. St Louis, MO: Facts and Comparisons, Inc; updated monthly.

The authors and publishers hope that this text fills a necessary void, and will allow health care professionals and students to provide better care to patients.

This handbook is intended to serve as a useful guide or quick reference and is not intended to be a complete source of information about prescription medications available in the United States. This handbook provides the reader with descriptive information about many of the most common generic and trade name products including their usual adult dosages as described in product labeling, contraindications, and major adverse effects/cautions/ precautions, as well as information that should be conveyed to a patient when the specific medication is dispensed. Due to the proliferation in the number of marketed medications and the information available about each, the authors and publishers cannot be responsible for the currency of the information provided. If there is a discrepancy between the information provided here and that provided in the product labeling, the reader is urged to use the information provided in the labeling.

Cardiovascular Agents

Table 1: Calcium Channel Blockers*

Generic Name and Selected Trade Names	Normal Adult Dosage	Major Adverse Effects/Cautions	Key Counseling Points	Miscellaneous Issues
Amlodipine Besylate Norvasc	Individualize dosage For hypertension, usually start with 5 mg QD with maximum of 10 mg QD; for angina usually 5 to 10 mg QD For hypertension, small/frail/ elderly and persons with hepatic insufficiency usually start with 2.5 mg QD	Considerations: Rarely, patients have developed increased angina or acute MI; use cautiously in patients with CHF or hepatic failure Most common AEs include headache, edema, flushing, and nausea but others such as arrhythmias and dizziness are possible Pregnancy category: C	Tell the prescriber if you have CHF, liver disease, or very low blood pressure; may be taken without regard for food; notify the prescriber if you feel an irregular heart beat, develop swelling of the feet or hands, become dizzy; if you miss a dose take it as soon as you remember, but if it is almost time for the next dose skip the missed one — do not double doses	

Generic Name and Selected Trade Names	Normal Adult Dosage	Major Adverse Effects/Cautions	Key Counseling Points	Miscellaneous Issues
Bepridil HCl Vascor	Individualize dosage Usually start with 200 mg QD, may increase after 10 days to 300 mg QD and then to a maximum of 400 mg/day	<u>Contraindications</u>: Patients with history of serious ventricular arrhythmias, sick sinus syndrome, second or third degree heart block, hypotension, uncompensated cardiac insufficiency (or CHF), congenital extension of QT interval on ECG, and use with other medications that prolong QT interval <u>Considerations</u>: Can induce life-threatening and other new arrhythmias (eg, torsades de pointes); avoid in post-MI period; use caution in sinus bradycardia, left bundle branch block, and renal or hepatic impairment; may increase hepatic enzymes Most common AEs include nausea, GI distress, diarrhea, dizziness, asthenia, nervousness Pregnancy category: C	Tell the prescriber if you have heart rhythm problems; it is very important to take potassium supplements or potassium-sparing diuretics if prescribed; ECG and serum potassium levels need to be checked routinely; may be taken with meals; notify the prescriber if you feel an irregular heart beat, develop swelling of the feet or hands, become dizzy; check your pulse rate while taking this medication and contact the prescriber if it is much slower than normal or is <50 beats/minute; if you miss a dose, take it as soon as you remember, but if it is almost time for the next dose skip the missed one and return to regular schedule — do not double doses	Usually reserved for patients who cannot use other agents; medication may cause life-threatening arrhythmias, monitor patient symptoms and ECG (eg, QT interval and heart rate); routinely check serum potassium levels

Generic Name and Selected Trade Names	Normal Adult Dosage	Major Adverse Effects/Cautions	Key Counseling Points	Miscellaneous Issues
Diltiazem HCl Cardizem Cardizem CD Cardizem SR Dilacor XR Tiazac	Individualize dosage Cardizem for angina: Start with 30 mg QID (ac and hs), increase every 1–2 days as needed; usual dosage 180 to 360 mg/day Cardizem CD for angina: Start with 120 or 180 mg QD and titrate over 7–14 days up to 480 mg QD Cardizem CD for hypertension: As monotherapy, start with 180 to 240 mg QD (some patients may respond to less) and titrate after 14 days if necessary up to 480 mg QD although usual dosage is 240 to 360 mg QD	Contraindications: Both sick sinus syndrome and second or third degree AV block unless ventricular pacemaker is present, hypotension, acute MI or pulmonary congestion Considerations: May decrease heart rate so be cautious if need to use with beta blockers or digitalis; can worsen CHF; can cause symptomatic hypotension; has caused acute hepatic injury; use caution in renal or hepatic impairment Most common AEs include edema, headache, bradycardia, first-degree AV block, nausea, dizziness, rash, asthenia Pregnancy category: C	Tell the prescriber if you recently had a heart attack, or have CHF, a heart rhythm problem or any other problem with your heart; notify the prescriber if you feel an irregular heart beat, develop swelling of the feet or hands, become dizzy; check your pulse rate and contact the prescriber if it is much slower than normal or is <50 beats/minute; if you miss a dose take it as soon as you remember, but if it is almost time for the next dose, skip the missed one and return to regular dosing schedule — do not double doses For Tablets: Take before meals For Extended-release Products: Swallow whole, do not open, crush, or chew	Diltiazem is metabolized by cytochrome P-450 mixed function oxidase. Co-administration with other agents that follow this method of biotransformation may require dosage adjustment

Generic Name and Selected Trade Names	Normal Adult Dosage	Key Counseling Points	Miscellaneous Issues
Diltiazem HCl (continued) Cardizem Cardizem CD Cardizem SR Dilacor XR Tiazac	Cardizem SR for hypertension: Start with 60 to 120 mg BID and titrate after 14 days if necessary; usual dosage 240 to 360 mg/day Dilacor XR for angina: Start with 120 mg once daily and titrate if necessary over 7–14 days up to 480 mg/day Dilacor XR for hypertension: Start with 180 mg or 240 mg QD (some patients may respond to less) and may titrate up to 540 mg QD Tiazac for hypertension: As monotherapy, start with 120–240 mg QD (some patients may respond to less) and titrate after 14 days if necessary up to 540 mg/day		

Generic Name and Selected Trade Names	Normal Adult Dosage	Major Adverse Effects/Cautions	Key Counseling Points	Miscellaneous Issues
Felodipine Plendil	Individualize dosage For hypertension, usually start with 5 mg QD and titrate if needed after at least two weeks; usual maintenance is 2.5 to 10 mg QD In patients over 65 years of age and those with hepatic impairment, start with 2.5 mg QD	<u>Considerations</u>: May cause significant hypotension and rarely syncope (fainting); may cause reflex tachycardia which can precipitate angina; use caution in CHF <u>Most common AEs with monotherapy</u> include peripheral edema, headache, dizziness, flushing, palpitations, asthenia (weakness) <u>Pregnancy category</u>: C	Notify the prescriber if you feel an irregular heart beat, develop swelling of the feet or hands, or become dizzy; swallow the tablet whole, do not break, crush or chew it; may cause gum swelling which may be prevented with good oral hygiene; if you miss a dose take it as soon as you remember, but if it is almost time for the next dose skip the missed one and return to regular schedule — do not double doses	Dosage >10 mg/day associated with large increase in rate of peripheral edema and other vasodilatory AEs; monitor blood pressure very closely in elderly and in patients with hepatic impairment because higher plasma felodipine levels may develop

Generic Name and Selected Trade Names	Normal Adult Dosage	Major Adverse Effects/Cautions	Key Counseling Points	Miscellaneous Issues
Isradipine DynaCirc DynaCirc CR	Individualize dosage <u>DynaCirc for hypertension</u>: Start with 2.5 mg BID alone or with a thiazide diuretic; may titrate in 5 mg/day increments every 2–4 weeks up to 20 mg/day <u>DynaCirc CR for hypertension</u>: Start with 5 mg QD alone or with a thiazide diuretic; may titrate upward in 5 mg/day increments every 2–4 weeks up to 20 mg/day	<u>Considerations</u>: May produce symptomatic hypotension; use caution in CHF Most common AEs include headache, dizziness, palpitations, fatigue, flushing, chest pain, nausea, dyspnea, abdominal discomfort, tachycardia, rash; edema, palpitations, fatigue, and flushing appear to be dose-related (especially at higher doses of 15 to 20 mg/day) <u>Pregnancy category</u>: C	Tell the prescriber if you have CHF; notify the prescriber if you feel an irregular heart beat, develop swelling of the feet or hands, become dizzy; if you miss a dose take it as soon as you remember, but if it is almost time for the next dose skip the missed one — do not double doses For Controlled-release Product: Swallow the tablet whole — do not bite, divide, crush or chew	Dosages above 10 mg/day are associated with increased frequency of AEs and may not produce greater antihypertensive effects; bioavailability increased in patients more than 65 years of age and in patients with hepatic or renal impairment

Generic Name and Selected Trade Names	Normal Adult Dosage	Major Adverse Effects/Cautions	Key Counseling Points	Miscellaneous Issues
Nicardipine HCl Cardene Cardene SR	Individualize dosage Cardene for angina or hypertension: Usually, start with 20 mg TID, and titrate upward if needed after at least three days; 20 to 40 mg TID have been shown to be effective; in hepatic impairment start with 20 mg BID and titrate as needed maintaining the BID regimen Cardene SR for hypertension: Start with 30 mg BID; doses in the range of 30 to 60 mg BID have been shown to be effective; not studied in patients with severe hepatic impairment	<u>Contraindications</u>: Patients with advanced aortic stenosis; may increase frequency/severity of angina <u>Considerations</u>: Use caution in CHF, impaired hepatic function or reduced hepatic blood flow, impaired renal function; may produce symptomatic hypotension Most common AEs include flushing, headache, pedal edema, asthenia, palpitations, dizziness, vasodilation, tachycardia, nausea, dyspepsia, dry mouth, somnolence, rash, increased angina <u>Pregnancy category</u>: C	Tell the prescriber if you have angina, CHF, liver disease, a problem with your aorta, or very low blood pressure; notify the prescriber if you feel an irregular heart beat, develop swelling of the feet or hands, become dizzy; if you miss a dose take it as soon as you remember, but if it is almost time for the next dose skip the missed one and return to regular schedule — do not double doses For Controlled-release Product: Swallow the capsule whole — do not bite, crush or chew	May be administered with thiazide diuretics or beta blockers <u>Cardene for hypertension</u>: To assess BP control, measure BP at end of dosing interval (8 hrs after dosing); peak effect is pronounced so measure BP 1–2 hrs after dosing, especially at initiation

Generic Name and Selected Trade Names	Normal Adult Dosage	Major Adverse Effects/Cautions	Key Counseling Points	Miscellaneous Issues
Nicardipine HCl (continued) Cardene Cardene SR				<u>Cardene SR for hypertension</u>: When starting therapy or changing dosages, monitor BP 2–4 hrs after the dose and at the end of the dosing interval

Generic Name and Selected Trade Names	Normal Adult Dosage	Major Adverse Effects/Cautions	Key Counseling Points	Miscellaneous Issues
Nifedipine Adalat Adalat CC Procardia Procardia XL	Individualize dosage Adalat/Procardia for angina: Start with 10 mg TID and titrate as needed over a 7–14 day period although shorter intervals have been used; usual dosage is 10 to 20 mg TID, some patients may require more but >180 mg/day is not recommended; excessive dosage may cause hypotension	Considerations: Do not use Adalat/Procardia for rapid reduction of BP or to treat essential hypertension; excessive and poorly controlled hypotension have been reported; do not use for 1 to 2 weeks following MI or when an MI may be imminent; increased frequency/severity of angina or acute MI reported; may exacerbate angina that occurs following acute withdrawal of beta blockers — taper beta blocker therapy; may cause CHF especially if patient has tight aortic stenosis, although rare, significant elevations of enzymes such as CPK, LDH, AST, ALT are reported	Tell the prescriber if you have angina or recently had a heart attack, if you have CHF, if you have a problem with your heart valves; notify the prescriber if you feel an irregular heart beat, develop swelling of the feet or hands, become dizzy or lightheaded; if you miss a dose take it as soon as you remember, but if it is almost time for the next dose skip the missed one and return to regular schedule — do not double doses For Sustained-release Product: Swallow the capsule whole — do not bite, crush, divide or chew it; take on an empty stomach not with food; do not be alarmed if you sometimes see something that looks like a tablet in the stool	If discontinuing Adalat CC/ Procardia XL reduce dosage gradually with close medical supervision

Generic Name and Selected Trade Names	Normal Adult Dosage	Major Adverse Effects/Cautions	Key Counseling Points	Miscellaneous Issues
Nifedipine (continued) Adalat Adalat CC Procardia Procardia XL	Adalat CC/Procardia XL for hypertension: Start with 30 mg QD and titrate over 7–14 days as needed; usual dosage is 30 mg or 60 mg QD; for Adalat CC doses above 90 mg/day not recommended, for Procardia XL doses above 120 mg/day not recommended	Most common AEs include dizziness, lightheadedness, flushing, heat sensation, fatigue, headache, weakness, nausea, peripheral edema (dose-dependent with Adalat CC/Procardia XL), muscle cramps, nervousness, cough, palpitations, dyspnea, nasal congestion, wheezing Pregnancy category: C		

Generic Name and Selected Trade Names	Normal Adult Dosage	Major Adverse Effects/Cautions	Key Counseling Points	Miscellaneous Issues
Nimodipine Nimotop	To improve neurological outcomes in patients with subarachnoid hemorrhage due to ruptured aneurysms, dosage is 60 mg (2 caps) Q4H for 21 consecutive days, preferably 1 hr ac or 2 hrs pc; begin therapy within 96 hrs of subarachnoid hemorrhage. In patients with hepatic cirrhosis, reduce dosage to 30 mg Q4H and monitor BP and heart rate closely	Considerations: Dose may need to be reduced in patients with impaired hepatic function — closely monitor blood pressure (BP) and pulse rate; may decrease BP. Most common AEs include decreased BP, abnormal liver function test, edema, rash, diarrhea, headache, hepatitis, itching, nausea, palpitations, bradycardia. Pregnancy category: C	This medication is used in the treatment of a burst blood vessel in the head; tell the prescriber if you have a liver disorder; notify the prescriber if you feel an irregular heart beat, develop swelling, become dizzy or lightheaded; try to take the medication 1 hr before meals or 2 hrs after meals; if you miss a dose take it as soon as you remember, but if it is almost time for the next dose skip the missed one — do not double doses	If the capsule cannot be swallowed, make a hole in both ends of the capsule with an 18 gauge needle, extract the medication into a syringe, empty the contents into the nasogastric tube and flush the tube with 30 mL of normal saline; nimodipine must not be administered parenterally

13

Generic Name and Selected Trade Names	Normal Adult Dosage	Major Adverse Effects/Cautions	Key Counseling Points	Miscellaneous Issues
Verapamil HCl Calan Calan SR Covera-HS Isoptin Isoptin SR Verelan	Individualize dosage <u>Calan/Isoptin for angina</u>: Usual dosage is 80 to 120 mg TID (patients with hepatic impairment and some others respond to 40 mg TID); titrate at daily or weekly intervals <u>Calan/Isoptin for arrhythmias</u>: In digitalized patients with atrial fibrillation, usual dosage is 240 to 320 mg/day in a TID or QID regimen; for prophylaxis of PSVT in nondigitalized patients, usual range is 240 to 480 mg/day in TID or QID regimen; maximal response to a dose is usually seen in 48 hrs	<u>Contraindications</u>: Severe left ventricular dysfunction, hypotension, both sick sinus syndrome and second or third degree AV block unless ventricular pacemaker is present, atrial flutter or fibrillation and an accessory bypass tract such as Wolff-Parkinson-White <u>Considerations</u>: Avoid in moderate to severe cardiac failure and in patients with a ventricular dysfunction receiving beta-adrenergic blocker; may elevate liver enzymes; use caution in liver impairment and adjust dose; use caution in renal impairment; reduce dosage in patients with decreased neuromuscular transmission	Tell the prescriber if you have a heart rhythm problem, a liver or kidney disorder, low blood pressure, CHF, or any other heart problem; teach patient to monitor pulse rate regularly — contact the prescriber if it is much slower than normal or is <50 beats/minute; notify the prescriber if you feel an irregular heart beat, or become constipated, dizzy or lightheaded; if you miss a dose take it as soon as you remember, but if it is almost time for the next dose skip the missed one and return to regular schedule — do not double doses For Sustained-release Product: Swallow the medication whole — do not bite, crush, divide or chew	Many drug interactions reported — refer to prescribing information Verelan: May be administered by opening the capsule and sprinkling the contents on a spoonful of applesauce; applesauce should be swallowed immediately and not chewed, and followed with a glass of cool water to ensure complete swallowing

Generic Name and Selected Trade Names	Normal Adult Dosage	Major Adverse Effects/Cautions
Verapamil HCl (continued) Calan Calan SR Covera-HS Isoptin Isoptin SR Verelan	Calan/Isoptin for essential hypertension: For monotherapy, usual starting dose is 80 mg TID (240 mg/day), dosages of 360 and 480 mg/day have been used but there is no evidence that >360 mg/day provide additional benefit; elderly and other persons who might respond to lower dosages should start with 40 mg TID Calan SR/Isoptin SR for essential hypertension: Start with 180 mg in AM with food, patients who may have an enhanced response to therapy (eg, elderly) should begin with 120 mg; titrate weekly based on response about 24 hrs after dose administration; for recommended titration — SEE Prescribing Information (PI) Covera-HS for angina or hypertension: Start with 180 mg hs; may titrate dosage as follows: 240 mg hs, 360 mg, then 480 mg hs Verelan for hypertension: Start with 240 mg in AM, but patients who may have an enhanced response to therapy (eg, the elderly) should begin with 120 mg; titrate weekly based on response about 24 hrs after administration; if adequate response is not obtained with 120 mg in the AM, may titrate as follows: 180 mg each morning, then 240 mg in AM, then 360 mg, then 480 mg in AM	Most common AEs include constipation, dizziness, nausea, dyspnea, bradycardia, hypotension, headache, edema, CHF, AV block, fatigue, rash, flushing Pregnancy category: C

*As a general rule, a medication should not be administered to a patient with a known hypersensitivity to it or a similar agent.

Table 2: Alpha-1 Blockers*

Generic Name and Selected Trade Names	Normal Adult Dosage	Major Adverse Effects/Cautions	Key Counseling Points	Miscellaneous Issues
Doxazosin Cardura	Individualize dosage For benign prostatic hyperplasia (BPH): Start with 1 mg QD in AM or PM; while monitoring BP, may titrate every 1–2 weeks to 2 mg, 4 mg, then maximum of 8 mg QD For hypertension: Start with 1 mg QD; while monitoring BP, may titrate dosage up to 16 mg QD — dosages >4 mg/day increase likelihood of excessive postural effects such as syncope	<u>Contraindication</u>: Patients allergic to quinazolines — eg, prazosin and terazosin <u>Considerations</u>: Orthostatic hypotension is most marked with first dose, increases in dosage, or when therapy stopped for a few days and restarted — initiate therapy with 1 mg at bedtime; use caution in hepatic impairment or if patient using other medication that influences hepatic metabolism Most common AEs include dizziness/vertigo, headache, fatigue, hypotension, edema, dyspnea, somnolence <u>Pregnancy category</u>: C	Medication could cause dizziness when you stand — especially after the first dose; avoid driving or using machinery for 24 hrs after starting therapy or a dosage change; if seated, stand up slowly; sit or lie down if dizzy; dizziness (etc) more common if you drink alcohol (minimize intake), stand for a long time, exercise, and if weather is hot; may cause drowsiness; notify the prescriber if you develop bothersome dizziness, lightheadedness, or heart palpitations; if miss a dose take it as soon as you remember, but if it is almost time for the next dose skip the missed one and return to regular schedule — do not double doses	If used for BPH, first ensure patient does not have prostate cancer; doxazosin will not shrink the size of the prostate; extensively metabolized in liver; monitor BP regardless of indication

16

Generic Name and Selected Trade Names	Normal Adult Dosage	Major Adverse Effects/Cautions	Key Counseling Points	Miscellaneous Issues
Prazosin HCl Minipress	Individualize dosage For hypertension, start with 1 mg BID or TID; usual maintenance range is 6 to 15 mg/day in divided doses; doses >20 mg/day usually do not increase efficacy, but some patients need 40 mg/day in divided doses; when adding a diuretic or another antihypertensive, reduce prazosin to 1 to 2 mg TID and re-titrate	Considerations: May cause syncope with sudden loss of consciousness usually due to excessive postural hypotension but sometimes has been preceded by severe tachycardia; may minimize syncope by initiating therapy with 1 mg, titrating slowly, and adding other antihypertensive therapies cautiously Most common AEs include dizziness, headache, drowsiness, lack of energy, weakness, palpitations, nausea, flu syndrome Pregnancy category: C	SEE doxazosin	Extensively metabolized in liver to active metabolites

Generic Name and Selected Trade Names	Normal Adult Dosage	Major Adverse Effects/Cautions	Key Counselling Points	Miscellaneous Issues
Tamsulosin HCl Flomax	Individualize dosage For benign prostatic hyperplasia (BPH), start with 0.4 mg QD one-half hour following the same meal each day; may increase dose 2–4 weeks later to 0.8 mg QD; if therapy stopped for a few days start again with 0.4 mg QD	<u>Considerations</u>: May produce orthostatic hypotension; do not use with other alpha-adrenergic blockers <u>Most common AEs</u> include signs and symptoms of orthostasis (eg, syncope, dizziness, vertigo), headache, rhinitis, abnormal ejaculation, asthenia, back pain <u>Pregnancy category</u>: B	Do not open, crush or chew capsule; also SEE doxazosin	Before using, ensure patient does not have prostate cancer; monitor BP

Generic Name and Selected Trade Names	Normal Adult Dosage	Major Adverse Effects/Cautions	Key Counseling Points	Miscellaneous Issues
Terazosin HCl Hytrin	Individualize dosage For benign prostatic hyperplasia (BPH): Start with 1 mg hs; increase dose to 2 mg, 5 mg, or 10 mg QD; maintain 10 mg QD for at least 4–6 weeks to assess results; some patients respond to 20 mg QD; if therapy stopped for a few days start again with initial regimen	Considerations: SEE prazosin Most common AEs include asthenia (weakness), postural hypotension, dizziness, somnolence, impotence, nasal congestion/rhinitis, blurred vision, headache, nausea, palpitations Pregnancy category: C	Although rare, if priapism develops seek medical attention immediately; also SEE doxazosin	If used for BPH, first ensure patient does not have prostate cancer; monitor BP for either indication

Generic Name and Selected Trade Names	Normal Adult Dosage	Major Adverse Effects/Cautions	Key Counseling Points	Miscellaneous Issues
Terazosin HCl (continued) Hytrin	For hypertension: Start with 1 mg hs; titrate dosage according to patient's BP; usual maintenance dosage is 1 to 5 mg QD, but some patients may require up to 20 mg QD; Q12H regimen also acceptable; if therapy stopped for a few days start again with initial regimen			

*As a general rule, a medication should not be administered to a patient with a known hypersensitivity to it or a similar agent.

Table 3: Alpha-2 Agonists*

Generic Name and Selected Trade Names	Normal Adult Dosage	Major Adverse Effects/Cautions	Key Counseling Points	Miscellaneous Issues
Clonidine Catapres Catapres-TTS	Individualize dosage for hypertension Tablets: Start with 0.1 mg AM and hs; titrate weekly in 0.1 mg/day increments if needed; usual maintenance is 0.2 to 0.6 mg/day; maximum dosage is 2.4 mg/day Decrease dosage in renal impairment — SEE Prescribing Information (PI)	Considerations: Sudden discontinuation has resulted in symptoms such as nervousness, agitation, headache, and tremor followed by rapid increase in BP and elevated catecholamine levels — must reduce dose gradually; use cautiously in persons with severe coronary insufficiency, conduction disturbances, recent MI, cerebrovascular disease, chronic renal failure Most common AEs include dry mouth, drowsiness, dizziness, constipation, sedation, weakness/fatigue, orthostasis, palpitations, tachycardia, bradycardia, nervousness, insomnia, rash, nausea, vomiting, headache Pregnancy category: C	Do not interrupt therapy without first discussing it with prescriber; tell the prescriber if you have a kidney or heart disease; may induce drowsiness, so know how you are affected before you drive or use machinery — sedation may be enhanced by other sedatives such as alcohol; may cause dryness of mouth, try sugarless gum/candy or ice but if problem persists, contact prescriber; before undergoing any type of surgery, tell the MD or dentist that you are taking this agent; if you miss a dose of the medication, take it as soon as possible then go back to regular schedule, but if you miss 2 or more doses of the tablets contact the prescriber	Tablets should be continued up to 4 hrs prior to surgery and re-instituted as soon as possible;

Generic Name and Selected Trade Names	Normal Adult Dosage	Major Adverse Effects/Cautions	Key Counseling Points	Miscellaneous Issues
Clonidine (continued) Catapres Catapres-TTS	<u>Transdermal system:</u> Apply Catapres-TTS-1 once every 7 days (SEE Key Counseling Points); may titrate after 1–2 weeks by adding another TTS-1 or starting a larger system; effect may not be noted for 2–3 days Decrease dosage in renal impairment — SEE (PI)		For transdermal: Apply each dose to a different hairless area of intact skin on upper outer arm or chest; if system loosens, apply the extra adhesive overlay directly over the system to ensure adhesion for full 7 days; contact prescriber if you feel that patch should be removed due to redness/rash or other skin change; do not trim or cut patches; after using, fold patch in half with the sticky sides together; keep used and unused patches away from children; if you missed changing the patch for 3 days, contact the prescriber	transdermal system should not be discontinued during surgical period

Generic Name and Selected Trade Names	Normal Adult Dosage	Major Adverse Effects/Cautions	Key Counseling Points	Miscellaneous Issues
Methyldopa Aldomet	Individualize dosage For hypertension, usually start with 250 mg BID or TID for 48 hrs; may titrate at intervals of at least two days; usual maintenance dosage is 500 mg to 2 g daily in 2–4 divided doses; maximum dosage 3 g/day Patients with impaired renal function may respond to lower doses — SEE Prescribing Information (PI)	<u>Contraindications</u>: Patients with active liver disease such as acute hepatitis or active cirrhosis as well as liver disorders associated with methyldopa therapy, and patients receiving monoamine oxidase inhibitors <u>Considerations</u>: Use caution in patients with renal impairment or history of liver disease/dysfunction; positive Coomb's test, hemolytic anemia, and liver disorders associated with therapy (could be lethal); fever has occurred within the first 3 weeks of therapy and may be associated with eosinophilia or liver test abnormalities; rarely, fatal hepatic necrosis and reversible decreases in WBC counts reported	Tell the prescriber if you have taken methyldopa in the past, have a liver or kidney disorder, and if you are allergic to sulfites; while taking the medication, tell the prescriber if you develop a fever and there is no clear reason, feel weak, develop swelling in your feet or legs, have dark or amber urine, develop diarrhea or stomach cramps, or have joint pain; this medication may make you sleepy/drowsy/tired, especially when you first start therapy or when the dosage is increased; if you miss a dose take it as soon as you remember, but if it is almost time for the next dose skip the missed one and return to regular schedule — do not double doses	If tolerance develops (usually between the second and third month of therapy) adding a diuretic or increasing the dose of methyldopa will frequently restore BP control; oral suspension contains sodium bisulfite which can induce severe allergic reactions and asthmatic episodes

23

Generic Name and Selected Trade Names	Normal Adult Dosage	Major Adverse Effects/Cautions	Key Counseling Points	Miscellaneous Issues
Methyldopa (continued) Aldomet		Most common AEs include sedation, headache, asthenia, weakness, dry mouth (dizziness, lightheadedness, and drowsiness more common in elderly) <u>Pregnancy category</u>: B		

*As a general rule, a medication should not be administered to a patient with a known hypersensitivity to it or a similar agent.

Table 4: Angiotensin II Receptor Antagonists*

Generic Name and Selected Trade Names	Normal Adult Dosage	Major Adverse Effects/Cautions	Key Counseling Points	Miscellaneous Issues
Candesartan Cilexetil Atacand	Individualize dosage For hypertension, as monotherapy in non-volume depleted patients the usual starting dose is 16 mg QD; maintenance is 8 to 32 mg daily in a QD or BID regimen; consider lower dosages in patients with depleted intravascular volume No initial dosage reduction in the elderly or patients with mildly impaired renal or hepatic function	<u>Considerations</u>: Use in second and third trimester of pregnancy can cause injury and perhaps death to fetus; symptomatic hypotension may occur in patients with intravascular volume depletion; use caution in patients who require renin-angiotensin-aldosterone system to maintain renal function (eg, patients with severe CHF) Most common AEs include back pain, dizziness, upper respiratory tract infection, pharyngitis, rhinitis <u>Pregnancy category</u>: C for first trimester, D for second and third trimester	Females of childbearing age should be warned about dangers of therapy during pregnancy, should consider an appropriate birth control method, and should notify the prescriber if they become pregnant; if you miss a dose take it as soon as you remember, but if it is almost time for the next dose skip the missed one and return to regular schedule— do not double doses	Not metabolized by the cytochrome P-450 system; if BP not well controlled with monotherapy, consider adding a low-dose diuretic; if pregnancy detected while on this medication, discontinue therapy as soon as possible (see "major adverse effects/cautions")

25

Generic Name and Selected Trade Names	Normal Adult Dosage	Major Adverse Effects/Cautions	Key Counseling Points	Miscellaneous Issues
Irbesartan Avapro	Individualize dosage For hypertension, usual initial dosage is 150 mg QD; may titrate to 300 mg QD Dosage adjustment not needed in elderly or patients with hepatic impairment or mild to severe renal impairment	<u>Considerations</u>: SEE candesartan <u>Most common AEs</u> include diarrhea, dyspepsia, fatigue, musculoskeletal trauma, upper respiratory infection <u>Pregnancy category</u>: C for first trimester, D for second and third trimester	Medication may be taken with or without food; also SEE candesartan	If BP not well controlled with monotherapy, consider adding a low-dose diuretic; if pregnancy detected while on this medication, discontinue therapy as soon as possible (see "major adverse effects/cautions")

Generic Name and Selected Trade Names	Normal Adult Dosage	Major Adverse Effects/Cautions	Key Counseling Points	Miscellaneous Issues
Losartan Potassium Cozaar	Individualize dosage For hypertension, usual starting dose is 50 mg QD, use 25 mg in patients who may be volume depleted; maintenance is 25 to 100 mg daily in a QD or BID regimen; if trough BP control not adequate with QD administer same total daily dose on a BID schedule before increasing dosage Dosage adjustment not needed in elderly or patients with renal impairment	Considerations: SEE candesartan Most common AEs include dizziness, cough, diarrhea, back and leg pain, muscle cramps, insomnia, upper respiratory infection, sinusitis, nasal congestion Pregnancy category: C for first trimester, D for second and third trimester	SEE irbesartan	SEE irbesartan

Generic Name and Selected Trade Names	Normal Adult Dosage	Major Adverse Effects/Cautions	Key Counseling Points	Miscellaneous Issues
Valsartan Diovan	For hypertension, as monotherapy in non volume-depleted patients start with 80 mg QD; maximum effect usually noted within 4 weeks, then titrate; maintenance regimen 80 to 320 mg QD although adding a diuretic may be more effective than valsartan dosages >80 mg QD No initial dosage adjustment in elderly or patients with mild/moderate renal or liver impairment; use cautiously in patients with hepatic or severe renal impairment	<u>Considerations</u>: SEE candesartan; also, use cautiously in patients with impaired hepatic or renal function; geriatric patients may be more sensitive to valsartan than younger persons Most common AEs include headache, dizziness, fatigue, abdominal pain <u>Pregnancy category</u>: C for first trimester, D for second and third trimester	SEE irbesartan	SEE irbesartan

*As a general rule, a medication should not be administered to a patient with a known hypersensitivity to it or a similar agent.

Table 5: Miscellaneous Antihypertensive Agents*

Generic Name and Selected Trade Names	Normal Adult Dosage	Major Adverse Effects/Cautions	Key Counselling Points	Miscellaneous Issues
Guanabenz Acetate Wytensin	Individualize dosage For hypertension, usually start with 4 mg BID alone or with a thiazide diuretic; may titrate in increments of 4 or 8 mg/day every 1–2 weeks; maximum studied dose is 32 mg BID	<u>Considerations</u>: Sudden discontinuation has resulted in symptoms such as nervousness, agitation, headache, and tremor followed by rapid increase in BP and elevated levels of catecholamines — must reduce dose gradually; use with caution in patients with recent MI, severe coronary insufficiency, or cerebrovascular disease; most AEs are dose related Most common AEs include sedation/drowsiness (VERY common), dry mouth, dizziness, weakness, headache <u>Pregnancy category</u>: C	SEE clonidine (tablets)	

Generic Name and Selected Trade Names	Normal Adult Dosage	Major Adverse Effects/Cautions	Key Counseling Points	Miscellaneous Issues
Guanadrel Hylorel	Individualize dosage For hypertension, start with one-half of a 10 mg tablet BID; monitor supine as well as standing BP and titrate weekly or monthly; usual maintenance 20 to 75 mg/day in twice daily doses — larger doses may be administered TID or QID but dosages >400 mg/day rarely needed Reduce dosage in patients with impaired renal function — SEE Prescribing Information (PI)	<u>Contraindications</u>: Frank CHF, use with monoamine oxidase inhibitors or within one week of receiving same <u>Considerations</u>: Orthostatic hypotension noted frequently (counsel patients) especially in patients with regional vascular disease (cerebral or coronary); discontinue therapy 48–72 hrs prior to elective surgery; if emergency, ensure surgical team knows patient taking this agent; may aggravate bronchial asthma; avoid sympathomimetic amines; salt and water retention may occur; use cautiously in patients with peptic ulcer disease and renal impairment	Tell the prescriber if you have a kidney disorder, are taking a monoamine oxidase inhibitor, or have CHF; use caution if driving or using machinery; may cause drowsiness/sedation, which may be enhanced by other sedatives such as alcohol; medication could cause dizziness when you stand; if seated, stand up slowly; sit or lie down if dizzy; dizziness (etc) more common if drink alcohol (minimize intake), stand for a long time, exercise, and if weather is hot; do not take any cold or allergy product without first discussing it with your physician and/or pharmacist;	

Generic Name and Selected Trade Names	Normal Adult Dosage	Major Adverse Effects/Cautions	Key Counseling Points	Miscellaneous Issues
Guanadrel (continued) Hylorel		Most common AEs include headache, SOB on exertion, fatigue, drowsiness, dizziness, weight gain/loss, nocturia, urinary frequency, and many others Pregnancy category: B	notify the prescriber if you develop bothersome dizziness, lightheadedness; notify MD or dentist that you are receiving this medication before any surgery; if miss a dose take it as soon as you remember, but if it is almost time for the next dose skip the missed one and return to regular schedule— do not double doses	

Generic Name and Selected Trade Names	Normal Adult Dosage	Major Adverse Effects/Cautions	Key Counseling Points	Miscellaneous Issues
Guanethidine Ismelin	Individualize dosage For hypertension in ambulatory patients: Start with 10 mg/day then titrate upward no more frequently than every 5–7 days — titrate only if no decrease in BP when patient stands; usual maintenance 25 to 50 mg QD For hypertensive hospitalized patients: Start with 25 to 50 mg QD and increase by 25 or 50 mg per day or every 2 days as needed — titrate only if no decrease in BP when patient stands; for severe hypertension, SEE Prescribing Information (PI)	<u>Contraindications</u>: Known or suspected pheochromocytoma, frank CHF not due to hypertension, patients using monoamine oxidase inhibitors <u>Considerations</u>: Orthostatic hypotension noted frequently (counsel patients); stop therapy 2 weeks prior to elective surgery, if emergency, ensure surgical team knows patient taking this agent and administer other therapies cautiously; fever may increase effects; may aggravate bronchial asthma; use very cautiously in renal or liver impairment, coronary artery disease, recent MI, history of peptic ulcer disease	Tell the prescriber if you have asthma, kidney or liver disease, a history of peptic ulcer disease, or are taking a monoamine oxidase inhibitor; medication could cause dizziness when you stand; if seated, stand up slowly; sit or lie down if dizzy; dizziness (etc) more common if drink alcohol (minimize intake), stand for a long time, exercise, and if weather is hot; notify the prescriber if develop bothersome dizziness, lightheadedness or if you develop severe diarrhea; notify MD or dentist that you are receiving this medication before any surgery;	Medication rarely used today; numerous drug interactions are possible

Generic Name and Selected Trade Names	Normal Adult Dosage	Major Adverse Effects/Cautions	Key Counseling Points	Miscellaneous Issues
Guanethidine (continued) Ismelin		Most common AEs include diarrhea (may be severe), orthostasis, fluid retention, dizziness, weakness, nausea, vomiting, inhibition of ejaculation, and many more Pregnancy category: C	If you miss a dose take it as soon as you remember, but if it is almost time for the next dose skip the missed one and return to regular schedule — do not double doses	

Generic Name and Selected Trade Names	Normal Adult Dosage	Major Adverse Effects/Cautions	Key Counseling Points	Miscellaneous Issues
Guanfacine HCl Tenex	Individualize dosage For hypertension, start with 1 mg hs; may increase after 3–4 weeks to 2 mg — but most of the effect noted with 1 mg; doses >3 mg/day associated with more AEs	<u>Considerations</u>: Sudden discontinuation has resulted in symptoms such as nervousness, agitation, headache, and tremor followed by rapid increase in BP and elevated catecholamine levels — must gradually reduce dose; use cautiously in persons with severe coronary insufficiency, recent MI, cerebrovascular disease, chronic renal or hepatic disease; causes sedation/drowsiness, especially when beginning therapy — dose related <u>Most common AEs</u> include dry mouth, somnolence/drowsiness, sedation, dizziness, constipation, weakness, headache, insomnia <u>Pregnancy category</u>: B	Ability to tolerate alcohol and other CNS depressants may be reduced; also SEE clonidine (tablets)	

Generic Name and Selected Trade Names	Normal Adult Dosage	Major Adverse Effects/Cautions	Key Counseling Points	Miscellaneous Issues
Hydralazine HCl Apresoline	Individualize dosage For oral therapy of hypertension in adults, start with 10 mg QID for 2–4 days, then 25 mg QID for remainder of week, then titrate as required up to 300 mg/day	Contraindications: Coronary artery disease, mitral valvular rheumatic heart disease Considerations: May produce a syndrome resembling systemic lupus erythematosus (SLE) — fever, arthralgia, enlarged spleen, etc; use cautiously in patients with advanced renal insufficiency, previous cerebral vascular accidents (strokes), and pulmonary hypertension; may produce blood dyscrasias (monitor CBC), orthostatic hypotension, palpitations Most common AEs include angina, general weakness, muscle/joint pain, headaches, dizziness, diarrhea, altered heart rate Pregnancy category: C	Take with food; tell the prescriber if you have a kidney or liver disease; while taking the medication, tell the prescriber if you develop a fever and there is no clear reason, feel weak, have joint or muscle pain; if you miss a dose take it as soon as you remember, but if it is almost time for the next dose skip the missed one and return to regular schedule — do not double doses	Some products may contain tartrazine so use with caution in patients with asthma or those who are sensitive

Generic Name and Selected Trade Names	Normal Adult Dosage	Major Adverse Effects/Cautions	Key Counseling Points	Miscellaneous Issues
Minoxidil Loniten	Individualize dosage For hypertension in adults (and children >12 years of age), start with 5 mg QD, may increase to 10 mg, 20 mg, then 40 mg in single or divided doses; usual maintenance 10 to 40 mg/day; maximum dosage 100 mg/day; if systolic BP decreased <30 mm Hg administer QD, >30 mm Hg administer BID Patients with renal impairment may require lower dosages — SEE Prescribing Information (PI)	<u>Contraindications</u>: Acute MI, pheochromocytoma, dissecting aortic aneurysm <u>Considerations</u>: Can produce pericardial effusion that can progress to cardiac tamponade; can worsen angina and CHF; may produce fluid retention, tachycardia, abnormal hair growth, breast tenderness, nausea, and vomiting; hematocrit, hemoglobin, and RBC count may decrease when therapy begun but usually will normalize Most common AEs include edema, tachycardia, rapid weight gain, abnormal hair growth <u>Pregnancy category</u>: C	Teach patient to monitor pulse rate regularly — report to prescriber if rate increases ≥20 beats/min; notify prescriber if there is weight gain of >5 pounds, swelling of any part of the body especially the feet or lower legs, difficulty breathing especially when lying down, new or worsened angina, dizziness, lightheadedness, fainting; if you miss a dose take it as soon as you remember, but if you remember when it is almost time for the next dose (for example, the next day) skip the missed one and return to regular schedule — do not double doses	May produce serious adverse events — reserve for hypertensive patients who do not respond to maximum doses of a diuretic and two other agents; administer under close supervision, usually along with a beta adrenergic blocking agent and a (loop) diuretic

Generic Name and Selected Trade Names	Normal Adult Dosage	Major Adverse Effects/Cautions	Key Counseling Points	Miscellaneous Issues
Reserpine	Individualize dosage For hypertension, in patients not receiving other therapy, usually start with 0.5 mg QD for 1–2 weeks — although data exist to recommend 0.05 to 0.1 mg initially; for maintenance 0.1 to 0.25 mg QD — high doses increase risk of AEs such as mental depression	<u>Contraindications</u>: Patients receiving electroconvulsive therapy, patients with or history of mental depression, active peptic ulcer disease, ulcerative colitis <u>Considerations</u>: May cause severe mental depression, bradycardia, Parkinson's disease like symptoms; some clinicians believe that it should be used cautiously in patients with epilepsy Most common AEs include nasal congestion, numerous CNS effects such as drowsiness, fatigue, and lethargy, and GI effects such as abdominal cramps, nausea, diarrhea, vomiting, and anorexia (loss of appetite) <u>Pregnancy category</u>: C	Tell the prescriber if you have a history of heart rhythm problems, Parkinson's disease, or mental depression, or if you have active peptic ulcer disease, ulcerative colitis, or a seizure disorder; may cause drowsiness/sedation that may be enhanced by other sedatives such as alcohol, medications for sleeping, and antihistamines; use caution if driving or using machinery; may cause dryness of mouth, try sugarless gum/candy or ice but if problem persists, contact prescriber; if nasal stuffiness occurs, do not self-treat without discussing it first with your physician or pharmacist; if you miss a dose, skip it and go back to regular schedule — do not double doses	Medication rarely used today

*As a general rule, a medication should not be administered to a patient with a known hypersensitivity to it or a similar agent.

Table 6: Angiotensin Converting Enzyme (ACE) Inhibitors*

Generic Name and Selected Trade Names	Normal Adult Dosage	Major Adverse Effects/Cautions	Key Counseling Points	Miscellaneous Issues
Benazepril Lotensin	Individualize dosage. For hypertension, in patients not receiving other therapy, usually start with 10 mg QD; usual maintenance 20 to 40 mg per day in a QD or BID regimen; if trough BP control not adequate with QD administer same total daily dose on a BID schedule or consider increasing dosage. Lower dosages required in renal impairment — SEE Prescribing Information (PI)	Contraindications: Patients allergic to any ACE inhibitor. Considerations: Anaphylactoid and other allergic reactions possible (SEE Prescribing Information); hypotension (especially in patients with CHF), hepatic failure, cough, neutropenia/agranulocytosis, hyperkalemia are possible; in patients with intra-vascular volume depletion symptomatic hypotension may occur; use caution in patients who require renin-angiotensin-aldosterone system to maintain renal function (eg, patients with severe CHF); use in second and third trimester of pregnancy may cause injury and perhaps death to fetus	Females of childbearing age should be warned about dangers of therapy during pregnancy, should consider an appropriate birth control method, and should notify the prescriber if they become pregnant; immediately report signs or symptoms of angioedema such as difficulty in breathing and swelling of the face, lips, and/or tongue; contact prescriber if develop an infection or fever without a clear cause, cough, lightheadedness or syncope, significant diarrhea or vomiting;	Adjust dosage based on peak (2–6 hrs after dosing) and trough effects; if BP not well controlled, consider addition of a diuretic; if patient receiving a diuretic, consider discontinuing same before starting benazepril — if cannot, start with benazepril 5 mg to avoid excessive hypotension;

Generic Name and Selected Trade Names	Normal Adult Dosage	Major Adverse Effects/Cautions	Key Counseling Points	Miscellaneous Issues
Benazepril (continued) Lotensin		Most common AEs include headache, dizziness, fatigue, somnolence, postural dizziness, nausea, cough <u>Pregnancy category</u>: C for first trimester, D for second and third trimester	maintain adequate fluid intake as dehydration (eg, from excessive perspiration, vomiting, or diarrhea) may increase chance of lightheadedness/syncope; do not take diuretics, potassium supplements, or salt substitutes, without first discussing it with prescriber; if you miss a dose take it as soon as you remember, but if it is almost time for the next dose skip the missed one — do not double doses	use of potassium supplements or potassium-sparing diuretics can increase risk of hyperkalemia

Generic Name and Selected Trade Names	Normal Adult Dosage	Major Adverse Effects/Cautions	Key Counseling Points	Miscellaneous Issues
Captopril Capoten	Individualize dosage For hypertension: Start with 25 mg BID or TID; may increase dosage 1–2 weeks later to 50 mg BID or TID; if not sufficient, consider adding low-dose thiazide diuretic before further dosage increase — SEE Prescribing Information (PI) For CHF: Usually, start with 25 mg TID which may be titrated; for patients vigorously treated with diuretics, start with 6.25 or 12.5 mg TID — SEE PI	Considerations: May cause proteinuria; also SEE benazepril for contraindications, cautions, etc Most common AEs include rash (often with pruritus), hypotension, tachycardia, chest pain, palpitations, taste impairment, cough, increases in serum potassium Pregnancy category: C for first trimester, D for second and third trimester	Take one hour before meals; also SEE benazepril	For hypertension, attempt to discontinue other antihypertensive for one week before starting captopril; use of potassium supplements or potassium-sparing diuretics can increase risk of hyperkalemia

Generic Name and Selected Trade Names	Normal Adult Dosage	Major Adverse Effects/Cautions	Key Counseling Points	Miscellaneous Issues
Captopril (continued) Capoten	For left ventricular dysfunction after MI: Start with 6.25 mg X 1, then 12.5 mg TID, then titrate upward to usual maintenance of 50 mg TID For diabetic nephropathy: Usual maintenance dosage is 25 mg TID Dosage adjustment in renal impairment: Lower dosages may be required — SEE PI			

Generic Name and Selected Trade Names	Normal Adult Dosage	Major Adverse Effects/Cautions	Key Counseling Points	Miscellaneous Issues
Enalapril Maleate Vasotec	Individualize dosage For hypertension: As monotherapy, start with 5 mg QD; usual range is 10 to 40 mg/day as a single dose or two equally divided doses; if not sufficient, consider adding low-dose thiazide diuretic If patient receiving a diuretic and it cannot be stopped, start with 2.5 mg QD with close supervision — SEE Prescribing Information (PI)	Considerations: SEE benazepril Most common AEs include hypotension, headache, dizziness, fatigue, orthostasis, syncope, chest pain, asthenia (weakness), diarrhea, cough Pregnancy category: C for first trimester, D for second and third trimester	SEE benazepril	When initiating therapy, reduce dose or stop diuretic if possible (SEE Prescribing Information); in some patients with hypertension treated QD, medication effect may diminish toward end of dosing interval — if this occurs, consider increase in dosage or change to a BID regimen; use of potassium supplements or potassium-sparing diuretics can increase risk of hyperkalemia

Generic Name and Selected Trade Names	Normal Adult Dosage	Major Adverse Effects/Cautions	Key Counseling Points	Miscellaneous Issues
Enalapril Maleate (continued) Vasotec	For <u>CHF</u>: Usually, start with 2.5 mg QD; maintenance is 2.5 to 20 mg BID; monitor patient closely For <u>asymptomatic left ventricular dysfunction</u>: Usually, start with 2.5 mg BID; usual maintenance is 20 mg/day in divided doses; monitor patient closely <u>Dosage adjustment in patients with renal impairment</u>: Lower dosages may be required — SEE PI			

43

Generic Name and Selected Trade Names	Normal Adult Dosage	Major Adverse Effects/Cautions	Key Counseling Points	Miscellaneous Issues
Fosinopril Monopril	Individualize dosage For hypertension: As monotherapy or when added to a diuretic, start with 10 mg QD; usual maintenance 20 to 40 mg/day but some patients may require 80 mg/day; if trough BP control not adequate with QD regimen, consider divided doses For CHF: Usually start with 10 mg QD and titrate to 20 to 40 mg QD; monitor patient very closely; start with 5 mg if patient has moderate to severe renal impairment	Considerations: SEE benazepril Most common AEs include cough, dizziness, nausea/vomiting, hypotension, orthostasis, musculoskeletal pain, diarrhea, chest pain, weakness Pregnancy category: C for first trimester, D for second and third trimester	SEE benazepril	Adjust dosage based on peak (2–6 hrs after dosing) and trough effects; if BP not well controlled, consider addition of a diuretic; if patient receiving a diuretic, consider discontinuing same for 2–3 days before starting fosinopril — if cannot, start with 10 mg to avoid excessive hypotension; use of potassium supplements or potassium-sparing diuretics can increase risk of hyperkalemia

Generic Name and Selected Trade Names	Normal Adult Dosage	Major Adverse Effects/Cautions	Key Counseling Points	Miscellaneous Issues
Lisinopril Prinivil Zestril	Individualize therapy For hypertension: As monotherapy, start with 10 mg QD; usual range is 20 to 40 mg QD, although up to 80 mg/day has been used; if not sufficient, consider adding low-dose thiazide diuretic If patient receiving a diuretic and it cannot be stopped, start with 5 mg QD with close supervision — SEE Prescribing Information (PI)	<u>Considerations</u>: SEE benazepril <u>Most common AEs</u> include headache, dizziness, cough, fatigue, diarrhea, nausea, upper respiratory infection <u>Pregnancy category</u>: C for first trimester, D for second and third trimester	SEE benazepril	Adjust dosage based on BP immediately before next dose — ie, trough effect; if BP not well controlled, consider addition of a diuretic; if patient receiving a diuretic, consider discontinuing same for 2–3 days before starting lisinopril; use of potassium supplements or potassium-sparing diuretics can increase risk of hyperkalemia

Generic Name and Selected Trade Names	Normal Adult Dosage	Major Adverse Effects/Cautions	Key Counseling Points	Miscellaneous Issues
Lisinopril (continued) Prinivil Zestril	For CHF: With a diuretic and digitalis, usually start with 5 mg QD and monitor closely (may need to decrease diuretic dose) — SEE PI; usual maintenance range is 5 to 20 mg QD For acute MI: Usually start with 5 mg, give 5 mg 24 hrs later, then 10 mg after 48 hrs, then 10 mg QD for 6 weeks; some patients require lower dosages — SEE PI Dosage adjustments: Lower dosages may be required in elderly patients, and patients with renal impairment or hyponatremia — SEE PI			

Generic Name and Selected Trade Names	Normal Adult Dosage	Major Adverse Effects/Cautions	Key Counseling Points	Miscellaneous Issues
Moexipril HCl Univasc	Individualize dosage For hypertension, if not on a diuretic, start with 7.5 mg QD 1 hr before a meal; usual range is 7.5 to 30 mg/day in a QD or BID regimen If patient receiving a diuretic and it cannot be stopped, start with 3.75 mg QD with close supervision — SEE Prescribing Information (PI) Lower dosages may be required in elderly, and patients with renal or hepatic impairment — SEE PI	<u>Considerations</u>: SEE benazepril Most common AEs include increased cough, dizziness, diarrhea, flu syndrome, fatigue, pharyngitis, flushing, rash, myalgia <u>Pregnancy category</u>: C for first trimester, D for second and third trimester	Take the medication 1 hr before eating a meal; also SEE benazepril	Adjust dosage based on BP immediately before next dose — ie, trough effect; if BP not well controlled, consider addition of a diuretic; if patient receiving a diuretic, consider discontinuing same for 2–3 days before starting moexipril; use of potassium supplements or potassium-sparing diuretics can increase risk of hyperkalemia

Generic Name and Selected Trade Names	Normal Adult Dosage	Major Adverse Effects/Cautions	Key Counseling Points	Miscellaneous Issues
Perindopril Erbumine Aceon	Individualize dosage For hypertension, usually start with 4 mg QD; usual maintenance dosage is 4 to 8 mg QD but up to 16 mg/day may be required; may be administered QD or BID; if BP control not sufficient, consider adding low-dose thiazide diuretic In the elderly, start with 4 mg/day in one or two divided doses and titrate to 8 mg/day if needed; patients with renal or hepatic impairment may need lower than usual dosages — SEE Prescribing Information (PI)	Considerations: SEE benazepril Most common AEs include cough, back pain, sinusitis, viral infection, upper extremity pain, dyspepsia, fever, proteinuria, palpitations Pregnancy category: C for first trimester, D for second and third trimester	SEE benazepril	Adjust dosage based on BP immediately before next dose — ie, trough effect; if BP not well controlled, consider addition of a diuretic; if patient receiving a diuretic, consider discontinuing same for 2–3 days before starting perindopril; use of potassium supplements or potassium-sparing diuretics can increase risk of hyperkalemia

Generic Name and Selected Trade Names	Normal Adult Dosage	Major Adverse Effects/Cautions	Key Counseling Points	Miscellaneous Issues
Quinapril HCl Accupril	Individualize therapy For hypertension: If not already receiving a diuretic, start with 10 or 20 mg QD; titrate at intervals of at least 2 weeks to a usual range of 20 to 80 mg/day on a QD or BID regimen; if dosage not sufficient, consider adding low-dose thiazide diuretic If patient receiving a diuretic and it cannot be stopped, start with 5 mg QD with close supervision — SEE Prescribing Information (PI)	Considerations: SEE benazepril Most common AEs include headache, dizziness, fatigue, cough, nausea/vomiting, chest pain, hypotension, dyspnea, diarrhea, myalgia, rash, back pain, hyperkalemia Pregnancy category: C for first trimester, D for second and third trimester	SEE benazepril	Adjust dosage based on peak (2–6 hrs after dosing) and trough effects; if patient receiving a diuretic, consider discontinuing same for 2–3 days before starting quinapril — if cannot, start with 5 mg (with supervision) to avoid excessive hypotension; in some hypertensive patients treated QD, medication effect may diminish toward end of dosing interval — if this occurs,

49

Generic Name and Selected Trade Names	Normal Adult Dosage	Major Adverse Effects/Cautions	Key Counseling Points	Miscellaneous Issues
Quinapril HCl (continued) Accupril	For CHF: With a diuretic and digitalis, usually start with 5 mg BID and monitor closely — SEE PI; may titrate weekly — usual maintenance range is 20 to 40 mg/day in 2 equally divided doses Dosage adjustments: Lower dosages may be required in the elderly and in patients with renal impairment or hyponatremia — SEE PI			consider increase in dosage or change to a BID regimen; if BP not well controlled, consider addition of a diuretic; use of potassium supplements or potassium-sparing diuretics can increase risk of hyperkalemia

Generic Name and Selected Trade Names	Normal Adult Dosage	Major Adverse Effects/Cautions	Key Counseling Points	Miscellaneous Issues
Ramipril Altace	Individualize therapy For hypertension: If not receiving a diuretic, usually start with 2.5 mg QD; usual maintenance is 2.5 to 20 mg/day on a QD or BID basis; if not sufficient, consider adding low-dose thiazide If patient receiving a diuretic that cannot be stopped, start with 1.25 mg QD — SEE Prescribing Information (PI)	<u>Considerations</u>: SEE benazepril Most common AEs include headache, dizziness, asthenia (weakness), nausea/vomiting, hypotension, cough, angina pectoris, syncope, postural hypotension <u>Pregnancy category</u>: C for first trimester, D for second and third trimester	SEE benazepril	Capsule usually swallowed whole, but it can be opened and the contents sprinkled on about 4 oz of applesauce or mixed with about 4 oz of water or apple juice; if patient taking a diuretic, consider stopping same for 2–3 days before starting ramipril — if cannot, start with 1.25 mg (with supervision) to avoid excessive hypotension;

Generic Name and Selected Trade Names	Normal Adult Dosage	Major Adverse Effects/Cautions	Key Counseling Points	Miscellaneous Issues
Ramipril (continued) Altace	For heart failure post-MI: Usually, start with 2.5 mg BID and titrate to 5 mg BID under close supervision Dosage adjustments: Lower dosages may be required in patients with hepatic or renal impairment — SEE PI			in some hypertensive patients treated QD, medication effect may diminish toward end of dosing interval — if this occurs, consider increase in dosage or change to a BID regimen; if BP not controlled, consider adding a diuretic; use of potassium supplements or potassium-sparing diuretics can increase risk of hyperkalemia

Generic Name and Selected Trade Names	Normal Adult Dosage	Major Adverse Effects/Cautions	Key Counseling Points	Miscellaneous Issues
Trandolapril Mavik	Individualize dosage For hypertension in patients not receiving a diuretic, usually start with 1 mg QD in non-black patients and 2 mg QD in black patients; titrate dosage at intervals of at least 1 week, usual range is 2 to 4 mg QD but up to 8 mg/day may be required; if BP control not sufficient, consider adding a diuretic If patient receiving a diuretic and it cannot be stopped, start with 0.5 mg QD — SEE Prescribing Information (PI)	<u>Considerations</u>: SEE benazepril <u>Most common AEs</u> include cough, dizziness, diarrhea, headache, fatigue <u>Pregnancy category</u>: C for first trimester, D for second and third trimester	SEE benazepril	If patient receiving a diuretic, consider discontinuing same for 2–3 days before starting trandolapril; if BP not well controlled, consider addition of a diuretic; use of potassium supplements or potassium-sparing diuretics can increase risk of hyperkalemia

Generic Name and Selected Trade Names	Normal Adult Dosage	Major Adverse Effects/Cautions	Key Counseling Points	Miscellaneous Issues
Trandolapril (continued) Mavik	In patients with creatinine clearance <30 mL/min or with hepatic cirrhosis start with 0.5 mg QD — SEE PI			

*As a general rule, a medication should not be administered to a patient with a known hypersensitivity to it or a similar agent.

Table 7: Beta Adrenergic Blocking Agents*

Generic Name and Selected Trade Names	Normal Adult Dosage	Major Adverse Effects/Cautions	Key Counseling Points	Miscellaneous Issues
Acebutolol HCl Sectral	Individualize dosage. For hypertension: In uncomplicated mild-to-moderate hypertension usually start with 400 mg QD or in two divided doses; usual maintenance 400 to 800 mg/day, although some patients respond to 200 mg/day and more severe hypertension may require 600 mg BID. For ventricular arrhythmias: Usually start with 200 mg BID and titrate gradually to usual maintenance of 600 to 1200 mg/day	Contraindications: Second and third degree heart block, persistently severe bradycardia, overt cardiac failure, cardiogenic shock Considerations: Use caution in aortic or mitral disease or decreased left ventricular function as CHF is possible, in diabetes mellitus or hypoglycemia, patients with thyroid, peripheral vascular or bronchospastic disease; use caution if patient on a calcium channel blocker; acute discontinuation could exacerbate angina pectoris or potentially cause an MI	Tell the prescriber if you have a heart, kidney, lung, liver, or thyroid disease, diabetes mellitus, or a blood circulation problem; while taking this medication tell the prescriber if you develop a breathing problem or swelling in your legs or ankle area; teach patient to monitor pulse rate and notify prescriber if it changes significantly; do not stop taking this medication without discussing it first with the prescriber; do not take any cold or allergy products without discussing it first with your physician and/or pharmacist;	Beta-1 selectivity diminshes as dosage increases; in general, persons with bronchospastic disease should <u>not</u> receive a beta blocker; discontinuation prior to surgery is controversial — SEE Prescribing Information

55

Generic Name and Selected Trade Names	Normal Adult Dosage	Major Adverse Effects/Cautions	Key Counseling Points	Miscellaneous Issues
Acebutolol HCl (continued) Sectral	<u>Dosage adjustments:</u> Avoid dosages >800 mg/day in elderly; reduce dosage in impaired renal and hepatic function — SEE Prescribing Information (PI)	Most common AEs include hypotension, heart failure, bradycardia, anxiety, impotence, pruritus, hyper/hypoesthesia, vomiting, abdominal pain, dysuria, nocturia, liver abnormalities, back/joint pain, pharyngitis, wheezing, development of antinuclear antibodies (ANA) <u>Pregnancy category:</u> B	try very hard not to miss any doses; if you miss a dose take it as soon as you remember, but if it is within 4 hrs of the next dose skip the missed one and return to regular schedule — do not double doses	

Generic Name and Selected Trade Names	Normal Adult Dosage	Major Adverse Effects/Cautions	Key Counseling Points	Miscellaneous Issues
Atenolol Tenormin	Individualize dosage For hypertension: Usually 50 mg QD alone or with a diuretic; may increase dosage in 1-2 weeks to 100 mg QD For angina: Usually 50 mg QD; may increase dosage in 1 week to 100 mg QD although some patients may require 200 mg QD For MI: Usually administered following atenolol IV regimen — SEE Prescribing Information (PI) Dosage adjustments: May need to reduce dosage in the elderly and in patients with impaired renal function — SEE PI	Contraindications: SEE acebutolol Considerations: Use caution in CHF, diabetes mellitus or hypoglycemia, and patients with thyroid, peripheral vascular and bronchospastic disease; bradycardia and heart block can occur and LVEDP can rise if used with verapamil or diltiazem; could cause CHF; acute stoppage could exacerbate angina pectoris or potentially cause an MI; may cause fetal injury Most common AEs include bradycardia, cold extremities, postural hypotension, leg pain, dizziness, vertigo, light-headedness, drowsiness, tiredness, depression, nausea, dyspnea, wheezing, diarrhea Pregnancy category: D	Tell the prescriber if you have a heart, kidney, lung, or thyroid disease, diabetes mellitus, or a blood circulation problem, or are taking a calcium channel blocker (eg, diltiazem and verapamil); while taking this medication tell the prescriber if you become pregnant, if you develop a breathing problem or swelling in your legs or ankle area; teach patient to monitor pulse rate and notify prescriber if it changes significantly; do not stop taking this medication without discussing it first with the prescriber; do not take any cold or allergy product without discussing it first with your physician and/or pharmacist;	SEE acebutolol

Generic Name and Selected Trade Names	Normal Adult Dosage	Major Adverse Effects/Cautions	Key Counseling Points	Miscellaneous Issues
Atenolol (continued) Tenormin			try very hard not to miss any doses; if you miss a dose take it as soon as you remember, but if it is within 8 hrs of the next dose skip the missed one and return to regular scheudule — do not double doses	

Generic Name and Selected Trade Names	Normal Adult Dosage	Major Adverse Effects/Cautions	Key Counselling Points	Miscellaneous Issues
Betaxolol HCl Kerlone	Individualize dosage For hypertension usually 10 mg QD alone or with a diuretic; may increase in 1–2 weeks to 20 mg QD; if monotherapy not sufficient, consider adding a diuretic or other antihypertensive agent Elderly or patients with impaired renal function may require lower dosages — SEE Prescribing Information (PI)	<u>Contraindications</u>: SEE acebutolol <u>Considerations</u>: Use cautiously in CHF, diabetes mellitus or hypoglycemia, and patients with thyroid, peripheral vascular and bronchospastic disease; use caution if patient receiving a calcium channel blocker; could cause CHF; acute discontinuation could exacerbate angina or potentially cause an MI Most common AEs include bradycardia, edema, headache, dizziness, fatigue, lethargy, dyspnea, chest pain, pharyngitis, dyspepsia, diarrhea, arthralgia <u>Pregnancy category</u>: C	SEE atenolol	SEE acebutolol

59

Generic Name and Selected Trade Names	Normal Adult Dosage	Major Adverse Effects/Cautions	Key Counseling Points	Miscellaneous Issues
Bisoprolol Fumarate Zebeta	Individualize dosage For hypertension usually start with 5 mg QD but some patients require less; may titrate to 10 then 20 mg QD Patients with impaired renal or hepatic function may require lower dosages — SEE Prescribing Information (PI)	Considerations: SEE betaxolol Most common AEs include dizziness, headache, fatigue, insomnia, arthralgia, diarrhea, nausea, dyspnea, pharyngitis, rhinitis, sinusitis, peripheral edema Pregnancy category: C	SEE atenolol	SEE acebutolol

Generic Name and Selected Trade Names	Normal Adult Dosage	Major Adverse Effects/Cautions	Key Counseling Points	Miscellaneous Issues
Carteolol HCl Cartrol	Individualize dosage For hypertension, usually start with 2.5 mg QD alone or added to a diuretic; may titrate to 5 then 10 mg QD Patients with impaired renal function may require lower dosages — SEE Prescribing Information (PI)	Contraindications: Bronchial asthma, severe bradycardia, greater than first degree heart block, cardiogenic shock, clinically evident CHF Considerations: Use cautiously in diabetes mellitus or hypoglycemia, and patients with renal, thyroid, peripheral vascular and bronchospastic disease; could cause CHF; acute discontinuation could exacerbate angina pectoris or potentially cause an MI Most common AEs include asthenia (weakness/tiredness/fatigue), insomnia, muscle cramps, somnolence, chest pain, arthralgia, back pain, paresthesia, diarrhea, nausea Pregnancy category: C	SEE atenolol	<u>Not</u> beta-1 selective; discontinuation prior to surgery is controversial — SEE Prescribing Information; in general, persons with bronchospastic disease should <u>not</u> receive a beta blocker

Generic Name and Selected Trade Names	Normal Adult Dosage	Major Adverse Effects/Cautions	Key Counseling Points	Miscellaneous Issues
Carvedilol[1] Coreg	Individualize dosage For hypertension: Usually start with 6.25 mg BID; may titrate every 1–2 weeks first to 12.5 mg BID then 25 mg BID For CHF: Monitor patient very closely and stabilize other therapies; usually start with 3.125 mg BID for 2 weeks; titrate by doubling dosage every 2 weeks to highest tolerated; maximum recommended dosage is 25 mg BID in patients <85 kg and 50 mg BID in patients >85 kg — SEE Prescribing Information (PI)	Contraindications: NYHA class IV decompensated cardiac failure requiring IV inotropic therapy, bronchial asthma, second- or third-degree heart block, sick sinus syndrome (unless pacemaker in place), cardiogenic shock, severe bradycardia Considerations: Not recommended in clinically manifest liver impairment; may cause liver injury; use caution in diabetes mellitus or hypoglycemia, and in patients with renal, thyroid, and peripheral vascular disease; could cause CHF and hypotension; acute discontinuation could worsen angina or potentially cause an MI; use in bronchospastic disease only if patient cannot take other therapies	Take with food; if you get dizzy or faint when standing, sit or lie down and contact the prescriber; if dizzy/drowsy don't drive a car or use hazardous machinery; contact lens wearers may develop decreased tearing; also SEE betaxolol	Not beta-1 selective; discontinuation prior to surgery is controversial — SEE Prescribing Information (PI); in general, persons with bronchospastic disease should not receive a beta blocker; adjust dosage based on standing systolic BP 1 hour after dose; may interact with other agents that affect cytochrome P-450 enzymes; many other drug interactions possible — see PI

Generic Name and Selected Trade Names	Normal Adult Dosage	Major Adverse Effects/Cautions	Key Counseling Points	Miscellaneous Issues
Carvedilol[1] **(continued)** Coreg		Most common AEs include fatigue, chest pain, edema, fever, bradycardia, syncope, hypotension, AV block, aggravation of angina, hyperglycemia, weight gain, back pain, sinusitis, bronchitis, arthralgia, vision abnormalities, dizziness, insomnia, diarrhea, nausea, vomiting Pregnancy category: C		

Generic Name and Selected Trade Names	Normal Adult Dosage	Major Adverse Effects/Cautions	Key Counseling Points	Miscellaneous Issues
Labetalol HCl[1] Normodyne Trandate	Individualize dosage For hypertension, as monotherapy or with a diuretic usually start with 100 mg BID for 2–3 days; may titrate in increments of 100 mg BID every 2–3 days; usual maintenance range is 200 to 400 mg BID; severe hypertension may require up to 2400 mg/day using a BID or TID regimen Elderly patients may require lower dosages — SEE Prescribing Information (PI) Parenteral dosage form available — SEE (PI)	<u>Contraindications</u>: Bronchial asthma, overt cardiac failure, severe bradycardia, greater than first degree heart block, cardiogenic shock, other conditions associated with severe and prolonged hypotension <u>Considerations</u>: Use cautiously in patients with pheochromocytoma, diabetes mellitus or hypoglycemia, history of CHF, and persons with liver disease; could cause CHF; acute discontinuation could exacerbate angina or potentially cause an MI Most common AEs include dizziness, fatigue, headache, nausea, vomiting, nasal stuffiness, ejaculation failure, dyspnea, vertigo <u>Pregnancy category</u>: C	Tell the prescriber if you have a lung, heart or liver disease, or diabetes mellitus; while taking this medication tell the prescriber if you develop a breathing problem or swelling in your legs or ankle area; do not stop taking this medication without discussing it first with the prescriber; do not take any cold or allergy product without discussing it first with your physician and/or pharmacist; try very hard not to miss any doses; if you miss a dose take it as soon as you remember, but if it is within 8 hrs of the next dose skip the missed one and return to regular schedule — do not double doses	Has both selective alpha-1 and non-selective beta adrenergic receptor blocking activity; if a diuretic is added the dose of labetalol may need to be decreased — SEE Prescribing Information (PI); in general, persons with bronchospastic disease should <u>not</u> receive a beta blocker; discontinuation prior to surgery is controversial — SEE PI

Generic Name and Selected Trade Names	Normal Adult Dosage	Major Adverse Effects/Cautions	Key Counseling Points	Miscellaneous Issues
Metoprolol Succinate Toprol-XL	Individualize dosage For hypertension: As monotherapy or with a diuretic, usually start with 50 to 100 mg QD; may titrate weekly up to 400 mg QD For angina: Usually start with 100 mg QD; may titrate weekly up to 400 mg QD, but if it is to be stopped, reduce gradually over 1–2 weeks — SEE Prescribing Information (PI)	<u>Contraindications</u>: Sinus bradycardia, greater than first degree heart block, overt cardiac failure, cardiogenic shock <u>Considerations</u>: Use caution in CHF, thyroid disease, diabetes mellitus or hypoglycemia, or in persons with impaired liver function or bronchospastic disease; could cause CHF; acute stoppage could exacerbate angina or potentially cause an MI — taper over a 1–2 week period Most common AEs include tiredness, dizziness, rash, depression, shortness of breath, bradycardia, dyspnea, wheezing, diarrhea, pruritus <u>Pregnancy category</u>: C	Tell the prescriber if you have a heart, lung or thyroid disease, diabetes mellitus, or a blood circulation problem; take with or immediately after meals; while taking this agent tell the prescriber if you develop a breathing problem or swelling in your legs or ankle area; if dizzy/drowsy don't drive a car or use hazardous machinery; teach patient to monitor pulse rate and notify prescriber if it changes significantly; do not stop taking this medication without discussing it first with the prescriber; if going for surgery, tell physician or dentist that you are taking this agent;	Extended release tablet; beta-1 selectivity diminishes as dosage increases; SEE Prescribing Information (PI) to convert patient from immediate-release metoprolol; in general, persons with bronchospastic disease should <u>not</u> receive a beta blocker; discontinuation prior to surgery is controversial — SEE PI

65

Generic Name and Selected Trade Names	Normal Adult Dosage	Major Adverse Effects/Cautions	Key Counseling Points	Miscellaneous Issues
Metoprolol Succinate (continued) Toprol-XL			do not take any cold or allergy product without discussing it first with your physician and/or pharmacist; try not to miss any doses; if you miss a dose take only the next scheduled one — do not double doses	

Generic Name and Selected Trade Names	Normal Adult Dosage	Major Adverse Effects/Cautions	Key Counseling Points	Miscellaneous Issues
Metoprolol Tartrate Lopressor	Individualize dosage For hypertension: As monotherapy or with a diuretic, usually start with 100 mg daily in a single or divided regimen; may titrate at weekly or longer intervals, usual maintenance is 100 to 450 mg/day For angina: Usually start with 100 mg daily given in two divided doses; may titrate at weekly intervals to usual range of 100 to 400 mg/day — if to be stopped, reduce gradually over 1–2 weeks — SEE Prescribing Information (PI)	<u>Contraindications</u>: *For hypertension and angina* — Sinus bradycardia, greater than first degree heart block, overt cardiac failure, cardiogenic shock; *For MI* — bradycardia <45 beats/min, second- and third-degree heart block, significant first degree heart block, systolic BP <100 mmHg, moderate-to-severe cardiac failure SEE metoprolol succinate for considerations, most common AEs, and pregnancy category	SEE metoprolol succinate	Once daily dosing may not provide effective BP control throughout 24 hour period; beta-1 selectivity diminishes as dosage increases; in general, persons with bronchospastic disease should <u>not</u> receive a beta blocker; discontinuation prior to surgery is controversial — SEE Prescribing Information (PI)

67

Generic Name and Selected Trade Names	Normal Adult Dosage	Major Adverse Effects/Cautions	Key Counseling Points	Miscellaneous Issues
Metoprolol Tartrate (continued) Lopressor	For MI: *Early phase* — if needed, 25 or 50 mg Q6h; *Late phase* — if no acute therapy, usually 100 mg BID for at least 3 months — SEE PI Parenteral dosage form available — SEE PI			

Generic Name and Selected Trade Names	Normal Adult Dosage	Major Adverse Effects/Cautions	Key Counseling Points	Miscellaneous Issues
Nadolol Corgard	Individualize dosage For hypertension: As monotherapy or with a diuretic, usually start with 40 mg QD; may titrate in 40 to 80 mg increments up to 320 mg QD For angina: Usually start with 40 mg/day; may titrate in 40 to 80 mg increments every 3–7 days up to 240 mg/day Dosage adjustment: May need reduced dosage in renal impairment — SEE Prescribing Information (PI)	Considerations: SEE carteolol Most common AEs include bradycardia, peripheral vascular insufficiency, cardiac failure, orthostatic hypotension, palpitations, dizziness, fatigue, nausea Pregnancy category: Not specified	SEE atenolol	Not beta-1 selective; in general, persons with bronchospastic disease should not receive a beta blocker; discontinuation prior to surgery is controversial — SEE Prescribing Information

Generic Name and Selected Trade Names	Normal Adult Dosage	Major Adverse Effects/Cautions	Key Counseling Points	Miscellaneous Issues
Penbutolol Sulfate Levatol	Individualize dosage For hypertension as monotherapy or with a diuretic, usual starting and maintenance dose is 20 mg QD; doses up to 80 mg/day have been used but may not be more effective; full effect of 20 mg QD or 40 mg QD seen after 2 weeks while full effect with 10 mg QD needs 4–6 weeks	Contraindications: Bronchial asthma, sinus bradycardia, second and third degree heart block, cardiogenic shock Considerations: Use cautiously in CHF, diabetes mellitus or hypoglycemia, and in patients with bronchospastic and thyroid disease; could cause CHF; acute stoppage could exacerbate angina or potentially cause an MI Most common AEs include headache, dizziness, fatigue, chest or limb pain, nausea, diarrhea, dyspepsia, cough, dyspnea, insomnia Pregnancy category: C	SEE atenolol	Not beta-1 selective; in general, persons with bronchospastic disease should not receive a beta blocker; discontinuation prior to surgery is controversial — SEE Prescribing Information

Generic Name and Selected Trade Names	Normal Adult Dosage	Major Adverse Effects/Cautions	Key Counseling Points	Miscellaneous Issues
Pindolol Visken	Individualize dosage For hypertension as monotherapy or with a diuretic, usual starting dose is 5 mg BID; may titrate after 3–4 weeks in 10 mg/day increments to maximum of 60 mg/day Reduce dosage in impaired liver function — SEE Prescribing Information (PI)	SEE carteolol Most common AEs include edema, dyspnea, weight gain, palpitations, cold extremities, dizziness, fatigue, insomnia, altered dreams, paresthesia, lethargy, nausea, abdominal discomfort, leg/muscle/joint pain, chest pain, wheezing <u>Pregnancy category</u>: Not specified	SEE acebutolol	<u>Not</u> beta-1 selective; in general, persons with bronchospastic disease should <u>not</u> receive a beta blocker; discontinuation prior to surgery is controversial — SEE Prescribing Information

Generic Name and Selected Trade Names	Normal Adult Dosage	Major Adverse Effects/Cautions	Key Counseling Points	Miscellaneous Issues
Propranolol HCl Inderal Inderal LA	Individualize dosage Inderal for hypertension: As monotherapy or with a diuretic, usually start with 40 mg BID; may titrate to usual maintenance range of 120 to 240 mg/day, although some patients need 640 mg/day Inderal for angina: Usually, a total daily dose of 80 to 320 mg/day on a BID, TID, or QID regimen; if therapy to be stopped, do so gradually over several weeks	Contraindications: Cardiogenic shock, bronchial asthma, sinus bradycardia and greater than first degree heart block, CHF Considerations: Use caution in diabetes mellitus or hypoglycemia, and patients with hepatic, renal, thyroid, peripheral vascular and bronchospastic disease, and in patients with Wolff-Parkinson-White syndrome; use caution if patient receiving a calcium channel blocker; could cause CHF; acute discontinuation could exacerbate angina pectoris or potentially cause an MI Most common AEs are generally mild, but are quite numerous — SEE Prescribing Information (PI) Pregnancy category: C	Inderal only: If you miss a dose take it as soon as you remember, but if it is within 4 hrs of the next dose skip the missed one — do not double doses Inderal LA only: Swallow the capsule whole — do not bite, crush, divide or chew it; if you miss a dose take it as soon as you remember, but if it is within 8 hrs of the next dose skip the missed one — do not double doses Inderal or Inderal LA: also SEE atenolol	Inderal and Inderal LA are NOT beta-1 selective; since all patients may have some coronary artery disease, it may be advisable to discontinue therapy slowly over a period of several weeks for all patients and not just those with known angina; in general, persons with bronchospastic disease should not receive a beta blocker;

Generic Name and Selected Trade Names	Normal Adult Dosage	Miscellaneous Issues
Propranolol HCl (continued) Inderal Inderal LA	Inderal for arrhythmias: Usually 10 to 30 mg TID or QID given ac and hs Inderal for MI: Usually 180 to 240 mg/day in divided doses Inderal for migraine: Usually start with 80 mg/day in divided doses; may titrate gradually to usual range of 160 to 240 mg/day; if therapy to be stopped, do so gradually over several weeks Inderal for hypertrophic subaortic stenosis: Usually 20 to 40 mg TID or QID given ac and hs Inderal for essential tremor: Usually start with 40 mg BID; may titrate to usual maintenance of 120 mg/day, although some patients need up to 320 mg/day Inderal for pheochromocytoma: Preoperatively — Usually 60 mg/day in divided doses for 3 days prior to surgery Manage inoperable tumor — Usually 30 mg/day in divided doses Parenteral dosage form available — SEE Prescribing Information (PI) Inderal LA for hypertension: As monotherapy or with a diuretic, usually start with 80 mg QD; may titrate to usual range of 120 to 160 mg QD, but some patients need 640 mg/day Inderal LA for angina: Usually start with 80 mg QD; may titrate at 3–7 day intervals to usual range of 160 mg QD; value and safety of doses >320 mg/day not established; if therapy to be stopped, do so gradually over a few weeks Inderal LA for migraine: Usually start with 80 mg QD; may titrate gradually to usual maintenance of 160 to 240 mg QD; if therapy to be stopped, do so gradually over several weeks Inderal LA for hypertrophic subaortic stenosis: Usually 80 to 160 mg QD	discontinuation prior to surgery is controversial — SEE Prescribing Information Inderal LA only: If patient switched from Inderal, may need to re-titrate — do not substitute on a mg per mg basis as pharmacokinetics are different

Generic Name and Selected Trade Names	Normal Adult Dosage	Major Adverse Effects/Cautions	Key Counseling Points	Miscellaneous Issues
Sotalol HCl[2] Betapace	Individualize dosage Initiate in a hospital and with close supervision — SEE Prescribing Information (PI) For ventricular arrhythmias, usually start with 80 mg BID; may titrate every 2–3 days to 120 to 160 mg BID although some patients may require up to 640 mg/day Reduce dosage in renal impairment — SEE PI	Contraindications: Bronchial asthma, sinus bradycardia, second- and third-degree heart block (unless pacemaker present), long QT syndrome, cardiogenic shock, uncontrolled CHF Considerations: May cause torsades de pointes (dose related) and other proarrhythmias; use caution in sick sinus syndrome associated with symptomatic arrhythmias; do not use in hypomagnesemia or hypokalemia; excessive prolongation of QT interval could cause serious arrhythmias and should be avoided; also SEE carteolol	While taking this medication, tell the prescriber if you develop any palpitations, feel dizzy, have difficulty breathing; if a potassium supplement or a special vitamin was prescribed, it is important to take it; make sure all your other physicians, dentists, etc know that you are taking this medication; also, SEE betaxolol	Not beta-1 selective; should be prescribed by a clinician with extensive experience with this agent; usually start in hospital; monitor patient very carefully; in general, persons with bronchospastic disease should not receive a beta blocker; discontinuation prior to surgery is controversial — SEE Prescribing Information

Generic Name and Selected Trade Names	Normal Adult Dosage	Major Adverse Effects/Cautions	Key Counseling Points	Miscellaneous Issues
Sotalol HCl[2] **(continued)** Betapace		Most common AEs include dyspnea, bradycardia, chest pain, palpitations, fatigue, dizziness, edema, asthenia (weakness), lightheadedness, nausea/vomiting, diarrhea, ECG abnormalities, and many others Pregnancy category: B		

Generic Name and Selected Trade Names	Normal Adult Dosage	Major Adverse Effects/Cautions	Key Counseling Points	Miscellaneous Issues
Timolol Maleate Blocadren	Individualize dosage For hypertension: As monotherapy or with a diuretic, usually start with 10 mg BID; may titrate in intervals of at least 7 days to 20 to 40 mg/day but some patients may need up to 60 mg/day in two divided doses For MI: Long-term, usually 10 mg BID For migraine: Usually start with 10 mg BID; long-term 10 or 20 mg QD or up to 30 mg/day in divided doses —SEE PI	Contraindications: Bronchial asthma or history of same, severe chronic obstructive pulmonary disease, sinus bradycardia, second and third degree heart block, overt cardiac failure, cardiogenic shock Considerations: SEE carteolol Most common AEs include bradycardia, fatigue, dyspnea, dizziness, arrhythmias Pregnancy category: C	SEE acebutolol	Not beta-1 selective; in general, persons with bronchospastic disease should not receive a beta blocker; discontinuation prior to surgery is controversial — SEE Prescribing Information

Generic Name and Selected Trade Names	Normal Adult Dosage	Major Adverse Effects/Cautions	Key Counseling Points	Miscellaneous Issues
Timolol Maleate (continued) Blocadren	<u>Dosage adjustment</u>: May need reduced dosage in renal and/or liver impairment — SEE PI			

*As a general rule, a medication should not be administered to a patient with a known hypersensitivity to it or a similar agent.
[1]Alpha/beta adrenergic blocker.
[2]Possesses other pharmacologic properties as well.

Table 8: Nitrates*

Generic Name and Selected Trade Names	Normal Adult Dosage	Major Adverse Effects/Cautions	Key Counseling Points	Miscellaneous Issues
Isosorbide Dinitrate Dilatrate-SR Isordil (Sub-lingual, Tembids, Titradose) Sorbitrate (Chewable, Oral Tablets, Sub-lingual)	Individualize dosage <u>Dilatrate-SR for angina</u>: Dosage ranges from 40 to 160 mg per day; do not exceed 160 mg per day <u>Isordil or Sorbitrate Sub-lingual for angina</u>: 2.5 or 5 mg about 15 minutes before starting an activity thought to cause angina <u>Isordil Tembids for angina</u>: Total daily dose ranges from 30 to 480 mg per day	<u>Considerations</u>: Benefits in acute MI or CHF not established; may cause tolerance — need nitrate-free interval daily; may cause severe hypotension, may aggravate angina due to hypertrophic cardiomyopathy Most common AEs include headache, cutaneous dilation with flushing, transient light-headedness/dizziness/ weakness, hypotension, syncope <u>Pregnancy category</u>: C	Tell the prescriber if you are allergic to nitrates or nitrites; anti-anginal effect strongly related to dosing regimen so follow schedule carefully; headaches may indicate nitrate efficacy, aspirin and/or acetaminophen may be used to treat headache if it lasts a long time or is troublesome, but first check with physician and/or pharmacist; when taking a dose, sit down and when you need to stand up do so slowly to avoid/ minimize dizziness; you may still need nitroglycerin tablets — check with the prescriber; extended-release tablets or capsules are not to be broken, crushed, or chewed before swallowed;	Nitrate-free interval needed to decrease risk of tolerance: <u>Dilatrate-SR</u>: To achieve an effective nitrate-free interval, at least one interdose interval must be >18 hrs <u>Isordil or Sorbitrate Sublingual</u>: At least one interdose interval must be >14 hrs <u>Isordil Tembids</u>: At least one interdose interval must be >14 hrs

Generic Name and Selected Trade Names	Normal Adult Dosage	Major Adverse Effects/Cautions	Key Counseling Points	Miscellaneous Issues
Isosorbide Dinitrate (continued) Dilatrate-SR Isordil (Sub-lingual, Tembids, Titradose) Sorbitrate (Chewable, Oral Tablets, Sub-lingual)	Isordil Titradose or Sorbitrate Oral Tablets for angina: Start with 5 to 20 mg two or three times daily; maintenance dose 10 to 40 mg two or three times daily Sorbitrate Chewable Tablet for angina: Take 5 mg about 15 minutes before starting an activity thought to cause angina		sublingual tablets should dissolve under the tongue and should not be swallowed, chewed, broken, or crushed; chewable tablets must be well chewed and then held in the mouth for about 2 minutes before swallowing	Isordil Titradose or Sorbitrate Oral Tablets: At least one interdose interval must be >14 hrs Sorbitrate Chewable Tablet: At least one interdose interval must be >14 hrs

Generic Name and Selected Trade Names	Normal Adult Dosage	Major Adverse Effects/Cautions	Key Counseling Points	Miscellaneous Issues
Isosorbide Mononitrate Imdur	Individualize dosage For angina start with 30 mg or 60 mg QD in the AM on arising; after several days may increase to 120 mg QD in AM, rarely, give 240 mg QD in AM	<u>Considerations</u>: Benefits in acute MI or CHF not established; may cause tolerance — need nitrate-free interval daily Most common AEs include headache and dizziness; for less commonly noted effects SEE Prescribing Information (PI) <u>Pregnancy category</u>: B	Medication is for long-term therapy and is not used to treat an acute episode of angina; swallow with a one-half glass of fluid, do not chew or crush; take the tablet on rising; therapy may be associated with light-headedness on standing especially just after rising from a recumbent or seated position — effect may be more frequent if alcoholic beverages consumed; also, SEE isosorbide dinitrate	

Generic Name and Selected Trade Names	Normal Adult Dosage	Major Adverse Effects/Cautions	Key Counseling Points	Miscellaneous Issues
Isosorbide Mononitrate ISMO	Individualize dosage For angina, usually 20 mg when rising then 20 mg 7 hrs later	<u>Considerations</u>: Benefits in acute MI or CHF not established; may cause tolerance — need nitrate-free interval daily Most common AEs include headache, dizziness, nausea/vomiting; for less commonly noted effects SEE Prescribing Information (PI) <u>Pregnancy category</u>: C	Medication is for long-term therapy and is not used to treat an acute episode of angina; take the tablet on rising and 7 hrs later as directed; therapy may be associated with light-headedness on standing especially just after rising from a recumbent or seated position — effect may be more frequent if alcoholic beverages consumed; also, SEE isosorbide dinitrate	

Generic Name and Selected Trade Names	Normal Adult Dosage	Major Adverse Effects/Cautions	Key Counselling Points	Miscellaneous Issues
Isosorbide Mononitrate Monoket	Individualize dosage For angina, usually 20 mg twice daily with doses 7 hrs apart; in small stature patients, start with 5 mg, but increase to at least 10 mg by second or third day of therapy	<u>Considerations</u>: Benefits in acute MI or CHF not established; may cause tolerance — need nitrate-free interval daily; may cause severe hypotension, may aggravate angina due to hypertrophic cardiomyopathy Most common AEs include headache, fatigue, dizziness, nausea, chest pain, diarrhea, flushing <u>Pregnancy category</u>: B	SEE isosorbide mononitrate, ISMO	

Generic Name and Selected Trade Names	Normal Adult Dosage	Major Adverse Effects/Cautions	Key Counseling Points	Miscellaneous Issues
Nitroglycerin, sublingual Nitrostat	Individualize dosage For acute angina: Dissolve tablet under tongue or in buccal pouch; may repeat every 5 minutes for maximum total of 15 minutes (3 tabs), and if pain persists promptly seek medical aid For angina prophylaxis: Dissolve one tablet under tongue or in buccal pouch about 5–10 minutes before starting an activity thought to cause angina	Contraindications: Early MI, severe anemia, increased intracranial pressure Considerations: Use lowest dose possible as excessive amounts may lead to tolerance; may cause severe hypotension, increased angina, blurred vision, paradoxical bradycardia; may aggravate angina caused by hypertrophic cardiomyopathy Most common AEs include headache, vertigo, weakness, palpitations, orthostatic hypotension, syncope, flushing, rash Pregnancy category: C	Tell the prescriber if you are allergic to nitrates or nitrites; headaches may indicate nitrate efficacy, aspirin and/or acetaminophen may be used to treat headache if it lasts a long time or is troublesome, but first check with physician and/or pharmacist; when taking a dose, sit down and when you need to stand up do so slowly to avoid/minimize dizziness; if you feel an anginal episode coming on, sit down and take one tablet, if pain not relieved within a few minutes, take another tablet and wait a few minutes, if not effective try a third — but if three tablets don't work,	

Generic Name and Selected Trade Names	Normal Adult Dosage	Major Adverse Effects/Cautions	Key Counseling Points	Miscellaneous Issues
Nitroglycerin, sublingual (continued) Nitrostat			seek immediate medical attention; may produce a burning or stinging sensation when taken sublingually, but this should NOT be used to determine if medication is potent; store in original container; do not store other medications with this one; first time container is opened, discard cotton; after removing tablet close container tightly	

Generic Name and Selected Trade Names	Normal Adult Dosage	Major Adverse Effects/Cautions	Key Counseling Points	Miscellaneous Issues
Nitroglycerin, translingual Nitrolingual Spray	Individualize dosage For acute angina: One or two metered doses sprayed onto or under the tongue; no more than three metered doses recommended in 15 minute period For angina prophylaxis: Use 5–10 minutes before starting an activity thought to cause angina	Considerations: Extra caution needed if used during early days of MI; may cause severe hypotension, increased angina Most common AEs include headache, hypotension, cutaneous dilation with flushing, transient dizziness and weakness, rash Pregnancy category: C	Tell the prescriber if you are allergic to nitrates or nitrites; headaches may indicate nitrate efficacy, aspirin and/or acetaminophen may be used to treat headache if it lasts a long time or is troublesome, but first check with physician and/or pharmacist; when taking a dose, sit down and when you need to stand up do so slowly to avoid/minimize dizziness; during use rest, hold, the canister vertically with the valve head uppermost and the spray orifice as close to the mouth as possible, preferably spray onto tongue and close mouth after each dose, do not inhale spray	

Generic Name and Selected Trade Names	Normal Adult Dosage	Major Adverse Effects/Cautions	Key Counseling Points	Miscellaneous Issues
Nitroglycerin, transdermals Deponit Minitran Nitro-Derm Nitro-Dur Nitrodisc Transderm-Nitro	Individualize dosage Products are similar but unique — refer to Prescribing Information (PI) for specific data For angina prophylaxis: Start with 0.2 to 0.4 mg/hr; usual maintenance dose 0.4 to 0.8 mg/hr	<u>Considerations</u>: SEE above nitrates and refer to Prescribing Information (PI)	Tell the prescriber if you are allergic to nitrates or nitrites; anti-anginal effect strongly related to dosing regimen so follow schedule carefully; medication is for long-term treatment, not for an acute episode of angina; headaches may indicate product efficacy, aspirin and/or acetaminophen may be used to treat headache if it lasts a long time or is troublesome, but first check with physician and/or pharmacist; when you need to stand up do so slowly to avoid/minimize dizziness; for acute attacks, you may still need nitroglycerin tablets; ensure patient knows how to apply product properly	After use, there is significant nitroglycerin in patch — discard properly; to achieve an effective nitrate-free interval, patients should wear the patch for 12–14 hrs and remove the patch for 10–12 hrs per day

Generic Name and Selected Trade Names	Normal Adult Dosage	Major Adverse Effects/Cautions	Key Counseling Points	Miscellaneous Issues
Nitroglycerin, topicals Nitro-Bid (oint) Nitrol (oint)	Individualize dosage. Start with 0.5 inches and administer another dose 6–8 hrs later; usual dose 0.5–2 inches although some patients require more	Considerations: SEE above and refer to Prescribing Information (PI)	SEE nitroglycerin, transdermals	To achieve effective nitrate-free interval remove dosage form for 10–12 hrs per day

*As a general rule, a medication should not be administered to a patient with a known hypersensitivity to it or a similar agent.

Table 9: Antihypertensive Agents*

Acebutolol	Cyclothiazide	Labetalol HCl	Polythiazide
Amiloride HCl	Diltiazem	Lisinopril	Prazosin HCl
Amlodipine Besylate	Doxazosin	Losartan Potassium	Propranolol HCl
Atenolol	Enalapril Maleate	Methyclothiazide	Quinapril
Benazepril HCl	Ethacrynic Acid	Methyldopa	Ramipril
Bendroflumethiazide	Felodipine	Metolazone	Reserpine
Benzthiazide	Fosinopril Sodium	Metoprolol Succinate	Sotalol HCl
Betaxolol	Furosemide	Metoprolol Tartrate	Spironolactone
Bisoprolol	Guanabenz Acetate	Minoxidil	Terazosin HCl
Bumetanide	Guanethidine Monosulfate	Moexipril HCl	Timolol Maleate
Candesartan Cilexetil	Guanfacine HCl	Nadolol	Torsemide
Captopril	Hydralazine HCl	Nicardipine HCl	Trandolapril
Carteolol	Hydrochlorothiazide	Nifedipine	Triamterene
Carvedilol	Hydroflumethiazide	Nitroglycerin	Trichlormethiazide
Chlorothiazide	Indapamide	Penbutolol Sulfate	Valsartan
Chlorthalidone	Irbesartan	Pindolol	Verapamil
Clonidine	Isradipine		

*Refer to the table dealing with the appropriate pharmacologic category for key information about each of the individual antihypertensive medications. When dispensing any antihypertensive medication, consider advising the patient about the following:
— This medication is used to *treat* your high blood pressure; it will *not cure* your hypertension. Left untreated, high blood pressure can lead to serious problems such as heart disease, strokes, kidney disease, and loss of vision.
— Treatment may include weight loss or control, and avoidance of foods rich in sodium.
— It is important to take the medication exactly as prescribed, even if you feel totally normal. Do not stop the medication unless directed by the prescriber.
— Do not take any non-prescription medication without discussing it first with your physician and/or pharmacist. This is especially important for medications used to treat colds, allergies, nasal congestion, hay fever, or sinus problems, and agents used for weight reduction/control.

Table 10: Antiarrhythmic Agents*

Generic Name and Selected Trade Names	Normal Adult Dosage	Major Adverse Effects/Cautions	Key Counseling Points	Miscellaneous Issues
Acebutolol[1]				
Amiodarone HCl Cordarone	Individualize dosage For life-threatening arrhythmias, load in hospital with 800 to 1600 mg per day for at least 1–3 weeks; if administering >1000 mg/day, use divided doses and give with food; when control reached, reduce dose to 600 to 800 mg/day for one month and then to usual maintenance dose of 400 mg/day, although some patients require up to 600 mg/day and some need less;	Contraindications: Severe sinus node dysfunction causing marked sinus bradycardia, second- and third-degree heart block, when episodes of bradycardia have caused syncope (unless artificial pacemaker present) Considerations: May cause fatal toxicities (the most important is pulmonary toxicity), liver disease, impairment or loss of vision, thyroid abnormalities, photosensitivity reactions, skin discoloration, and exacerbate arrhythmias	Tell the prescriber if you have a heart, liver, or thyroid disease; you may be more sensitive to sunlight so wear sunblock, a hat, and clothing that covers your skin; contact the prescriber if you notice that your skin is developing a blue-gray color, you develop a cough or any type of a breathing problem, if your pulse slows, if you develop palpitations, changes in your vision, numbness or tingling in your fingers, difficulty walking; if you miss a dose of this medication, do not take the missed dose at all and do not double doses — go back to usual dosage regimen;	Should be administered only by a physician with experience in treatment of life-threatening arrhythmias; important drug interactions are possible — SEE Prescribing Information (PI); attempt to stop other antiarrhythmics when initiating amiodarone

89

Generic Name and Selected Trade Names	Normal Adult Dosage	Major Adverse Effects/Cautions	Key Counseling Points	Miscellaneous Issues
Amiodarone HCl (continued) Cordarone	important to use lowest effective dose Parenteral dosage form available, SEE Prescribing Information (PI)	Most common AEs include neurologic abnormalities (eg, malaise, fatigue, tremor, gait abnormalities), ophthalmic abnormalities, GI effects, photosensitivity reactions, CHF, arrhythmias, taste and smell disturbances, flushing, and many more — SEE Prescribing Information (PI) Pregnancy category: D	If you miss two or more doses in a row, contact the prescriber	
Atenolol[1]				
Diltiazem[2]				

Generic Name and Selected Trade Names	Normal Adult Dosage	Major Adverse Effects/Cautions	Key Counseling Points	Miscellaneous Issues
Disopyramide Phosphate Norpace Norpace CR	Individualize dosage. For arrhythmias, the usual dosage of either the immediate or extended release product is 400 to 800 mg per day in divided doses; most adults use 600 mg/day; if body weight <50 kg, usual dosage is 400 mg/day in divided doses	<u>Contraindications</u>: Cardiogenic shock, preexisting second or third degree AV block if pacemaker not present, congenital Q-T prolongation <u>Considerations</u>: May worsen or cause CHF; may cause hypotension, QRS widening or prolongation of Q-T interval on ECG, hypoglycemia; avoid in glaucoma, myasthenia gravis, and urinary retention due to anticholinergic effect; avoid use with other Type 1A agents; use caution in renal or liver impairment, sick sinus, potassium imbalance	Tell the prescriber if you have a heart or kidney disease, glaucoma, difficulty with urination, diabetes mellitus or myasthenia gravis; this medication may make you tired/dizzy, so do not drive a car or use hazardous machinery until you know how you are affected; contact the prescriber if you develop swelling (edema), gain weight, notice blurred vision, difficulty in breathing or urinating; if you miss a dose take it as soon as you remember, but if it is within 4 hrs of the next dose skip the missed one and return to regular dosing schedule — do not double doses	Studies (eg, CAST) revealed that certain antiarrhythmics are associated with increased mortality or non-fatal cardiac arrest if administered soon after an MI ("black-box warning"); numerous drug interactions are possible, SEE Prescribing Information (PI)

Generic Name and Selected Trade Names	Normal Adult Dosage	Major Adverse Effects/Cautions	Key Counseling Points	Miscellaneous Issues
Disopyramide Phosphate (continued) Norpace Norpace CR	For patients with renal insufficiency, cardiomyopathy or possible cardiac decompensation, or to transfer patient from one dosage form to the other, or for pediatric dosage, SEE Prescribing Information (PI)	Most common AEs include anticholinergic effects (eg, dry mouth, urinary hesitancy, constipation, blurred vision), hypotension, CHF, cardiac conduction abnormalities, edema, anorexia, diarrhea, dizziness, fatigue, rash, nervousness, hypokalemia Pregnancy category: C	Controlled release form: Do not crush, break, chew, or cut — swallow whole	

Generic Name and Selected Trade Names	Normal Adult Dosage	Major Adverse Effects/Cautions	Key Counseling Points	Miscellaneous Issues
Flecainide Acetate Tambocor	Individualize dosage For PSVT or PAF: Start with 50 mg Q12H and may titrate in increments of 50 mg BID every 4 days For sustained VT: Start with 100 mg Q12H and titrate; dosing regimens are complex, SEE Prescribing Information (PI) Dosage adjustments: May need reduced dosage in renal impairment and may be used in children — SEE PI	Contraindications: Pre-existing second or third-degree heart block, right bundle branch block associated with left hemiblock unless pacemaker present, cardiogenic shock Considerations: May cause (or worsen) CHF, supraventricular/ventricular arrhythmias, QRS widening, prolongation of Q-T and/or PR interval; use caution in renal or liver impairment, sick sinus syndrome, potassium imbalance; may adversely affect artificial pacemaker	Tell the prescriber if you have a heart, kidney, or liver disease, or had a recent heart attack; this medication may make you tired/dizzy, so do not drive a car or use machinery until you know how you are affected; contact the prescriber if you develop swelling (edema), shortness of breath, or chest pain, gain weight, notice palpitations; do not stop taking this agent without discussing it first with the prescriber; it is best to take the doses 12 hrs apart; very important to take the medication as directed; if you miss a dose take it as soon as you remember, but if it is within 6 hrs of the next dose skip the missed one and return to regular dosing schedule — do not double doses	For patients with ventricular tachycardia, initiate therapy in a hospital with appropriate monitoring facilities; medication has a long half-life — increase dosage no more frequently than once every four days; monitor plasma levels during therapy — peak levels >1 mcg/mL associated with increased risk of adverse effects; also, SEE disopyramide phosphate

Generic Name and Selected Trade Names	Normal Adult Dosage	Major Adverse Effects/Cautions	Key Counseling Points	Miscellaneous Issues
Flecainide Acetate (continued) Tambocor		Most common AEs include heart block, new or worsened arrhythmias, CHF, sinus bradycardia, dizziness, visual disturbances, dyspnea, headache, nausea, fatigue, palpitations, chest pain, tremor, asthenia (weakness), constipation, edema, abdominal pain, and many others Pregnancy category: C		

Generic Name and Selected Trade Names	Normal Adult Dosage	Major Adverse Effects/Cautions	Key Counselling Points	Miscellaneous Issues
Lidocaine HCl Xylocaine	Individualize dosage For ventricular arrhythmias, administer usual loading dose of 50 to 100 mg IV at rate of 25 to 50 mg/min followed by another if necessary; for maintenance, use continuous IV infusion of 20–50 mcg/kg/min — SEE Prescribing Information (PI) For IM self-injection, SEE PI	<u>Contraindications</u>: Stokes-Adams syndrome, Wolff-Parkinson-White syndrome, severe heart block if pacemaker not present <u>Considerations</u>: Use caution in patients with CHF, reduced cardiac function, digitalis toxicity, sinus bradycardia, renal or liver impairment; amide agents reported to cause malignant hyperthermia Most common AEs include CNS effects (eg, dizziness, confusion, disorientation, lightheadedness, tinnitus, and hallucinations), hypotension, bradycardia, cardiovascular depression Pregnancy category: B	Not applicable	When used IV, must be diluted; should be administered with constant monitoring
Metoprolol[1]				

Generic Name and Selected Trade Names	Normal Adult Dosage	Major Adverse Effects/Cautions	Key Counseling Points	Miscellaneous Issues
Mexiletine HCl Mexitil	Individualize dosage For arrhythmias, start with 200 mg Q8H; may titrate every 2–3 days in 50 or 100 mg increments; most patients require 200 to 300 mg Q8H with food or antacid; some patients who respond to Q8H regimen may change to Q12H; maximal dose recommended is 1200 mg/day For loading dose and methods to transfer patients from other agents to mexiletine, SEE Prescribing Information (PI)	<u>Contraindications</u>: Cardiogenic shock, pre-existing second- or third-degree AV block if pacemaker not present <u>Considerations</u>: May worsen arrhythmias; use caution in hypotension, severe CHF, liver impairment; may increase AST (SGOT) levels Most common AEs include nausea/vomiting, dizziness/lightheadedness, tremor, palpitations, diarrhea, constipation, coordination difficulties, changes in sleep habits, weakness, nervousness, visual disturbances, headache, dyspnea, rash <u>Pregnancy category</u>: C	Take with food or antacid; tell the prescriber if you have a heart or liver disease; this medication may make you tired/dizzy/lightheaded, so do not drive a car or use hazardous machinery until you know how you are affected; contact the prescriber if you develop chest pain, a change in your heartbeat, or difficulty in breathing; very important to take the medication as directed; if you miss a dose take it as soon as you remember, but if it is within 4 hrs of the next dose skip the missed one and return to regular dosing schedule — do not double doses	SEE disopyramide phosphate

Generic Name and Selected Trade Names	Normal Adult Dosage	Major Adverse Effects/Cautions	Key Counseling Points	Miscellaneous Issues
Moricizine HCl Ethmozine	Individualize dosage For arrhythmias, usual dose is 600 to 900 mg per day in 3 equally divided doses on a Q8H regimen; may titrate within this range every 3 days in 150 mg/day increments; some patients who respond to Q8H regimen may change to Q12H May need reduced dosage in renal or liver impairment — SEE Prescribing Information (PI) To transfer patients from other agents to moricizine, SEE (PI)	Contraindications: SEE flecainide Considerations: May worsen or cause arrhythmias; use extreme caution in sick sinus syndrome; use caution in renal or hepatic impairment, CHF; hypomagnesemia, hypokalemia, hyperkalemia, may alter effects of Type I agents; may increase PR and QRS interval on ECG Most common AEs include proarrhythmias, nausea/vomiting, ECG abnormalities, CHF, dizziness, headache, pain, dyspnea, fatigue Pregnancy category: B	Tell the prescriber if you have a heart/kidney/ or liver disease, or have an artificial pacemaker; this medication may make you tired/dizzy/lightheaded, so do not drive a car or use hazardous machinery until you know how you are affected; contact the prescriber if you develop chest pain, a change in your heartbeat, or difficulty in breathing; very important to take the medication as directed; if you miss a dose take it as soon as you remember, but if it is within 4 hrs of the next dose skip the missed one and return to regular dosing schedule — do not double doses	SEE disopyramide phosphate
Nadolol[1]				

Generic Name and Selected Trade Names	Normal Adult Dosage	Major Adverse Effects/Cautions	Key Counseling Points	Miscellaneous Issues
Phenytoin Sodium[3] Dilantin				
Procainamide HCl Procanbid-extended release Procan SR Pronestyl Pronestyl-SR	Individualize dosage For arrhythmias, usually start with 50 mg/kg of body weight per day in divided doses; depending on need and dosage form selected, a dose may be given Q3H to Q12H — SEE Prescribing Information (PI) for individual products; older persons and those with renal, hepatic, or cardiac insufficiency require lower dosages — SEE PI	<u>Contraindications</u>: Complete heart block (prudent to avoid in second-degree heart block and hemiblock), systemic lupus erythematosus (SLE), torsades de pointes <u>Considerations</u>: May cause severe blood dyscrasias including agranulocytosis and bone marrow depression as well as positive antinuclear antibody (ANA) titers with or without symptoms of SLE; use caution in first-degree heart block, digitalis intoxication, CHF, acute ischemic heart disease, renal insufficiency, myasthenia gravis, use with other antiarrhythmic agents; may widen QRS complex and prolong QT interval	Tell the prescriber if you are allergic to any "caine" medications, or if you have a heart/kidney/liver disease, myasthenia gravis, SLE; contact the prescriber if you develop muscle aches, joint pain, fever, chills, skin rash, easy bruising, an infection that lingers, muscle weakness, dizziness, nausea/vomiting; do not stop taking this agent without first discussing it with the prescriber; it is very important to adhere to the prescribed regimen;	Monitor laboratory tests and ECG frequently; may need to monitor serum levels of procainamide and metabolite; also, SEE disopyramide phosphate

Generic Name and Selected Trade Names	Normal Adult Dosage	Major Adverse Effects/Cautions	Key Counseling Points	Miscellaneous Issues
Procainamide HCl (continued) Procanbid-extended release Procan SR Pronestyl Pronestyl-SR	Parenteral form available — SEE PI	Most common AEs include SLE-like syndrome, hypotension, hematologic abnormalities such as thrombocytopenia and neutropenia, urticaria, rash, anorexia, abdominal pain, nausea/vomiting, increase in liver transaminase enzymes, taste disturbances, dizziness, weakness <u>Pregnancy category:</u> C	If you miss a dose take it as soon as you remember, but if it is within 2 hrs of the next dose for short-acting product or 4 hrs for extended release product skip the missed one and return to regular dosing schedule — do not double doses <u>Extended-release products:</u> Should be swallowed whole and should not be bitten or chewed	

Generic Name and Selected Trade Names	Normal Adult Dosage	Major Adverse Effects/Cautions	Key Counseling Points	Miscellaneous Issues
Propafenone HCl Rythmol	Individualize dosage For arrhythmias, start with 150 mg Q8H; may titrate at a minimum of 3–4 day intervals to 225 mg Q8H and then if necessary to 300 mg Q8H; titrate more slowly in elderly or those with previous myocardial damage May need reduced dosage in renal and liver impairment — SEE Prescribing Information (PI)	Contraindications: Uncontrolled CHF, cardiogenic shock, cardiac conduction abnormalities such as sick sinus syndrome and AV block in the absence of a pacemaker, bradycardia, marked hypotension, bronchospastic disease, electrolyte imbalances Considerations: May cause or worsen arrhythmias and CHF; may alter artificial pacemaker; use caution in liver or kidney impairment; may cause heart block and positive antinuclear antibody (ANA) titers Most common AEs include dizziness, unusual taste, dry mouth, proarrhythmia, rash, nausea/vomiting, dyspepsia, constipation, blurred vision, headache, fatigue, angina, CHF, palpitations Pregnancy category: C	Tell the prescriber if you have asthma or any other type of lung disorder, or SLE; notify the prescriber if you develop any muscle/joint pain or alterations in your taste perception; also, SEE moricizine	SEE disopyramide phosphate

Generic Name and Selected Trade Names	Normal Adult Dosage	Major Adverse Effects/Cautions	Key Counseling Points	Miscellaneous Issues
Propranolol HCl[1]				
Quinidine Gluconate Quinaglute Dura-Tabs	Individualize dosage For arrhythmias, the dosage varies widely depending upon the general condition and cardiovascular state of the patient; one initial regimen is 1 tab Q8H or Q12H, which is then titrated as needed — SEE Prescribing Information (PI); 324 mg tablets = 202 mg of quinidine base Parenteral dosage form available — SEE PI	Contraindications: Patients who developed thrombocytopenia during prior therapy with quinidine or quinine, patients who require an artificial pacemaker (eg, patients with complete heart block) but do not have one yet, myasthenia gravis or any other condition that might be worsened by an anticholinergic agent Considerations: In certain populations, associated with increased mortality; may cause proarrhythmia, syncope, hepatotoxicity, exacerbate bradycardia in sick sinus syndrome;	Tell the prescriber if you had any problem while taking quinidine or quinine previously, if you have myasthenia gravis or a heart/liver/kidney disorder; contact the prescriber if you develop a breathing problem, become dizzy, notice a change in vision, feel palpitations; the number of doses you take depends on the strength of the specific product and the specific arrhythmia being treated — take exactly what was prescribed;	Monitor laboratory tests, patient symptomatology, and ECG frequently; may need to monitor serum levels of quinidine; many drug interactions possible — SEE Prescribing Information (PI)

Generic Name and Selected Trade Names	Normal Adult Dosage	Major Adverse Effects/Cautions	Key Counseling Points	Miscellaneous Issues
Quinidine Gluconate (continued) Quinaglute Dura-Tabs		use caution in heart block in persons without implanted pacemaker; CHF, renal or liver impairment; may widen QRS complex and prolong QT interval Most common AEs include diarrhea, fever, rash, arrhythmias, abnormal ECG, nausea/vomiting, dizziness, headache, cerebral ischemia, asthenia (weakness) Pregnancy category: C	do not stop taking this medication without discussing it first with the prescriber; if medication bothers your stomach, take with food; medication may be broken in half, but should not be crushed or chewed; if you miss a dose take it as soon as you remember, but if it is close to the time that you would take the next dose, skip the missed one and return to regular dosing schedule — do not double doses	

Generic Name and Selected Trade Names	Normal Adult Dosage	Major Adverse Effects/Cautions	Key Counseling Points	Miscellaneous Issues
Quinidine Poly-galacturonate Cardioquin	Individualize dosage. For arrhythmias, the dosage varies widely depending upon the general condition and cardiovascular state of the patient; one initial regimen is 1 tab Q6H or Q8H, which is then titrated as needed — SEE Prescribing Information (PI); 275 mg tablets = 166 mg of quinidine base	<u>Considerations</u>: SEE quinidine gluconate	Do not crush, break, chew tablets; also, SEE quinidine gluconate	SEE quinidine gluconate

Generic Name and Selected Trade Names	Normal Adult Dosage	Major Adverse Effects/Cautions	Key Counseling Points	Miscellaneous Issues
Quinidine Sulfate Quinidex Extentabs (and tabs) Quinora	Individualize dosage For arrhythmias, the dosage varies widely depending upon the general condition and cardiovascular state of the patient — SEE Prescribing Information (PI); 300 mg Extentabs = 249 mg of quinidine base; 200 mg tablets = 166 mg of quinidine base	<u>Considerations</u>: SEE quinidine gluconate	SEE quinidine polygalacturonate	SEE quinidine gluconate
Sotalol HCl[1]				
Timolol[1]				

Generic Name and Selected Trade Names	Normal Adult Dosage	Major Adverse Effects/Cautions	Key Counselling Points	Miscellaneous Issues
Tocainide HCl Tonocard	Individualize dosage For arrhythmias, start with 400 mg Q8H; usual maintenance dosage is between 1200 and 1800 mg/day in three equally divided doses although some patients require less; some patients who do well on TID regimen may be changed to BID May need to reduce dosage in renal or liver impairment — SEE Prescribing Information (PI)	Contraindications: Second- or third-degree AV block without an artificial pacemaker, hypersensitivity to local anesthetics of amide type Considerations: Has caused blood dyscrasias such as agranulocytosis and bone marrow depression, pulmonary fibrosis, and proarrhythmias; use caution in CHF or minimal cardiac reserve, severe liver or kidney disease Most common AEs include dizziness/vertigo, nausea, vomiting, paresthesia, tremor, rash, hypotension, diarrhea/ loose stools, headache, altered mood Pregnancy category: C	Tell the prescriber if you are allergic to any "caine" medications, have an artificial pacemaker, or if you have a heart/ kidney/liver disease; notify the prescriber if you develop easy bruising, bleeding, signs of infection such as fever and chills, difficulty in breathing or wheezing, a rash; this agent may make you lightheaded/ tired, so do not drive a car or use hazardous machinery until you know how you are affected; it is very important to take the medication as directed; if you miss a dose but remember within 4 hrs take the tablet but if it is more than 4 hrs late, skip the missed dose and return to regular schedule — do not double doses	SEE disopyramide phosphate

Generic Name and Selected Trade Names	Normal Adult Dosage	Major Adverse Effects/Cautions	Key Counseling Points	Miscellaneous Issues
Verapamil[2]				

*As a general rule, a medication should not be administered to a patient with a known hypersensitivity to it or a similar agent.
[1]See Beta Adrenergic Blocking Agents.
[2]See Calcium Channel Blockers.
[3]See Antiepileptics.

Table 11: Digitalis Glycosides*

Generic Name and Selected Trade Names	Normal Adult Dosage	Major Adverse Effects/Cautions	Key Counseling Points	Miscellaneous Issues
Digitoxin Crystodigin	Individualize dosage. The dosages below are averages that may need to be altered significantly for individual patients; other dosing regimens exist — refer to specific references. <u>Slow digitalization</u>: 0.2 mg BID for 4 days. <u>Rapid digitalization</u>: 0.6 mg initially followed by 0.4 mg and then 0.2 mg at intervals of 4–6 hrs. <u>Maintenance</u>: 0.05 to 0.3 mg QD; 0.15 mg QD most common	<u>Contraindications</u>: Toxic response or idiosyncrasy to digitalis, ventricular tachycardia, beriberi, heart disease, some instances of the hypersensitive carotid sinus syndrome. <u>Considerations</u>: May cause many of the same arrhythmias it is used to treat; use cautiously in the elderly and monitor carefully; hypokalemia predisposes to toxicity. Most common AEs include anorexia, nausea, vomiting, abdominal discomfort, diarrhea, altered mental status, bradycardia and other arrhythmias, visual disturbances. <u>Pregnancy category</u>: C	Tell the prescriber if you have a liver, heart, kidney, lung, or thyroid problem/disease; if a potassium supplement or a potassium-sparing diuretic is prescribed, be sure to take it; ECG, serum potassium levels, and drug serum levels need to be checked routinely; do not take any other prescription or non-prescription medication without first discussing it with your physician or pharmacist; while taking this medication, contact the prescriber if you develop a loss of appetite, palpitations, nausea, vomiting; teach patient to monitor pulse rate and notify prescriber if it decreases significantly;	Monitor serum levels as well as ECG and clinical effects; may interact with agents that stimulate liver microsomal enzymes and numerous other drug interactions are possible — SEE Prescribing Information (PI) and other sources

107

Generic Name and Selected Trade Names	Normal Adult Dosage	Major Adverse Effects/Cautions	Key Counseling Points	Miscellaneous Issues
Digitoxin (continued) Crystodigin	<u>Dosage adjustment:</u> May need reduced dosage in liver impairment		if you miss a dose and remember it within 12 hrs take it as soon as you remember, but if more than 12 hrs skip the dose and go back to regular dosing regimen — do not double doses	

Generic Name and Selected Trade Names	Normal Adult Dosage	Major Adverse Effects/Cautions	Key Counseling Points	Miscellaneous Issues
Digoxin Lanoxicaps Lanoxin Lanoxin Elixir	Individualize dosage. Recommended dosages are average values that may require considerable modification when treating an individual; diminished renal function probably is the most important factor requiring dosage adjustment; a common digitalizing or loading dose is 8 to 15 mcg/kg depending on condition being treated (eg, 560 mcg–1 mg for a 70 kg patient), with one-half the dose given immediately and fractions of the rest in 6–8 hr intervals with close monitoring	<u>Contraindications</u>: Toxic response or idiosyncrasy to any digitalis preparation, ventricular tachycardia <u>Considerations</u>: May cause many of the same arrhythmias it is used to treat; use cautiously in patients with renal impairment and monitor carefully; hyperkalemia, hypokalemia, hypomagnesemia predispose patient to toxicity; hypocalcemia may nullify digoxin effects; may worsen AV block and sinus node diseases Most common AEs include ventricular tachycardia, AV block, bradycardia, ventricular premature contractions, anorexia, nausea, vomiting, visual disturbances (eg, yellow vision), headache, weakness, dizziness <u>Pregnancy category</u>: C	SEE digitoxin	Frequency and severity of adverse effects are dependent on dose and route of administration; certain adverse effects such as anorexia, nausea and vomiting, may be due to CHF or overdose — monitor digoxin serum levels (monitor ECG and clinical effects too); numerous drug interactions are possible — SEE Prescribing Information and other sources

Generic Name and Selected Trade Names	Normal Adult Dosage	Major Adverse Effects/Cautions	Key Counseling Points	Miscellaneous Issues
Digoxin Lanoxicaps Lanoxin Lanoxin Elixir	Refer to Prescribing Information (PI), specific references, and pharmacokinetic dosing regimens for loading and maintenance doses; note that dosage adjustments may need to take place when changing digoxin preparations due to differences in bioavailability Parenteral dosage form is available — SEE PI			

*As a general rule, a medication should not be administered to a patient with a known hypersensitivity to it or a similar agent.

Table 12: Diuretics — Thiazides and Related Agents*

Generic Name and Selected Trade Names	Normal Adult Dosage	Major Adverse Effects/Cautions	Key Counseling Points	Miscellaneous Issues
Bendroflume-thiazide Naturetin	Individualize dosage For edema: Usually start with 5 mg QD, preferably in AM although up to 20 mg once daily or in two doses can be given; maintenance dose is 2.5 to 5 mg daily; intermittent therapy — eg, 3–5 days/week may be advantageous For hypertension: Usually start with 5 to 20 mg daily; usual maintenance dose is 2.5 to 15 mg daily	Contraindications: Anuria; allergy to sulfonamide derivatives Considerations: Use caution in renal disease, liver disease, decreased liver function; may increase effect of other antihypertensives; sensitivity reactions may occur in persons with history of allergy or bronchial asthma; may cause abnormalities such as hypokalemia, hyponatremia, hyperuricemia, hypomagnesemia, and hyperglycemia; may increase cholesterol and triglyceride levels; may cause or exacerbate systemic lupus erythematosus (SLE)	Tell the prescriber if you are allergic to any other water pill or sulfonamide, have gout, a kidney/liver/ lung disease, diabetes mellitus; medication will increase urination — take it early in the day; if ordered, remember to take potassium supplement or potassium-sparing diuretic; you may be more sensitive to sunlight than normal so stay out of direct sunlight as much as possible, wear protective clothing including a hat, and apply sunblock; do not take other medications without first discussing it with your physician or pharmacist;	In general, avoid routine use of diuretics in pregnancy — SEE Prescribing Information (PI); frequently monitor patient for hypokalemia and dehydration; drug interactions may occur, SEE PI

111

Generic Name and Selected Trade Names	Normal Adult Dosage	Major Adverse Effects/Cautions	Key Counseling Points	Miscellaneous Issues
Bendroflume-thiazide Naturetin		Most common AEs include dehydration, electrolyte and metabolic abnormalities (see above) as well as hypotension; others, see Prescribing Information (PI) Pregnancy category: C	when standing up, do so slowly; contact prescriber if you become very thirsty/dizzy/lightheaded as you may be dehydrated, or develop severe diarrhea or vomiting as this may lead to a loss of too much liquid; if you miss a dose take it as soon as you remember, but if it is almost time for the next dose, skip the missed one and go back to regular dosing regimen — do not double doses	

Generic Name and Selected Trade Names	Normal Adult Dosage	Major Adverse Effects/Cautions	Key Counseling Points	Miscellaneous Issues
Benzthiazide Exna	Individualize dosage For edema: Usually start with 50 to 200 mg daily for several days; if using >100 mg/day, consider divided doses; maintenance 50 to 150 mg daily For hypertension: Usually 50 to 100 mg daily, administered as 25 to 50 mg after breakfast and lunch; maintenance up to 200 mg daily	Considerations: SEE bendroflumethiazide	SEE bendroflumethiazide	SEE bendroflumethiazide

113

Generic Name and Selected Trade Names	Normal Adult Dosage	Major Adverse Effects/Cautions	Key Counseling Points	Miscellaneous Issues
Chlorothiazide Diuril Diurigen	Individualize dosage For edema: Usually start with 0.5 to 1 G QD or BID; intermittent therapy — eg, alternate day therapy or 3–5 days/week may be preferred For hypertension: Usually start with 0.5 to 1 G/day in single or divided doses; some patients require up to 2 G/day in divided doses Parenteral dosage form is available — SEE Prescribing Information (PI)	Considerations: SEE bendroflumethiazide	SEE bendroflumethiazide	SEE bendroflumethiazide

Generic Name and Selected Trade Names	Normal Adult Dosage	Major Adverse Effects/Cautions	Key Counseling Points	Miscellaneous Issues
Chlorthalidone Hygroton Thalitone	Individualize dosage For edema: Start with 30 to 60 mg daily on alternate days, although some patients require up to 120 mg daily; maintenance doses should be titrated and are usually lower than initial dose For hypertension: Usually start with 15 mg daily, which may then be titrated as needed up to 45 to 50 mg daily; if greater antihypertensive effect needed, add another agent	Considerations: SEE bendroflumethiazide Pregnancy category: B	SEE bendroflumethiazide	Increases in serum uric acid levels and decreases in serum potassium levels are dose-related over the 15 to 50 mg/day range and beyond; also SEE bendroflumethiazide

Generic Name and Selected Trade Names	Normal Adult Dosage	Major Adverse Effects/Cautions	Key Counseling Points	Miscellaneous Issues
Hydrochlorothiazide Esidrix Ezide HydroDiuril Hydro-Par Oretic	Individualize dosage For edema: Usually 25 to 200 mg daily in single or divided doses; maintenance, usually 25 to 100 mg daily; intermittent therapy — eg, alternate day therapy or 3–5 days/week may be preferred For hypertension: Usually start with 25 mg QD and may increase to 50 mg QD although maximum doses of 100 mg BID have been used	<u>Considerations</u>: SEE bendroflumethiazide <u>Pregnancy category</u>: B	SEE bendroflumethiazide	Doses above 50 mg/day usually not needed when additional antihypertensive therapy used and may produce marked reductions in serum potassium; also SEE bendroflumethiazide

Generic Name and Selected Trade Names	Normal Adult Dosage	Major Adverse Effects/Cautions	Key Counseling Points	Miscellaneous Issues
Hydroflume-thiazide Diucardin Saluron	Individualize dosage For edema: Average dose is 25 to 200 mg daily For hypertension: Average dose is 50 to 100 mg daily	Considerations: SEE bendroflumethiazide	SEE bendroflumethiazide	SEE bendroflumethiazide
Indapamide Lozol	Individualize dosage For edema associated with CHF: Start with 2.5 mg in morning; may titrate after 1 week to 5 mg QD For hypertension: Start with 1.25 mg in AM; may titrate after 4 weeks to 2.5 mg QD and then to 5 mg QD before consider adding another agent	Considerations: SEE bendroflumethiazide Pregnancy category: B	SEE bendroflumethiazide	SEE bendroflumethiazide

Generic Name and Selected Trade Names	Normal Adult Dosage	Major Adverse Effects/Cautions	Key Counseling Points	Miscellaneous Issues
Methyclo-thiazide Aquatensen Enduron	Individualize dosage For edema: Usual range is 2.5 to 10 mg QD; single doses >10 mg offer no additional benefit For hypertension: Usual range is 2.5 to 5 mg QD; if after 8–12 weeks 5 mg not sufficient, add another antihypertensive agent	Considerations: SEE bendroflumethiazide Pregnancy category: B	SEE bendroflumethiazide	SEE bendroflumethiazide

Generic Name and Selected Trade Names	Normal Adult Dosage	Major Adverse Effects/Cautions	Key Counseling Points	Miscellaneous Issues
Metolazone Mykrox Zaroxolyn	Individualize dosage Mykrox for mild-to-moderate hypertension: Start with 0.5 mg QD, usually in morning; may titrate to 1 mg QD; if not sufficient, add another agent as higher doses of Mykrox provide no additional benefit Zaroxolyn for edema: Usually, 5 to 20 mg QD Zaroxolyn for mild-to-moderate hypertension: Usually, 2.5 to 5 mg QD; to switch patients from Zaroxolyn to Mykrox, SEE Prescribing Information (PI)	Contraindications: Anuria, hepatic coma, precoma; cross-allergy with sulfonamide-derived medications and thiazide diuretics is possible Considerations: Use caution in renal disease, liver disease, decreased liver function; may increase effect of other antihypertensives; sensitivity reactions may occur in persons with history of allergy or bronchial asthma; may cause abnormalities such as hypokalemia, hyponatremia, hyperuricemia, hypomagnesemia, and hyperglycemia; may increase cholesterol and triglyceride levels; may cause or exacerbate systemic lupus erythematosus (SLE)	SEE bendroflumethiazide	Mykrox is a "rapidly available" dosage form, and is NOT equivalent to Zaroxolyn which is a "slow formulation" of metolazone; if changing metolazone products, re-titrate patient; only thiazide-like agent that produces diuresis when glomerular filtration rate is <20 mL/min; also SEE bendroflumethiazide

Generic Name and Selected Trade Names	Normal Adult Dosage	Major Adverse Effects/Cautions	Key Counseling Points	Miscellaneous Issues
Metolazone (continued) Mykrox Zaroxolyn		Most common AEs with Mykrox include dehydration, electrolyte and metabolic abnormalities (see above) orthostatic hypotension, dizziness/ lightheadedness, headache, muscle cramps, fatigue, joint pain, chest pain Most common AEs with Zaroxolyn, SEE bendroflumethiazide Pregnancy category: B		

Generic Name and Selected Trade Names	Normal Adult Dosage	Major Adverse Effects/Cautions	Key Counseling Points	Miscellaneous Issues
Polythiazide Renese	Individualize dosage For edema: Usual range is 1 to 4 mg as a single dose in AM For hypertension: Usual range is 2 to 4 mg QD	Considerations: SEE bendroflumethiazide	SEE bendroflumethiazide	SEE bendroflumethiazide
Quinethazone Hydromox	Individualize dosage For edema or hypertension, range is 50 to 200 mg daily in single or divided into two doses	Considerations: SEE bendroflumethiazide	SEE bendroflumethiazide	SEE bendroflumethiazide
Trichlorme-thiazide Diurese Metahydrin Naqua	Individualize dosage For edema and hypertension, usually 1 to 4 mg QD	Considerations: SEE bendroflumethiazide	SEE bendroflumethiazide	SEE bendroflumethiazide

*As a general rule, a medication should not be administered to a patient with a known hypersensitivity to it or a similar agent.

Table 13: Diuretics — Loop*

Generic Name and Selected Trade Names	Normal Adult Dosage	Major Adverse Effects/Cautions	Key Counseling Points	Miscellaneous Issues
Bumetanide Bumex	Individualize dosage For edema, usual total daily dose is 0.5 to 2 mg QD; if response to initial dose not sufficient, may administer a second or third at 4-5 hr intervals up to a total daily dose of 10 mg; for maintenance, may administer on alternate days or several times per week only Parenteral dosage form is available — SEE Prescribing Information (PI)	Contraindications: Anuria, oliguria during therapy of patient with progressive renal disease, hepatic coma, severe electrolyte depletion Considerations: Excessive use may lead to volume and electrolyte loss; may cause hypokalemia, ototoxicity, thrombocytopenia (reduced platelets); for patients with hepatic cirrhosis and ascites, initiate therapy in a hospital; patients allergic to sulfonamides may exhibit sensitivity; may cause laboratory abnormalities such as hyperuricemia, hypochloremia, hyponatremia, hyperglycemia, and increased BUN and serum creatinine; use extreme caution when administering with other agents that may cause renal or ototoxicity	Tell the prescriber if you are allergic to any other water pill or sulfonamide, have a kidney or liver disease, gout, diabetes mellitus, or have difficulty in hearing; medication will increase urination — take it early in the day; if prescribed remember to take the potassium supplement or potassium-sparing diuretic; do not take other medications without first discussing it with your physician or pharmacist; when standing up, do so slowly; contact the prescriber if you become dizzy or lightheaded, or develop severe diarrhea or vomiting as this may lead to a loss of too much liquid;	Many drug interactions are possible — SEE Prescribing Information; frequently monitor patient for hypokalemia and dehydration

122

Generic Name and Selected Trade Names	Normal Adult Dosage	Major Adverse Effects/Cautions	Key Counseling Points	Miscellaneous Issues
Bumetanide (continued) Bumex		Most common AEs include muscle cramps, dizziness, hypotension, headache, nausea Pregnancy category: C	If you miss a dose take it as soon as you remember, but if it is almost time for the next dose, skip the missed one and go back to regular dosing schedule — do not double doses	

Generic Name and Selected Trade Names	Normal Adult Dosage	Major Adverse Effects/Cautions	Key Counseling Points	Miscellaneous Issues
Ethacrynic Acid Edecrin	Individualize dosage For diuresis, usually start with 50 mg (single dose) after a meal and may titrate in 25 to 50 mg increments up to 200 mg BID; after diuresis achieved, the minimally effective dose (usually 50 to 200 mg daily) may be given on continuous or intermittent regimen — SEE Prescribing Information (PI) Parenteral dosage form is available — SEE PI	<u>Contraindications</u>: Anuria, increasing electrolyte imbalance, azotemia and/or oliguria during treatment of severe renal disease, if severe diarrhea develops <u>Considerations</u>: Excessive use may lead to volume and electrolyte loss; too vigorous diuresis may cause hypotension; may cause hypokalemia, hyperuricemia, and many other electrolyte abnormalities, ototoxicity, weakness, muscle cramps, paresthesia, anorexia; use extreme caution when administering with other agents that can cause ototoxicity <u>Most common AEs</u> include anorexia, malaise, nausea, vomiting, diarrhea, and others related to electrolyte abnormalities <u>Pregnancy category</u>: B	SEE bumetanide	Is a potent diuretic, which in excessive amounts may lead to profound diuresis with water and electrolyte disturbances — regulate dosage carefully and monitor closely; many drug interactions are possible — SEE Prescribing Information

Generic Name and Selected Trade Names	Normal Adult Dosage	Major Adverse Effects/Cautions	Key Counseling Points	Miscellaneous Issues
Furosemide Lasix	Individualize dosage For edema: Usually start with 20 to 80 mg as a single dose; if needed, give same dose or increase dose by 20 to 40 mg 6–8 hrs later; long-term, dose may be given once or twice daily; may titrate up to 600 mg/day; long term, may be given 2–4 consecutive days/week — SEE Prescribing Information (PI)	Contraindication: Anuria Considerations: For patients with hepatic cirrhosis and ascites, initiate therapy in a hospital; do not use in hepatic coma until condition stabilized; stop therapy if azotemia and/or oliguria occur during treatment of severe progressive renal disease; may cause ototoxicity and many electrolyte abnormalities such as hypokalemia, hyperglycemia, and hyperuricemia Most common AEs include pancreatitis, jaundice, tinnitus and hearing loss, dizziness, orthostatic hypotension, glycosuria, and others related to electrolyte abnormalities Pregnancy category: C	The skin of some patients may be more sensitive to the effects of sunlight — avoid exposure to sun; also SEE bumetanide	If patient receives >80 mg/day for prolonged periods, monitor patient carefully clinically and via laboratory tests; many drug interactions are possible — SEE Prescribing Information

Generic Name and Selected Trade Names	Normal Adult Dosage	Major Adverse Effects/Cautions	Key Counseling Points	Miscellaneous Issues
Furosemide (continued) Lasix	For hypertension: Usually start with 40 mg BID; titrate based upon response; dosage of other antihypertensives should be reduced by at least 50% when furosemide added. Parenteral dosage form is available — SEE PI			

Generic Name and Selected Trade Names	Normal Adult Dosage	Major Adverse Effects/Cautions	Key Counseling Points	Miscellaneous Issues
Torsemide Demadex	Individualize dosage For edema due to CHF: Usually start with 10 or 20 mg QD; may titrate by approximately doubling dose; doses >200 mg not studied adequately For edema due to chronic renal failure: Usually start with 20 mg QD; may titrate by approximately doubling dose; doses >200 mg not studied adequately	Contraindication: Anuria Considerations: Excessive use may lead to volume and electrolyte loss; for patients with hepatic cirrhosis and ascites, initiate therapy in a hospital; may cause hypotension, electrolyte disturbances such as hypokalemia and hyperuricemia, ototoxicity, weakness, muscle cramps, paresthesia, anorexia Most common AEs include excessive urination, headache, rhinitis, asthenia (weakness), diarrhea, ECG abnormality, increase cough, constipation, nausea, arthralgia, dyspepsia, myalgia, electrolyte abnormalities Pregnancy category: B	May be taken with, before, or after a meal; also SEE bumetanide	Parenteral and oral forms are therapeutically equivalent — patients may be switched from injectable to oral form without a change in dose; special dosage adjustments in elderly not needed; frequently monitor patient for hypokalemia and dehydration

Generic Name and Selected Trade Names	Normal Adult Dosage	Major Adverse Effects/Cautions	Key Counseling Points	Miscellaneous Issues
Torsemide (continued) Demadex	For edema due to hepatic cirrhosis: Usually start with 5 to 10 mg QD with an aldosterone antagonist or a potassium-sparing diuretic; may titrate by approximately doubling dose; doses >40 mg not studied adequately; chronic use not studied For hypertension: Usually start with 5 mg; if response not acceptable within 4-6 weeks, may increase to 10 mg QD Parenteral dosage form is available — SEE Prescribing Information			

*As a general rule, a medication should not be administered to a patient with a known hypersensitivity to it or a similar agent.

Table 14: Diuretics — Potassium Sparing*

Generic Name and Selected Trade Names	Normal Adult Dosage	Major Adverse Effects/Cautions	Key Counseling Points	Miscellaneous Issues
Amiloride Midamor	Individualize dosage Start with 5 mg QD; may titrate to 10 mg QD, and if persistent hypokalemia persists, may increase to 15 mg and then 20 mg QD	<u>Contraindications</u>: Hyperkalemia (serum potassium >5.5 mEq/L), patients receiving other potassium-sparing diuretics, usually patients receiving potassium supplements, patients with anuria, acute or chronic renal insufficiency, diabetic nephropathy <u>Considerations</u>: May cause hyperkalemia (incidence increased in renal impairment, diabetes mellitus, in the elderly, and in patients taking other potassium-conserving agents, ACE inhibitors, and potassium supplements); use caution when other electrolyte imbalances are present	Tell the prescriber if you have a kidney disorder; take with food; medication will increase urination so take it early in the day; do not eat extra potassium-rich foods, or take potassium supplements or salt substitutes without discussing it first with the prescriber; especially when starting therapy, may cause tiredness/fatigue or dizziness, so be cautious when driving a car, using machinery, or doing other tasks that require alertness; if you miss a dose take it as soon as you remember, but if it is almost time for the next dose, skip the missed one and go back to regular dosing schedule — do not double doses	Monitor serum potassium levels and ECG; if hyperkalemia develops, treat promptly

Generic Name and Selected Trade Names	Normal Adult Dosage	Major Adverse Effects/Cautions	Key Counseling Points	Miscellaneous Issues
Amiloride (continued) Midamor		Most common AEs include headache, nausea/anorexia, diarrhea, vomiting, abdominal pain, flatulence, hyperkalemia, mild skin rash, those associated with diuresis Pregnancy category: B		

Generic Name and Selected Trade Names	Normal Adult Dosage	Major Adverse Effects/Cautions	Key Counselling Points	Miscellaneous Issues
Spironolactone Aldactone	Individualize dosage. For edema in adults: Usually start with 100 mg daily in single or divided doses, but may range from 25 to 200 mg daily; when used alone for diuresis continue dose for at least 5 days before consider adding another diuretic. For essential hypertension: Start with 50 to 100 mg daily in single or divided doses; may not see maximal effect for two weeks	Contraindications: Anuria, acute renal insufficiency, significant impairment of renal excretory function, hyperkalemia. Considerations: May cause hyperkalemia (and other electrolyte imbalances); generally should not be administered with potassium supplements or other potassium-sparing diuretics; ACE inhibitors may increase risk of hyperkalemia; may cause gynecomastia; shown to be a tumorigen in rats	For males: Sometimes, this medication causes breasts to enlarge, especially when taken for a long time (if you notice this, contact the prescriber), but breast size usually decreases over time after the medication is stopped; also SEE amiloride	Monitor serum potassium levels and ECG; if hyperkalemia develops, treat promptly

Generic Name and Selected Trade Names	Normal Adult Dosage	Major Adverse Effects/Cautions	Key Counseling Points	Miscellaneous Issues
Spironolactone (continued) Aldactone	For hypokalemia: 25 to 100 mg daily For diagnosing primary hyperaldosteronism and use in children: SEE Prescribing Information (PI)	Most common AEs include gynecomastia, GI symptoms such as cramping and diarrhea, drowsiness, lethargy, headache, rash, urticaria, drug fever, ataxia, hirsutism, irregular menses or amenorrhea, postmenopausal bleeding, mental confusion Pregnancy category: Not specified		

Generic Name and Selected Trade Names	Normal Adult Dosage	Major Adverse Effects/Cautions	Key Counseling Points	Miscellaneous Issues
Triamterene Dyrenium	Individualize dosage. For hypertension, when used as monotherapy start with 100 mg BID pc; when combined with another agent, the dosage of each should be reduced and then titrated as needed; total daily dosage should not exceed 300 mg	Contraindications: Anuria, severe or progressive kidney disease or dysfunction (with possible exception of nephrosis), severe hepatic disease. Considerations: Do not use in patients with hyperkalemia; may cause photosensitivity; also SEE amiloride. Most common AEs include rash, hyperkalemia, azotemia, elevated BUN and serum creatinine, jaundice, elevation in liver enzymes, thrombocytopenia, megaloblastic anemia, weakness, fatigue, dizziness, headache. Pregnancy category: B	You may be more sensitive to sunlight than normal so stay out of direct sunlight as much as possible, wear protective clothing including a hat, and apply sunblock; if you develop a severe reaction to sunlight, contact the prescriber; contact the prescriber if sore throat, mouth sores, unusual bleeding, or unexplained fever develop; also SEE amiloride	Monitor serum potassium levels and ECG; if hyperkalemia develops, treat promptly

*As a general rule, a medication should not be administered to a patient with a known hypersensitivity to it or a similar agent.

Lipid Lowering Agents

Table: Antilipemics*,1

Generic Name and Selected Trade Names	Normal Adult Dosage	Major Adverse Effects/Cautions	Key Counseling Points	Miscellaneous Issues
Atorvastatin Calcium Lipitor	Individualize dosage <u>For hypercholesterolemia and mixed dyslipidemia</u>: Start with 10 mg QD; range for maintenance is 10 to 80 mg QD <u>For homozygous familial hypercholesterolemia</u>: Administer 80 mg QD	<u>Contraindications</u>: Active liver disease or unexplained persistent elevations of serum transaminases, pregnancy, and nursing <u>Considerations</u>: May elevate serum transaminases so liver function tests should be conducted prior to and during therapy and when doses increased; rhabdomyolysis with acute renal failure has occurred; patients should be warned to report signs of myalgia, which is increased when co-administered with certain agents — SEE Prescribing Information Most common AEs include constipation, flatulence, dyspepsia, abdominal pain <u>Pregnancy category</u>: X	Inform the prescriber if you have a history of alcohol abuse, liver disease, seizures, recent major surgery or organ transplantation; patient should be aware of the importance of maintaining a low fat/cholesterol diet; should not be used during pregnancy or by women who plan on becoming pregnant, effective form of birth control should be used during therapy; notify the physician or pharmacist before taking other medications; if you experience unexplained muscle pain, tenderness or weakness check with the prescriber; inform the physician or dentist that you are receiving this medication;	

Generic Name and Selected Trade Names	Normal Adult Dosage	Major Adverse Effects/Cautions	Key Counseling Points	Miscellaneous Issues
Atorvastatin Calcium (continued) Lipitor			it is important that you take this medication as directed and that the prescriber checks your progress; do not stop taking without consulting the prescriber; may be given with or without food; if you miss a dose take it as soon as possible, but if it is almost time for the next dose skip the missed dose and return to regular schedule — do not double doses	

Generic Name and Selected Trade Names	Normal Adult Dosage	Major Adverse Effects/Cautions	Key Counseling Points	Miscellaneous Issues
Cerivastatin Sodium Baycol	Individualize dosage For hypercholesterolemia and mixed dyslipidemia, usually start with 0.3 mg in the evening; start with 0.2 mg in patients with renal dysfunction (ie, creatinine clearance below 60 mL/min)	<u>Contraindications and Considerations</u>: SEE atorvastatin calcium Most common AEs include dyspepsia, diarrhea, asthenia, arthralgia, myalgia, insomnia, sinusitis <u>Pregnancy category</u>: X	SEE atorvastatin calcium	

Generic Name and Selected Trade Names	Normal Adult Dosage	Major Adverse Effects/Cautions	Key Counseling Points	Miscellaneous Issues
Cholestyramine LoCholest Powder LoCholest Light Powder Questran Powder Questran Light	Individualize dosage For primary hypercholesterolemia or relief of pruritus associated with partial biliary obstruction, start with 1 packet or 1 level scoopful once or twice a day; maintenance dose 2 to 4 packets or scoopfuls daily in two divided doses; increase in dosage should occur at intervals of at least 4 weeks and with monitoring of lipid levels	<u>Contraindication</u>: Complete biliary obstruction <u>Considerations</u>: Chronic use can lead to vitamin K deficiency and subsequent hypoprothrombinemia and increased bleeding; folic acid deficiency can occur; may aggravate constipation (lower dosage); complete lipid profile should be determined before and during therapy Most common AEs include constipation, abdominal pain or cramps, bloating, flatulence <u>Pregnancy category</u>: C	Inform the prescriber if you have bleeding problems, constipation, gallstones, heart or blood vessel disorders, hemorrhoids, ulcers, underactive thyroid, kidney disease; patient should be aware of the importance of maintaining a low fat/cholesterol diet; notify the physician or pharmacist before taking other medications; take other agents at least 1 hr before or 4–6 hrs after ingesting this agent; contact prescriber if you experience black, tarry stools, severe stomach pain or nausea/vomiting;	Questran Light contains 16.8 mg phenylalanine per 5-G dose; not to be taken in dry form, always mix with water or other fluids before ingesting; many drug interactions are possible SEE Prescribing Information

Generic Name and Selected Trade Names	Normal Adult Dosage	Major Adverse Effects/Cautions	Key Counseling Points	Miscellaneous Issues

Cholestyramine (continued)
  LoCholest Powder
  LoCholest Light Powder
  Questran Powder
  Questran Light
			it is important that you take this medication as directed and that your prescriber checks your progress regularly; do not stop taking without consulting your prescriber; this medication should never be taken in its dry form, mix in 2 ounces of any beverage, then add 2–4 more ounces and mix again, drink the liquid then add a little more liquid to the glass and drink that also; may also be mixed with thin broth, pulpy fruits, or cereals; if you miss a dose take it as soon as possible, but if it is almost time for the next dose skip the missed dose and return to regular schedule — do not double doses	

Generic Name and Selected Trade Names	Normal Adult Dosage	Major Adverse Effects/Cautions	Key Counseling Points	Miscellaneous Issues
Colestipol Colestid (micronized) Flavored Colestid	Individualize dosage For primary hypercholesterolemia, start with 1 dose (1 packet or 1 teaspoonful) QD or BID; then, may titrate by 1 dose per day at 1–2 month intervals; usual range is 1–6 packets/teaspoonfuls daily, which can be given QD or in divided doses	<u>Considerations and most common AEs</u>: SEE cholestyramine <u>Pregnancy category</u>: Not specified	SEE cholestyramine	Not to be taken in dry form, always mix with water or other fluids before ingesting
Fluvastatin Sodium Lescol	Individualize dosage For primary hypercholesterolemia, start with 20 to 30 mg HS; maintenance dosage is 20 to 80 mg/day; 80 mg should be given as 40 mg BID	<u>Contraindications and considerations</u>: SEE atorvastatin calcium Most common AEs include dyspepsia, diarrhea, nausea, insomnia, headache <u>Pregnancy category</u>: X	SEE atorvastatin calcium	

Generic Name and Selected Trade Names	Normal Adult Dosage	Major Adverse Effects/Cautions	Key Counseling Points	Miscellaneous Issues
Gemfibrozil Lopid	Individualize dosage For hypertriglyceridemia, 1200 mg BID, 30 min prior to morning and evening meal For specific limitations and guidelines — SEE Prescribing Information (PI)	Contraindications: Hepatic or sever renal dysfunction, biliary cirrhosis, preexisting gallbladder disease Considerations: Complete lipid profile should be measured; clinical studies suggest patients may be at risk for gallbladder disease and certain malignancies so risk vs. benefit must be determined — SEE Prescribing Information Most common AEs include dyspepsia, abdominal pain, acute appendicitis, diarrhea Pregnancy category: C	Inform the prescriber if you have a history of gallbladder problems, liver or kidney disease; agent may be associated with increased risk of cancer, patient should discuss risks with prescriber; patient should be aware of the importance of maintaining a low fat/cholesterol diet; notify the physician or pharmacist before taking any other medication; contact the prescriber if you experience cough, fever, chills, lower back or side pain, painful urination, stomach pain, or nausea/vomiting;	

Generic Name and Selected Trade Names	Normal Adult Dosage	Major Adverse Effects/Cautions	Key Counseling Points	Miscellaneous Issues
Gemfibrozil (continued) Lopid			it is important to take this agent as directed and that the prescriber checks your progress regularly; do not stop taking this without consulting the prescriber; best if taken 30 min before meals; if you miss a dose take it as soon as possible, but if it is almost time for the next dose skip the missed one and return to regular schedule — do not double doses	

Generic Name and Selected Trade Names	Normal Adult Dosage	Major Adverse Effects/Cautions	Key Counseling Points	Miscellaneous Issues
Lovastatin Mevacor	Individualize dosage For primary hypercholesterolemia, start with 20 mg QD with evening meal; maintenance dosage is 10 to 80 mg/day in single or divided doses, administer doses >20 mg in patients with renal impairment (ie, creatinine clearance <30 mL/min) with caution	<u>Contraindications and considerations</u>: SEE atorvastatin calcium <u>Most common AEs</u> include headache, diarrhea, constipation, flatulence, abdominal pain/cramps <u>Pregnancy category</u>: X	SEE atorvastatin calcium, except best if taken with food	

Generic Name and Selected Trade Names	Normal Adult Dosage	Major Adverse Effects/Cautions	Key Counseling Points	Miscellaneous Issues
Pravastatin Sodium Pravachol	Individualize dosage For primary hypercholesterolemia, primary prevention of coronary events, and atherosclerosis, usually start with 10 to 20 mg HS; maintenance dosage is 10 to 40 mg/day; in elderly, renal or hepatic patients start with 10 mg HS	<u>Contraindications and considerations</u>: SEE atorvastatin calcium <u>Most common AEs</u> include nausea/vomiting, headache, rash Pregnancy category: X	SEE atorvastatin calcium	

Generic Name and Selected Trade Names	Normal Adult Dosage	Major Adverse Effects/Cautions	Key Counseling Points	Miscellaneous Issues
Simvastatin Zocor	Individualize dosage For primary hypercholesterolemia and patients with coronary heart disease and hypercholesterolemia, usually start with 5 to 10 mg in the evening; maintenance dosage is 5 to 40 mg/day	<u>Contraindications and considerations</u>: SEE atorvastatin calcium <u>Most common AEs</u> include constipation, flatulence <u>Pregnancy category</u>: X	SEE atorvastatin calcium	

*As a general rule, a medication should not be administered to a patient with a known hypersensitivity to it or a similar agent.
†A lipid lowering agent should be started only in patients who have attempted appropriate diet and exercise regimens.

Blood Modifiers

Table 1: Anticoagulants*

Generic Name and Selected Trade Names	Normal Adult Dosage	Major Adverse Effects/Cautions	Key Counseling Points	Miscellaneous Issues
Ardeparin Sodium Normiflo	Individualize dosage For prevention of DVT due to knee replacement surgery, administer 50 anti-Xa U/kg of body weight Q12H by deep (intra-fat) subcutaneous injection, begun the evening of the day of surgery or the next morning and continued for up to 14 days or until the patient is fully ambulatory To calculate volume to be administered — SEE Prescribing Information (PI)	Contraindications: Patients with active major bleeding or thrombocytopenia associated with positive tests for anti-platelet antibody in the presence of the agent, hypersensitivity to heparin or pork products Considerations: Not intended for intramuscular or intravenous use; use with caution in patients with heparin-induced thrombocytopenia; signs of bleeding should be assessed, thrombocytopenia can occur	Tell the prescriber if you have any unusual bleeding or previously had a bad reaction to heparin or pork, and tell him/her all other medications you are taking; do not take any new medication without first discussing it with your physician or pharmacist; ensure all your physicians, pharmacists, dentists, and other health care providers know you are taking this agent; if patient or caregiver is injecting, ensure he/she is familiar with proper injection technique — in part, SEE Prescribing Information (PI);	Cannot be used interchangeably with heparin sodium or other low molecular weight heparins

151

Generic Name and Selected Trade Names	Normal Adult Dosage	Major Adverse Effects/Cautions	Key Counseling Points	Miscellaneous Issues
Ardeparin Sodium (continued) Normiflo		Most common AEs include hemorrhage, thrombocytopenia, fever, anemia, nausea <u>Pregnancy category</u>: C	rotate injection sites including the abdomen, anterior aspect of thighs, and outer aspect of upper arm; if you miss a dose, take it as soon as you remember, but if it is almost time for the next dose, skip the missed one and return to regular dosing schedule — do not double doses	

Generic Name and Selected Trade Names	Normal Adult Dosage	Major Adverse Effects/Cautions	Key Counseling Points	Miscellaneous Issues
Dalteparin Sodium Fragmin	For patient undergoing abdominal surgery with a risk of thromboembolic complications: Administer 2500 International Units (I.U.) by deep subcutaneous (SC) injection 1–2 hrs prior to surgery and then QD for 5–10 days post-operatively For patient undergoing abdominal surgery with a high risk of thromboembolic complications: Give 5000 I.U. (deep) SC on the evening prior to the surgery and then QD for 5–10 days post-operatively	Contraindications: SEE ardeparin sodium Considerations: Not for IM use; use with caution in patients at risk for hemorrhage (eg, hypertension, GI disease), and with extreme caution in patients with history of heparin-induced thrombocytopenia; monitor patient for thrombocytopenia Most common AEs include hematoma and pain at injection site, allergic reactions Pregnancy category: B	SEE ardeparin sodium except that injection sites are the u-shaped area around the navel, upper outer side of the thigh, or the upper outer quadrant of the buttock	Cannot be interchanged unit for unit with other types of heparin

Generic Name and Selected Trade Names	Normal Adult Dosage	Major Adverse Effects/Cautions	Key Counseling Points	Miscellaneous Issues
Danaparoid Sodium Orgaran	For prevention of DVT due to hip replacement surgery, administer 750 anti-Xa units BID by deep subcutaneous (SC) injection beginning 1–4 hrs pre-operatively, and then not sooner than 2 hrs after surgery; average duration is 7–10 days	Contraindications: Severe hemorrhagic diathesis; active major bleeding; thrombocytopenia associated with positive tests for anti-platelet antibody in the presence of danaparoid; hypersensitivity to pork products Considerations: Not intended for IM injection; may cause hemorrhage; use caution in patients with serum creatinine levels ≥ 2 mg/dL Most common AEs include hemorrhage, fever, nausea, constipation, pain at injection site, rash, pruritus, edema, insomnia Pregnancy category: B	SEE ardeparin sodium except that injection sites should be rotated between the left and right anterolateral and posterolateral abdominal wall	Not equivalent to heparin or other low-molecular weight heparin products so cannot be used interchangeably

Generic Name and Selected Trade Names	Normal Adult Dosage	Major Adverse Effects/Cautions	Key Counseling Points	Miscellaneous Issues
Enoxaparin Sodium Lovenox	For prevention of DVT due to hip or knee replacement surgery: Give 30 mg BID by deep subcutaneous (SC) injection starting 12–24 hrs following surgery; average duration is 7–10 days For prevention of DVT due to abdominal surgery: Administer 40 mg QD via a SC injection, initial dose given 2 hrs prior to surgery; usual duration is 7–10 days	Contraindications: Patients with active bleeding, thrombocytopenia associated with a positive test for anti-platelet antibodies in the presence of enoxaparin, patients with heparin or pork hypersensitivity Considerations: Not intended for IM injection; use with caution in patients with heparin induced thrombocytopenia or patients at risk for hemorrhage Most common AEs include hemorrhage, thrombocytopenia, fever, nausea, edema Pregnancy category: B	SEE danaparoid sodium	Cannot be used interchangeably with heparin sodium or other low molecular weight heparins

Generic Name and Selected Trade Names	Normal Adult Dosage	Major Adverse Effects/Cautions	Key Counselling Points	Miscellaneous Issues
Heparin Sodium	Individualize dosage Dosage is determined and adjusted based upon the patient's coagulation test results, body weight, and condition being treated; for dosage recommendations — SEE Prescribing Information (PI)	Contraindications: Patients with severe thrombocytopenia and patients who cannot undergo periodic laboratory testing Considerations: Not intended for IM use; may cause hemorrhage and thrombocytopenia that can lead to complications; any decrease in hematocrit, blood pressure, or unexplained symptom of a hemorrhagic condition should be considered; use with caution in any patient with condition that puts him/her at risk for hemorrhage (eg, severe hypertension, surgery, hemophilia, women over 60) Most common AEs include hemorrhage, irritation at injection site, hypersensitivity reactions, thrombocytopenia Pregnancy category: C	SEE ardeparin sodium; except injection sites vary, product may be used IV or SC; you will need to be evaluated by the prescriber and undergo laboratory tests on a regular basis	Not to be used interchangeably with low molecular weight heparins

Generic Name and Selected Trade Names	Normal Adult Dosage	Major Adverse Effects/Cautions	Key Counseling Points	Miscellaneous Issues
Warfarin Sodium Coumadin	Individualize dosage Dosage is individualized and is dependent upon the indication as well as individual patient factors; dosage must be adjusted according to the patient's PT/INR — SEE Prescribing Information (PI)	Contraindications: Any condition where the hazard of hemorrhage or other toxicity might be greater than the potential benefit (eg, pregnancy, patients with bleeding tendencies, surgery, inadequate laboratory facilities, unsupervised patients) Considerations: There is a risk of hemorrhage and less frequently necrosis; patient must have PT/INR monitored on a routine basis; effects can be altered by diet and concomitant drug therapy; risk of atheromatous plaque emboli (ie, purple toe syndrome); use caution in elderly or debilitated patients	Tell the prescriber about all medical conditions that you have and all other medications (prescription and non-prescription that you are taking); while taking this medication, contact the prescriber if you notice any bleeding; do not take any new medication (prescription or non-prescription) or change your diet without first discussing it with your physician or pharmacist; usually, do not begin this medicine during pregnancy and do not become pregnant while taking it; take this medication exactly as directed, do not take it less or more often;	Many drug-drug and drug-food interactions are possible — SEE Prescribing Information (PI)

157

Generic Name and Selected Trade Names	Normal Adult Dosage	Major Adverse Effects/Cautions	Key Counseling Points	Miscellaneous Issues
Warfarin Sodium (continued) Coumadin		Most common AEs include hemorrhage, necrosis, allergy, liver injury, rash, fever, abdominal pain and cramping, fatigue, lethargy Pregnancy category: X	you will need to be evaluated by the prescriber and undergo laboratory tests on a regular basis; carry an ID bracelet or other type of identification to indicate that you are taking this agent; avoid sports and other activities that could produce injuries; avoid cutting yourself and do not shave with a straight razor blade; if you miss a dose, take it as soon as you remember and go back to regular dosing schedule, but if it is almost time for the next dose, skip the missed one entirely and return to regular dosing schedule only — do not double doses; notify the prescriber about doses you missed	

*As a general rule, a medication should not be administered to a patient with a known hypersensitivity to it or a similar agent.

Table 2: Antiplatelet Agents*

Generic Name and Selected Trade Names	Normal Adult Dosage	Major Adverse Effects/Cautions	Key Counseling Points	Miscellaneous Issues
Clopidogrel Bisulfate Plavix	For antiplatelet effects, 75 mg QD	Contraindications: Active bleeding such as with intracranial hemorrhage or peptic ulcer Considerations: May cause neutropenia and/or agranulocytosis so monitor patient routinely; use caution in patients with severe liver impairment, and in patients at risk for bleeding (eg, acute trauma, surgery); prolongs bleeding time Most common AEs include the same ones caused by aspirin — for a complete list, SEE Product Information (PI) Pregnancy category: B	Tell the prescriber if you have any type of blood disorder, ulcer, or a liver disease; contact the prescriber if you develop an infection or easy bruising; may take this medication with or without food; take this medication exactly as directed, do not take it less or more often; you will need to be evaluated by the prescriber and undergo laboratory tests on a regular basis; do not take any new medication without first discussing it with your physician or pharmacist;	Many drug interactions are possible — SEE Prescribing Information (PI)

159

Generic Name and Selected Trade Names	Normal Adult Dosage	Major Adverse Effects/Cautions	Key Counseling Points	Miscellaneous Issues
Clopidogrel Bisulfate (continued) Plavix			tell all your physicians, dentists, and pharmacists that you are taking this agent; if you miss a dose, take it as soon as you remember, but if it is almost time for the next dose, skip the missed one and go back to regular dosing schedule — do not double doses	

Generic Name and Selected Trade Names	Normal Adult Dosage	Major Adverse Effects/Cautions	Key Counseling Points	Miscellaneous Issues
Ticlopidine HCl Ticlid	To reduce the risk of thrombotic stroke in patients who have experienced stroke precursors and in patients who have had a completed stroke, 250 mg BID Dosage adjustment may be required in patients with liver or kidney impairment — SEE Prescribing Information (PI)	Contraindications: Presence of hematopoietic disorders (neutropenia, thrombocytopenia), bleeding or severe liver impairment Considerations: Neutropenia may occur, CBC should be measured at least every 2 weeks during the first 3 months of therapy; rarely thrombocytopenia has occurred; may elevate liver enzymes; use with caution in patients at risk for bleeding Most common AEs include diarrhea, rash, nausea/vomiting, GI pain, neutropenia Pregnancy category: B	Tell the prescriber if you have any type of blood disorder or a liver disease; contact the prescriber if you develop an infection or easy bruising; take with food; provide patient and/or caregiver with the information leaflet provided by the manufacturer; take this medication exactly as directed, do not take it less or more often; you will need to be evaluated by the prescriber and undergo laboratory tests on a regular basis;	Reserved for patients intolerant of aspirin

Generic Name and Selected Trade Names	Normal Adult Dosage	Major Adverse Effects/Cautions	Key Counseling Points	Miscellaneous Issues
Ticlopidine HCl (continued) Ticlid			do not take any new medication without first discussing it with your physician or pharmacist; tell all your physicians, dentists, and pharmacists that you are taking this agent; if you miss a dose, take it as soon as you remember, but if it is almost time for the next dose, skip the missed one and go back to regular dosing schedule — do not double doses	

*As a general rule, a medication should not be administered to a patient with a known hypersensitivity to it or a similar agent.

Respiratory Agents

Table 1: Antiinflammatory Agents for the Respiratory Tract*

Generic Name and Selected Trade Names	Normal Adult Dosage	Major Adverse Effects/Cautions	Key Counseling Points	Miscellaneous Issues
Beclometh-asone Dipropionate Beclovent Vanceril Vanceril Double Strength	Individualize dosage *Beclovent and Vanceril* For asthma in patients over 12 years of age: 2 inhalations TID or QID, or 4 inhalations BID; patients with severe asthma may be started on 12–16 inhalations/day, then titrate downward For asthma in patients 6–12 years of age: 1 to 2 inhalations TID or QID, or 4 inhalations BID *Vanceril Double Strength* For asthma in patients over 12 years of age: Usually, 2 inhalations BID;	Contraindications: Primary treatment of acute asthma attacks where intensive measures are required Considerations: Patients switched from oral corticosteroids to inhalation may experience adrenal insufficiency when exposed to trauma, surgery, infections stress, or severe asthma attacks, patients should be warned that they may require oral therapy during these periods and they should carry a warning card and contact their physician immediately if any of these events occur (SEE Prescribing Information for details); localized fungal infections in the throat and pharynx may occur and occasionally require therapy;	Tell the prescriber if you have any type of bone disease such as osteoporosis or a chronic infection like tuberculosis, and tell him/her all other asthma medications you are taking; use this medication as prescribed, do not take any more and do not stop taking this agent without discussing it first with the prescriber; if you are taking an oral corticosteroid, do not stop taking it without first discussing it with the prescriber; it may take up to four weeks before you begin to feel better; contact the prescriber if you get an asthma attack that does not improve readily, if your symptoms are not improving or are getting worse,	

Generic Name and Selected Trade Names	Normal Adult Dosage	Major Adverse Effects/Cautions	Key Counseling Points
Beclomethasone Dipropionate (continued) Beclovent Vanceril Vanceril Double Strength	patients with severe asthma may be started on 6–8 inhalations/day, then titrate; do not exceed 10 inhalations/day For asthma in patients 6–12 years of age: Usually, 2 inhalations BID; do not exceed 5 inhalations/day; not recommended for use in children under 6 years of age SEE Prescribing Information (PI) for details on patients also receiving systemic corticosteroids Other dosage forms are available — SEE PI	use with caution in patients with tuberculosis, and untreated systemic infections; chronic use in children should be accompanied by monitoring of growth and adrenal suppression Most common AEs include headache, dizziness, unpleasant taste or smell, suppression of adrenal function has occurred at high doses Pregnancy category: Not specified	if you go through a time of unusual stress such as surgery, a bad infection, or a severe injury, and if you have signs of a mouth/throat/lung infection; after each dose of this medication, gargle and rinse your mouth with water and then spit the water out to help prevent throat irritation, hoarseness, and mouth infection; this medication is not used to treat an acute asthmatic episode, but rather to prevent them from happening; if recommended, remember to use the spacer device; ensure patient knows the proper technique of using the metered dose inhaler and a spacer device if suggested; if you miss a dose of this medication, use it as soon as possible and then take the remaining doses for that day at regularly spaced times

Generic Name and Selected Trade Names	Normal Adult Dosage	Major Adverse Effects/Cautions	Key Counseling Points	Miscellaneous Issues
Budesonide Pulmicort Turbuhaler	Individualize dosage For asthma in adults previously receiving bronchodilators alone: Start with 200 to 400 mcg BID; highest recommended dose is 400 mcg BID For asthma in adults previously receiving inhaled corticosteroids: Start with 200 to 400 mcg BID; highest recommended dose is 800 mcg BID For asthma in children previously receiving bronchodilators alone: Start with 200 mcg BID; highest recommended dose is 400 mcg BID	Contraindications: SEE beclomethasone dipropionate Considerations: Not recommended for use in patients under 6 years of age; also, SEE beclomethasone dipropionate Most common AEs include headache, pain, oral candidiasis, respiratory infection, sinusitis/rhinitis, asthenia Pregnancy category: C	SEE beclomethasone dipropionate	

Generic Name and Selected Trade Names	Normal Adult Dosage	Major Adverse Effects/Cautions	Key Counseling Points	Miscellaneous Issues
Budesonide (continued) Pulmicort Turbuhaler	For asthma in children previously receiving inhaled corticosteroids: Start with 200 to 400 mcg BID, highest recommended dose is 800 mcg BID SEE Prescribing Information (PI) for details on patients also receiving systemic corticosteroids			

Generic Name and Selected Trade Names	Normal Adult Dosage	Major Adverse Effects/Cautions	Key Counselling Points	Miscellaneous Issues
Cromolyn Sodium Intal Intal Nebulizer Solution	Individualize dosage Inhaler for bronchial asthma: Start with 2 metered inhalations QID at regular intervals Inhaler for prevention of acute bronchospasm that follows exercise or exposure to environmental agents: 2 metered inhalations 10–15 min before exposure to the precipitating factor Nebulizer for bronchial asthma: Contents of 1 ampule via nebulizer QID at regular intervals	Considerations: Not for use in the treatment of acute asthma attacks; severe allergic reactions can occur; discontinue if patient develops eosinophilic pneumonia; due to the propellants, use with caution in patients with coronary artery disease or arrhythmias; occasionally, administration may produce bronchospasm or cough; not recommended for use in patients under 5 years of age Most common AEs include throat irritation or dryness, bad taste, cough, wheezing, nausea, rarely bronchospasm, laryngeal edema, nasal congestion Pregnancy category: B	Tell the prescriber if you have a liver or kidney disorder, and tell him/her all other medications you are taking; this medication is used to prevent an asthma attack not treat one; use this medication as prescribed, do not take any more and do not stop taking this agent without discussing it first with the prescriber; if you are taking another asthma medication, do not stop taking it without first discussing this with the prescriber; contact the prescriber if you do not begin to feel better (or feel worse) within four weeks;	

Generic Name and Selected Trade Names	Normal Adult Dosage	Major Adverse Effects/Cautions	Key Counseling Points	Miscellaneous Issues
Cromolyn Sodium (continued) Intal Intal Nebulizer Solution	Dosage adjustments: May need to decrease dosage in patients with renal or hepatic dysfunction — SEE Prescribing Information (PI) Other dosage forms are available — SEE PI		after each dose of this medication, gargle and rinse your mouth with water and then spit the water out to help prevent throat irritation; ensure patient knows how to use the inhaler, (and if appropriate a spacer device) or the inhalation solution properly; if you miss a dose of this medication, use it as soon as possible and then take the remaining doses for that day at regularly spaced times	

Generic Name and Selected Trade Names	Normal Adult Dosage	Major Adverse Effects/Cautions	Key Counseling Points	Miscellaneous Issues
Dexamethasone Sodium Phosphate Dexacort	Individualize dosage For asthma in adults: Initially 3 inhalations TID or QID; maximum of 3 inhalations per dose and 12/day For asthma in children: Initially 2 inhalations TID or QID, maximum of 2 inhalations per dose and 8/day Other dosage forms are available — SEE Prescribing Information (PI)	Contraindications: Systemic fungal infections; persistently positive cultures for *Candida albicans* Considerations: SEE beclomethasone dipropionate Most common AEs include throat irritation, hoarseness, coughing, laryngeal and pharyngeal fungal infections Pregnancy category: Not specified	SEE beclomethasone dipropionate	May be more likely than some others to cause systemic effects

Generic Name and Selected Trade Names	Normal Adult Dosage	Major Adverse Effects/Cautions	Key Counseling Points	Miscellaneous Issues
Flunisolide Aerobid	Individualize dosage For asthma in patients 6 years of age and older, 2 inhalations BID, maximal dose should not exceed 4 inhalations BID SEE Prescribing Information (PI) for details on patients also receiving systemic corticosteroids Other dosage forms are available — SEE PI	<u>Contraindications and considerations</u>: SEE beclomethasone dipropionate <u>Most common AEs</u> include diarrhea, nausea/vomiting, flu, sore throat, headache, cold symptoms, upper respiratory tract infections, unpleasant taste <u>Pregnancy category</u>: C	SEE beclomethasone dipropionate	If used at 4 inhalations BID, monitor for suppression of adrenal function

Generic Name and Selected Trade Names	Normal Adult Dosage	Major Adverse Effects/Cautions	Key Counseling Points	Miscellaneous Issues
Fluticasone Propionate Flovent 44 mcg Flovent 110 mcg Flovent 220 mcg	Individualize dosage For asthma in patients previously receiving bronchodilators alone: Start with 88 mcg BID; highest recommended dose is 440 mcg BID For asthma in patients previously receiving inhaled corticosteroids: Start with 88 to 220 mcg BID; highest recommended dose is 440 mcg BID SEE Prescribing Information (PI) for details on patients also receiving systemic corticosteroids Other dosage forms are available — SEE PI	Contraindications: SEE beclomethasone dipropionate Considerations: Only recommended for use in patients 12 years of age and older; also, SEE beclomethasone dipropionate Most common AEs include those that affect the ear, nose and throat such as pharyngitis, nasal congestion, dysphonia, oral candidiasis, upper respiratory tract infection, and influenza; headache, nausea/vomiting Pregnancy category: C	SEE beclomethasone dipropionate	

173

Generic Name and Selected Trade Names	Normal Adult Dosage	Major Adverse Effects/Cautions	Key Counseling Points	Miscellaneous Issues
Nedocromil Sodium Tilade	Individualize dosage For mild to moderate asthma, usually, 2 inhalations QID at regular intervals	<u>Considerations</u>: Not for use in the treatment of acute asthma attacks Most common AEs include bad taste, headache, nausea/vomiting, rhinitis, abdominal pain <u>Pregnancy category</u>: B	This medication is used to prevent an asthma attack not treat one; use this medication as prescribed, do not take any more and do not stop taking this agent without discussing it first with the prescriber; if you are taking another asthma medication, do not stop taking it without first discussing this with the prescriber; it may take 2–4 weeks for this medication to reach its full effect; after each dose of this medication, gargle and rinse your mouth with water and then spit the water out to help prevent throat irritation and unpleasant taste;	

Generic Name and Selected Trade Names	Normal Adult Dosage	Major Adverse Effects/Cautions	Key Counseling Points	Miscellaneous Issues
Nedocromil Sodium (continued) Tilade			ensure patient knows how to use the inhaler properly; if you miss a dose of this medication, use it as soon as possible and then take the remaining doses for that day at regularly spaced times	

Generic Name and Selected Trade Names	Normal Adult Dosage	Major Adverse Effects/Cautions	Key Counseling Points	Miscellaneous Issues
Triamcinolone Acetonide Azmacort	Individualize dosage For asthma in adults: 2 inhalations TID or QID, or 4 inhalations BID; maximum should not exceed 16 inhalations/day; For asthma in children 6–12 years of age: 1 to 2 inhalations TID or QID; maximum should not exceed 12 inhalations/ day SEE Prescribing Information (PI) for details on patients also receiving systemic corticosteroids	<u>Contraindications and considerations</u>: SEE beclomethasone dipropionate Most common AEs include facial edema, pain, abdominal pain, diarrhea, dry mouth, rash, chest congestion, voice alteration, urogenital infections <u>Pregnancy category</u>: C	SEE beclomethasone dipropionate	

Generic Name and Selected Trade Names	Normal Adult Dosage	Major Adverse Effects/Cautions	Key Counseling Points	Miscellaneous Issues
Zafirlukast Accolate	For asthma in patients 12 years of age and older, 20 mg BID	<u>Considerations</u>: Not indicated for use in acute reversal of bronchospasm; rarely, liver enzyme elevation has occurred; not recommended for use in patients who are breast-feeding <u>Most common AEs</u> include headache, infections (more common in elderly), nausea, diarrhea <u>Pregnancy category</u>: B	This medication is used to prevent an asthma attack not treat one; use this medication as prescribed, do not take any more and do not stop taking this agent without discussing it first with the prescriber; if you are taking another asthma medication, do not stop taking it without first discussing this with the prescriber; do not take any other medication without first discussing this with your physician or pharmacist; tell the prescriber if you develop pain on the right side above (or near) the belly button area, nausea, fatigue, itchiness, yellow color of your skin or the white part of your eyes, or flu-like symptoms;	Bioavailability may be decreased if taken with food; many drug interactions are possible — SEE Prescribing Information (PI)

Generic Name and Selected Trade Names	Normal Adult Dosage	Major Adverse Effects/Cautions	Key Counseling Points	Miscellaneous Issues
Zafirlukast (continued) Accolate			take the medication on an empty stomach, about 1 hour before or 2 hrs after meals; if you miss a dose of this medication take it as soon as possible but if it is almost time for the next dose, skip the missed one and return to regular schedule — do not double doses	

Generic Name and Selected Trade Names	Normal Adult Dosage	Major Adverse Effects/Cautions	Key Counseling Points	Miscellaneous Issues
Zileuton Zyflo	For asthma, 600 mg QID	Contraindications: Active liver disease or patients with elevations of transaminase levels equal to or greater than 3 times the upper limit of normal Considerations: Not for use in the treatment of acute asthma attacks, but therapy may be continued during treatment of acute attacks; co-administration with agents such as theophylline, warfarin, and propranolol require dosage adjustments; elevation of liver enzymes has occurred, enzyme levels should be measured prior to and during therapy Most common AEs include dyspepsia, arthralgia, constipation, dizziness, fever, insomnia, urinary tract infection, vaginitis, chest pain Pregnancy category: C	SEE zafirlukast except that agent may be taken with meals, and patient should tell prescriber if he/she has or had liver disease The most serious adverse effect of this agent is on your liver so you must have periodic testing of your blood to make sure you are not experiencing any liver toxicity	Many drug interactions are possible — SEE Prescribing Information (PI)

*As a general rule, a medication should not be administered to a patient with a known hypersensitivity to it or a similar agent.

Table 2: Bronchodilators*

Generic Name and Selected Trade Names	Normal Adult Dosage	Major Adverse Effects/Cautions	Key Counseling Points	Miscellaneous Issues
Albuterol Sulfate Airet Proventil Proventil Repetabs Ventolin Ventolin Nebules Ventolin Rotacaps **Albuterol** Ventolin	Individualize dosage Solution in patients 12 years of age and older: 2.5 mg (1 vial) TID or QID via nebulizer Aerosol in patients 12 years of age and older for treatment of bronchospasm or prevention of asthma symptoms: 2 inhalations repeated Q4 to 6H; in some patients 1 inhalation Q4H may be sufficient Aerosol in patients 12 years of age and older for prevention of exercise-induced bronchospasm: 2 inhalations 15 min prior to exercise	Considerations: May produce paradoxical bronchospasm; deaths have been associated with overuse, patient should be warned if symptoms get worse to contact their prescriber; use caution in patients with diabetes mellitus and with cardiovascular, convulsive, or hyperthyroid disorders; transient hypokalemia and allergic reactions have occurred Most common AEs include tremors, bronchospasm, dizziness, nervousness, headache, nausea, cough Pregnancy category: C	Tell the prescriber if you had an allergic reaction to any medication for asthma, are allergic to sulfites, or have a heart disease, epilepsy, a thyroid disease, or diabetes mellitus; use this medication as prescribed, do not take any more and do not stop taking this agent without discussing it first with the prescriber; if you are taking another asthma medication, do not stop taking it without speaking with the prescriber; do not take any other medication without first discussing this with your physician or pharmacist;	

Generic Name and Selected Trade Names	Normal Adult Dosage	Key Counseling Points	Miscellaneous Issues
Albuterol Sulfate (continued) Airet Proventil Proventil Repetabs Ventolin Ventolin Nebules Ventolin Rotacaps **Albuterol** Ventolin	Syrup in patients over 14 years of age: 2 or 4 mg TID or QID; use caution if dose is increased — SEE Prescribing Information (PI) Syrup in patients 6–14 years of age: 2 mg TID or QID; use caution if dose is increased — SEE PI Syrup in patients 2–6 years of age: 0.1 mg/kg TID; use caution if dose is increased — SEE PI Repetabs in patients 12 years of age and over: 4 or 8 mg Q12H; use caution if dose is increased or when switching from regular release to extended release preparations — SEE PI Proventil or Ventolin tablets in patients 12 years of age and over: 2 or 4 mg TID or QID; use caution if dose is increased or when switching from regular release to extended release preparations — SEE PI Proventil tablets in patients 6–12 years of age: 2 mg TID or QID; use caution if dose is increased — SEE PI For proper use of Ventolin Rotacaps — SEE PI Lower doses recommended in elderly patients or those with a history of sensitivity to beta-adrenergic agonists	if you have difficulty breathing after using this medication or your symptoms are getting worse, contact the prescriber as soon as possible; if you are using this medication regularly and miss a dose, take it as soon as possible and then take the remaining doses for that day at regularly spaced times — do not double doses If patient is using an inhaler, a spacer, or a nebulizer, ensure he/she knows how to use it properly If patient is taking extended-release tablets, do not break, crush, or chew before swallowing	

181

Generic Name and Selected Trade Names	Normal Adult Dosage	Major Adverse Effects/Cautions	Key Counseling Points	Miscellaneous Issues
Bitolterol Mesylate Tornalate	Individualize dosage For relief of bronchospasm in patients over 12 years of age: 2 inhalations at an interval of 1–3 min followed by a 3rd inhalation if needed For prevention of bronchospasm: 2 inhalations Q8H; do not exceed 3 inhalations every 6 hrs or 2 inhalations every 4 hrs	Considerations: SEE albuterol sulfate Most common AEs include tremors, dizziness, nervousness, headache, palpitations, cough, nausea, throat irritation Pregnancy category: C	SEE albuterol sulfate	

Generic Name and Selected Trade Names	Normal Adult Dosage	Major Adverse Effects/Cautions	Key Counseling Points	Miscellaneous Issues
Ipratropium Bromide Atrovent	Individualize dosage Inhaler for chronic obstructive pulmonary disease: Start with 2 inhalations QID; patients may take additional inhalations as required, but do not exceed 12 per 24 hrs Solution for chronic obstructive pulmonary disease: 1 vial administered via nebulizer TID or QID (doses should be 6–8 hrs apart) Other dosage forms available — SEE Prescribing Information (PI)	Contraindications: Hypersensitivity to atropine Contraindications for aerosol only: Hypersensitivity to soya lecithin, soybean, or peanut food substances Considerations: Not for use in the initial treatment of acute episodes of bronchospasm; use with caution in patients with narrow-angle glaucoma, prostatic hypertrophy, or bladder neck obstruction Most common AEs include nausea, dry mouth, cough, exacerbation of symptoms, allergic reactions (urticaria, angioedema, rash), for nasal spray: nasal irritation Pregnancy category: B	Tell the prescriber if you are allergic to atropine or atropine-like products such as belladonna, or are allergic to soybeans, peanuts, or soya lecithin, and if you have glaucoma or difficulty in urinating (eg, due to a prostate or bladder disease); also, SEE albuterol sulfate	Solution may be mixed with albuterol or metaproterenol if used within one hour; spray pump requires priming

Generic Name and Selected Trade Names	Normal Adult Dosage	Major Adverse Effects/Cautions	Key Counseling Points	Miscellaneous Issues
Isoetharine Bronkometer Bronkosol	Individualize dosage For Bronkometer: 1 to 2 inhalations, may be repeated in 4 hrs if needed For Bronkosol: SEE Prescribing Information (PI) for details on dosage and methods of administration	Considerations: SEE albuterol sulfate Most common AEs include tachycardia, blood pressure changes, nausea, headache, restlessness, insomnia, tremor Pregnancy category: C	SEE albuterol sulfate	

Generic Name and Selected Trade Names	Normal Adult Dosage	Major Adverse Effects/Cautions	Key Counseling Points	Miscellaneous Issues
Isoproterenol HCl Isuprel Medihaler-Iso Mistometer	Individualize dosage Agent may be administered via a variety of devices such as metered dose inhalers and nebulizers, SEE Prescribing Information (PI) Other dosage forms available — SEE PI	<u>Contraindications</u>: Cardiac arrhythmias associated with tachycardia <u>Considerations</u>: SEE albuterol sulfate Most common AEs include nervousness, headache, nausea/vomiting, tachycardia/ palpitations, flushing, tremor <u>Pregnancy category</u>: C	SEE albuterol sulfate	

Generic Name and Selected Trade Names	Normal Adult Dosage	Major Adverse Effects/Cautions	Key Counselling Points	Miscellaneous Issues
Metaproterenol Sulfate Alupent Metaprel	Individualize dosage Inhalation aerosol: Usually, a single dose is 2 to 3 inhalations; should not be repeated more frequently than every 3–4 hrs — SEE Prescribing Information (PI) Inhalation solution: Usually, a single dose is 1 vial via nebulizer, should not be repeated more frequently than every 4 hrs — SEE PI	Contraindications: Cardiac arrhythmias associated with tachycardia Considerations: SEE albuterol sulfate Most common AEs include nervousness, headache, dizziness, palpitations, tremor, throat irritation, nausea/vomiting, cough, asthma exacerbation Pregnancy category: C	SEE albuterol sulfate	

Generic Name and Selected Trade Names	Normal Adult Dosage	Major Adverse Effects/Cautions	Key Counseling Points	Miscellaneous Issues
Metaproterenol Sulfate (continued) Alupent Metaprel	Syrup for adults: Usually, 2 teaspoonfuls TID or QID; dosage in children is based on age and weight — SEE PI Tablets for adults: Usually, 20 mg TID or QID; dosage in children is based on age and weight — SEE PI			

Generic Name and Selected Trade Names	Normal Adult Dosage	Major Adverse Effects/Cautions	Key Counselling Points	Miscellaneous Issues
Pirbuterol Acetate Maxair	Individualize dosage For asthma in patients 12 years of age and older, administer 1 to 2 inhalations; dosage may be repeated every 4–6 hrs; do not exceed 12 inhalations/day	<u>Considerations</u>: SEE albuterol sulfate Most common AEs include nervousness, headache, dizziness, palpitations, tremor, nausea/vomiting, cough <u>Pregnancy category</u>: C	SEE albuterol sulfate	

Generic Name and Selected Trade Names	Normal Adult Dosage	Major Adverse Effects/Cautions	Key Counseling Points	Miscellaneous Issues
Salmeterol Xinafoate Serevent	Individualize dosage For asthma in patients 12 years of age and older: Administer 2 inhalations BID (12 hrs apart) For prevention of exercise-induced bronchospasm: 2 inhalations at least 30–60 minutes before exercise; additional doses should not be used for 12 hrs; for patients receiving this agent Q12H a different medication should be used for prevention of acute attacks	Considerations: Do not initiate in patients with significantly worsening or acutely deteriorating asthma, which may be a life-threatening condition; not for treatment of acute symptoms; not a substitute for corticosteroids; do not exceed recommended doses; acute bronchospasm has occurred; use with caution in patients with cardiovascular, convulsive, hyperthyroid disorders, diabetes mellitus; transient hypokalemia and allergic reactions have occurred Most common AEs include tachycardia/palpitations, headache, tremor, cough, nervousness, respiratory infection Pregnancy category: C	This medication is used to prevent an acute asthma attack, it should not be used to treat an attack that has already started; if you do not have another medication to treat an acute attack, contact the prescriber; if you miss a dose of this medication, use it as soon as possible then go back to regular schedule — do not double doses, but, if you have wheezing or difficulty in breathing before the next dose is due, use a different bronchodilator to relieve the acute symptoms; also, SEE albuterol sulfate except for missed dose instructions	Agent has a much slower onset of action than other beta agonists; safety and efficacy with spacers has not been studied

Generic Name and Selected Trade Names	Normal Adult Dosage	Major Adverse Effects/Cautions	Key Counseling Points	Miscellaneous Issues
Terbutaline Sulfate Brethine Bricanyl	Individualize dosage Tablets for adults: Usually, 5 mg Q6H while patient is awake; may decrease dose to 2.5 mg if adverse effects are problematic Tablets for patients 12–15 years of age: Usually, 2.5 mg Q6H while patient is awake Other dosage forms available — SEE Prescribing Information (PI)	<u>Considerations</u>: SEE albuterol sulfate and not recommended for use in children under 12 years of age form <u>Most common AEs include</u> nervousness, tremor, headache, tachycardia/ palpitations, drowsiness, nausea/vomiting, sweating, muscle cramps <u>Pregnancy category</u>: B	SEE albuterol sulfate	

Generic Name and Selected Trade Names	Normal Adult Dosage	Major Adverse Effects/Cautions	Key Counseling Points	Miscellaneous Issues
Theophylline Aerolate Elixophyllin Respbid Slo-Bid Slo-Phyllin Theobid Theo-Dur Theo-24 Extended-Release Theo-X Extended-Release Theolair Uni-Dur Extended-Release Uniphyl Unicontin	Individualize dosage based upon peak and trough serum levels to achieve maximum benefit with minimum risk of adverse effects Various formulations have different dosage and/or frequency requirements; SEE Prescribing Information (PI) for details, as theophylline can have life-threatening toxicities; dosing must be done with caution in many patients with constant monitoring	Contraindications: Hypersensitivity to xanthine derivatives, active peptic ulcer disease, seizure disorders (unless receiving appropriate anticonvulsant medication) Considerations: Reduced clearance (eg, elderly, patients with renal/hepatic impairment, cardiac failure, or sustained high fever, and in neonates and infants, co-administration of some pharmacologic agents, SEE Prescribing Information for others) may result in elevated serum levels of theophylline and toxicity; toxicity is not always preceded by less severe AEs, therefore monitoring of blood levels is recommended;	Tell the prescriber if you have a heart, kidney or liver disease, a seizure disorder, or an ulcer; you may need to undergo blood tests from time to time to ensure that you are getting the right dose; if you are breast feeding, speak with the prescriber; use this medication as prescribed, do not take any more and do not stop taking this agent without discussing it first with the prescriber; if you are taking another asthma medication, do not stop taking it without speaking with the prescriber; do not take any other medication without first discussing this with your physician or pharmacist; if your symptoms are getting worse, contact the prescriber;	Not to be taken with other xanthine derivatives; many drug interactions are possible — SEE Prescribing Information (PI); AEs are more common with levels about 20 mcg/mL

Generic Name and Selected Trade Names	Normal Adult Dosage	Major Adverse Effects/Cautions	Key Counselling Points	Miscellaneous Issues
Theophylline (continued) Aerolate Elixophyllin Respbid Slo-Bid Slo-Phyllin Theobid Theo-Dur Theo-24 Extended-Release Theo-X Extended-Release Theolair Uni-Dur Extended-Release Uniphyl Unicontin		may worsen arrhythmias; half-life may be shorter in smokers; use with caution in patients with hypertension, hypoxemia, history of peptic ulcer Most common AEs include nausea/vomiting, epigastric pain, hematemesis, diarrhea, headaches, insomnia, reflex hyperexcitability, nervousness <u>Pregnancy category:</u> C	If you miss a dose of this medication take it as soon as possible, but if it is almost time for the next dose skip the missed one and return to regular dosing schedule — do not double doses If using extended release or enteric coated product, do not break, crush, or chew before swallowing If using capsules, tablets, liquids, it may be best taken with water on an empty stomach unless otherwise directed; may need to take it immediately after meals due to GI distress; Slo-Bid may be given without regard to meals	

*As a general rule, a medication should not be administered to a patient with a known hypersensitivity to it or a similar agent.

Antihistamines

Table: Antihistamines (H$_1$ Receptors)*

Generic Name and Selected Trade Names	Normal Adult Dosage	Major Adverse Effects/Cautions	Key Counseling Points	Miscellaneous Issues
Astemizole Hismanal	Individualize dosage Usually, 10 mg QD	Contraindications: Use with erythromycin, ketoconazole, itraconazole, quinine Considerations: Prolongation of the QT interval on the ECG has occurred in patients taking higher than recommended doses; avoid in patients with liver impairment and in patients prone to prolongation of QT interval; use with caution in patients with lower airway disease or renal dysfunction Most common AEs include weight gain, fatigue, nervousness, dry mouth Pregnancy category: C	Tell the prescriber if you have prostate or urinary problems, glaucoma, a heart problem, or a liver disorder; while taking this medication, if you experience dizziness stop taking it and contact the prescriber immediately; do not increase the dose under any circumstances; do not take any other medications without discussing it first with your physician or pharmacist; some people get drowsy on this agent, so do not drive or use machines until you know how you are affected;	Arrhythmias generally occur in overdose situations, due to drug interactions, and/or in patients with an underlying cardiac condition; patient must not exceed recommended doses; medication has minimal anticholinergic effects

Generic Name and Selected Trade Names	Normal Adult Dosage	Major Adverse Effects/Cautions	Key Counseling Points	Miscellaneous Issues
Astemizole (continued) Hismanal			take on an empty stomach at least 2 hrs after a meal and 1 hr before the next; if you miss a dose take it as soon as you remember, but if it is almost time for the next dose skip the missed one and return to normal dosing schedule — do not double doses	

Generic Name and Selected Trade Names	Normal Adult Dosage	Major Adverse Effects/Cautions	Key Counseling Points	Miscellaneous Issues
Azatadine Maleate Optimine	Individualize dosage Usually, 1 to 2 mg Q8–12H	<u>Considerations</u>: Use with caution in patients with urinary hesitancy (eg, BPH, obstruction), or closed angle (narrow angle) glaucoma Most common AEs include somnolence, fatigue, dry mouth, changes in vision, urinary hesitancy, headache, nausea <u>Pregnancy category</u>: B	Tell the prescriber if you have any type of a urination problem, benign prostatic hyperplasia, or glaucoma; some people become drowsy on this agent, so do not drive or use machinery until you know how you are affected; drowsiness may be increased if taken with other CNS depressants such as alcohol, tranquilizers, and barbiturates so avoid if possible; if this agent bothers your stomach, it may be taken with food or a full glass of water or milk; if you are taking this agent regularly and miss a dose take it as soon as you remember, but if it is almost time for the next dose skip the missed one and return to normal dosing schedule — do not double doses	

Generic Name and Selected Trade Names	Normal Adult Dosage	Major Adverse Effects/Cautions	Key Counseling Points	Miscellaneous Issues
Brompheniramine Maleate Bromphen (Elixir) Diamine TD Dimetapp Allergy Dimetapp Extentabs (major ingredient) Veltane	<u>Capsules, elixir, tablets</u>: Usually, 4 mg Q4–6H up to 24 mg/day <u>Extended release dosage form</u>: Usually, 8 mg Q8–12H Parenteral form available —SEE Prescribing Information (PI)	<u>Considerations and most common AEs</u>: SEE azatadine maleate <u>Pregnancy category</u>: B	For extended release dosage form, swallow tablets whole do not break, crush, or chew; also, SEE azatadine maleate	Sedation is reported to be less than with some of the other "sedating" antihistamines

Generic Name and Selected Trade Names	Normal Adult Dosage	Major Adverse Effects/Cautions	Key Counselling Points	Miscellaneous Issues
Cetirizine HCl Zyrtec	Individualize dosage Usually administer 5 to 10 mg QD Dosage adjustment required for patient's with renal or liver dysfunction — SEE Prescribing Information (PI)	Most common AEs include somnolence, fatigue, dry mouth, headache, increased appetite and weight gain Pregnancy category: B	Tell the prescriber if you have liver or kidney disease; do not use in the first few months of pregnancy; also, SEE azatadine maleate	Has minimal anticholinergic effects
Chlorpheniramine Maleate Chlorspan-12 Chlortab-4 Chlor-Trimeton Phenetron Lanacaps Phenetron Syrup	Individualize dosage Syrup or tablets: Usually, 4 mg Q4–6H Extended release capsules/ tablets: Usually, 8 to 12 mg Q8–12H Parenteral form available — SEE Prescribing Information (PI)	Considerations and most common AEs: SEE azatadine maleate Pregnancy category: B	For extended release dosage form, swallow whole do not break, crush, or chew; also, SEE azatadine maleate	Sedation is reported to be less than some of the other "sedating" antihistamines

Generic Name and Selected Trade Names	Normal Adult Dosage	Major Adverse Effects/Cautions	Key Counselling Points	Miscellaneous Issues
Clemastine Fumarate Tavist	Individualize dosage For antihistamine: Usually administer 1.34 to 2.68 mg QD to TID For dermatologic conditions: Usually administer 2.68 mg QD to TID	<u>Considerations and most common AEs</u>: SEE azatadine maleate <u>Pregnancy category</u>: B	For extended release dosage form, swallow tablets whole do not break, crush, or chew; also, SEE azatadine maleate	
Cyprohep-tadine Periactin	Individualize dosage Usually, initiate with 4 mg Q8H; may increase as needed to 20 mg/day	<u>Contraindications</u>: Not for use in newborn or premature infants, nursing mothers <u>Considerations</u>: SEE azatadine maleate Most common AEs include increased appetite and weight gain (sometimes used therapeutically for this use); also, SEE azatadine maleate <u>Pregnancy category</u>: B	Do not use if breast feeding; also, SEE azatadine maleate	

Generic Name and Selected Trade Names	Normal Adult Dosage	Major Adverse Effects/Cautions	Key Counseling Points	Miscellaneous Issues
Dexchlorpheniramine Maleate Dexchlor Polaramine Polaramine Repetabs Poladex T.D.	Individualize dosage <u>Syrup and tablets:</u> Usually, 2 mg Q4–6H <u>Extended release dosage form:</u> Usually, 4 to 6 mg Q 8–12 H	SEE chlorpheniramine maleate	For extended release dosage form, swallow tablets whole do not break, crush, or chew; also, SEE azatadine maleate	Sedation is reported to be less than some of the other "sedating" antihistamines

Generic Name and Selected Trade Names	Normal Adult Dosage	Major Adverse Effects/Cautions	Key Counseling Points	Miscellaneous Issues
Dimenhydrinate Dimetabs Dramamine Dramamine Liquid Nico-Vert	Individualize dosage <u>Capsules, elixir, tablets, or syrup for anti-emetic or anti-vertigo</u>: Usually, administer 50 to 100 mg Q4H <u>Extended release capsules for anti-emetic or anti-vertigo</u>: Usually, 1 capsule Q12H Parenteral form available — SEE Prescribing Information (PI)	<u>Consideration</u>: Geriatric patients may be more sensitive to this agent <u>Most common AEs</u>: SEE azatadine maleate <u>Pregnancy category</u>: B	If using for motion sickness, take this medicine at least 30 minutes or even better 1–2 hrs before you begin to travel; for extended release dosage form, swallow whole, do not break, crush, or chew; also, SEE azatadine maleate	

Generic Name and Selected Trade Names	Normal Adult Dosage	Major Adverse Effects/Cautions	Key Counseling Points	Miscellaneous Issues
Diphenhydramine HCl Benadryl Benadryl Allergy Benadryl Kapseals Genahist Tusstat	Individualize dosage Capsules, elixir, syrup, or tablets for antihistamine, antiemetic or anti-vertigo: Usually, 25 to 50 mg Q4-6H For antidyskinetic: Usually, administer 25 mg TID; may gradually titrate dosage to 50 mg QID if needed For sedation: Usually, 50 mg 20-30 minutes before bedtime Syrup only for cough: Usually, 25 mg Q4-6H Parenteral form available — SEE Prescribing Information (PI)	Contraindications: Not for use in newborn or premature infants, nursing mothers Considerations: Geriatric patients may be more sensitive to effects; also, SEE azatadine maleate Most common AEs: SEE azatadine maleate Pregnancy category: B	If using for motion sickness, take this medicine at least 30 minutes or preferably 1-2 hrs before you begin to travel; also, SEE azatadine maleate	

203

Generic Name and Selected Trade Names	Normal Adult Dosage	Major Adverse Effects/Cautions	Key Counseling Points	Miscellaneous Issues
Fexofenadine HCl Allegra	Individualize dosage Usually administer 60 mg BID Lower doses required for patients with renal dysfunction — SEE Prescribing Information (PI)	Most common AEs include viral infection, nausea, dysmenorrhea, drowsiness, dyspepsia <u>Pregnancy category</u>: C	Inform the prescriber if you have kidney disease; also, SEE azatadine maleate	Developed to replace terfenadine
Hydroxyzine HCl Atarax	Individualize dosage <u>For pruritus</u>: Usually give 25 mg TID or QID <u>For anxiety</u>: Usually, 50 to 100 mg QID <u>For sedation</u>: Usually, 50 to 100 mg Parenteral form available — SEE Prescribing Information (PI)	<u>Contraindication</u>: Early pregnancy <u>Considerations</u>: Effect potentiated when taken with other CNS depressants Most common AEs include dry mouth, drowsiness, at higher doses tremors and convulsions have occurred <u>Pregnancy category</u>: Not specified	SEE azatadine maleate	CNS depression is enhanced when used with agents such as alcohol, narcotics, and barbiturates; combining injectable form with narcotics is common in certain clinical situations such as surgery

Generic Name and Selected Trade Names	Normal Adult Dosage	Major Adverse Effects/Cautions	Key Counseling Points	Miscellaneous Issues
Hydroxyzine Pamoate Vistaril	SEE hydroxyzine HCl	SEE hydroxyzine HCl	SEE azatadine maleate	SEE hydroxyzine HCl
Loratadine Claritin Claritin Reditabs	Individualize dosage Usually give 10 mg QD Dosage adjustment required for patients with renal or liver dysfunction — SEE Prescribing Information (PI)	Most common AEs include headache, fatigue, somnolence, dry mouth, increased appetite, weight gain Pregnancy category: B	SEE azatadine maleate, except usually take on an empty stomach For Reditabs, place on tongue and allow to disintegrate, administer with or without water	Medication has minimal anticholinergic effects

Generic Name and Selected Trade Names	Normal Adult Dosage	Major Adverse Effects/Cautions	Key Counseling Points	Miscellaneous Issues
Promethazine HCl Phenergan	Individualize dosage Syrup, tablets, or suppositories for allergy: Administer 25 mg HS, or 12.5 mg before meals and HS if needed For motion sickness: Initial dose of 25 mg taken 30 min to 1 hr before travel then repeated 8–12 hrs later; on succeeding days of travel give 25 mg BID For anti-emesis: Administer 25 mg once; 12.5 to 25 mg may be repeated Q4–6H as needed	Contraindication: Treatment of lower respiratory tract symptoms including asthma Considerations: Additive CNS depression occurs with other agents; may lower seizure threshold; use with caution in patients with narrow angle glaucoma, stenosing peptic ulcer, pyloroduodenal obstruction, urinary bladder obstruction, or BPH; cholestatic jaundice has occurred; elderly patients may be more sensitive to effects Most common AEs include sedation, blurred vision, nausea/vomiting, rash Pregnancy category: C	Tell the prescriber if you have asthma, a seizure disorder, a GI disorder such as ulcers, or a liver disease; may cause marked drowsiness or impair the mental and/or physical abilities required for performance of potentially hazardous tasks, such as driving a vehicle or operating heavy machinery; report any involuntary muscle movements to the physician; the agent may sensitize your skin to sunlight, so stay out of the sun as much as possible, and wear protective clothing and sunblock; if using for motion sickness, take this agent 30 minutes to 1 hour before you begin to travel;	Despite additive CNS depression, combining this agent with narcotics is common in certain clinical situations

Generic Name and Selected Trade Names	Normal Adult Dosage	Major Adverse Effects/Cautions	Key Counseling Points	Miscellaneous Issues
Promethazine HCl (continued) Phenergan	For sedation: 25 to 50 mg Parenteral form available — SEE Prescribing Information (PI)		if using suppository, ensure patient knows proper administration technique such as remove packaging, insert rectally, and retain until medication dissolves; also, SEE azatadine maleate	
Pyrilamine Maleate Nisaval	Individualize dosage Usually, 25 to 50 mg Q8H	Considerations: Geriatric patients may be more sensitive to effects; also SEE azatadine maleate Most common AEs: SEE azatadine maleate Pregnancy category: B	SEE azatadine maleate	

207

Generic Name and Selected Trade Names	Normal Adult Dosage	Major Adverse Effects/Cautions	Key Counseling Points	Miscellaneous Issues
Terfenadine Seldane	Individualize dosage Usually, 60 mg BID Dosage adjustment required in patients with impaired renal function — SEE Prescribing Information (PI)	Contraindications: Use with erythromycin, clarithromycin, ketoconazole, itraconazole, and troleandomycin; significant hepatic dysfunction Considerations: Prolongation of the QT interval on ECG has occurred in patients taking higher than recommended doses; avoid in patients with liver dysfunction and in patients prone to prolongation of QT interval Most common AEs include GI distress, dry mouth, headache; arrhythmias generally occur in overdose situations, due to drug interactions, and/or in patients with an underlying cardiac condition Pregnancy category: C	Tell the prescriber if you have a liver disease; while taking this agent, if you experience dizziness stop taking the medication and contact the prescriber immediately; do not increase the dose under any circumstances; take no more than one tablet every 12 hrs; ask your physician or pharmacist before taking any other medication with this agent; do not take this agent with ketoconazole, itraconazole, erythromycin, clarithromycin, or troleandomycin; also SEE azatadine maleate	Medication has minimal anticholinergic effects

Generic Name and Selected Trade Names	Normal Adult Dosage	Major Adverse Effects/Cautions	Key Counseling Points	Miscellaneous Issues
Tripelenna-mine HCl PBZ PBZ-SR	Individualize dosage <u>Tablets</u>: 25 to 50 mg Q4–6H <u>Extended release tablets</u>: 100 mg Q8–12H	<u>Considerations and most common AEs</u>: SEE azatadine maleate <u>Pregnancy category</u>: Not specified	SEE azatadine maleate	
Triprolidine HCl Myidil	Individualize dosage Usually, administer 2.5 mg Q4–6H	<u>Consideration and most common AEs</u>: SEE azatadine maleate <u>Pregnancy category</u>: B	SEE azatadine maleate	

*As a general rule, a medication should not be administered to a patient with a known hypersensitivity to it or a similar agent.

Antiinfectives

Table 1: Tetracyclines*[1,2]

Generic Name and Selected Trade Names	Normal Adult Dosage	Major Adverse Effects/Cautions	Key Counseling Points	Miscellaneous Issues
Demeclocycline HCl Declomycin	Usually, 150 mg QID or 300 mg BID, but regimens vary with the type of infection — SEE Prescribing Information (PI)	Considerations: May discolor teeth if used during tooth development (not recommended for use in children up to 8 years of age); lower doses required in patients with renal disease; photosensitivity and superinfections can occur Most common AEs include anorexia, nausea/vomiting, diarrhea, glossitis, dysphagia, rash, rise in BUN, hypersensitivity reactions Pregnancy category: D	Inform the prescriber if you have diabetes insipidus, kidney disease, or have had an unusual or allergic reaction to any of the tetracyclines; notify the physician or pharmacist before taking any other medication; if symptoms do not improve within a few days, or if they become worse check with the prescriber; while on this medication skin may be more sensitive to sunlight, avoid direct sunlight, wear protective clothing and sun block; it is important to take this medication for the full time of treatment even if you feel better; take with a full glass of water, one hour before or two hours after meals;	

213

Generic Name and Selected Trade Names	Normal Adult Dosage	Major Adverse Effects/Cautions	Key Counselling Points	Miscellaneous Issues
Demeclocycline HCl (continued) Declomycin			it is best not to miss any doses and to take the doses at evenly spaced intervals; if you miss a dose take it as soon as possible, but if it is almost time for the next dose skip the missed one — do not double doses	

Generic Name and Selected Trade Names	Normal Adult Dosage	Major Adverse Effects/Cautions	Key Counselling Points	Miscellaneous Issues
Doxycycline Calcium Vibramycin Calcium	Usually, 100 mg Q12H for 1 day then 100 mg/day as a single or divided dose, but regimens vary with the type of infection — SEE Prescribing Information (PI)	SEE demeclocycline	SEE demeclocycline, except inform the prescriber if you have liver disease (rather than kidney); may be taken with food or milk if you experience stomach upset For syrup, use specially marked measuring spoon or other device to measure each dose	
Doxycycline Hyclate Doryx Vibramycin Hyclate Vibra-Tabs	Usually, 100 mg Q12H for 1 day then 100 mg/day as a single or divided dose, but regimens vary with the type of infection — SEE Prescribing Information (PI)	SEE demeclocycline	SEE doxycycline calcium	

Generic Name and Selected Trade Names	Normal Adult Dosage	Major Adverse Effects/Cautions	Key Counselling Points	Miscellaneous Issues
Doxycycline Monohydrate Monodox Vibramycin Monohydrate	Usually, 100 mg Q12H for 1 day then 100 mg/day as a single or divided dose, but regimens vary with the type of infection — SEE Prescribing Information (PI)	SEE demeclocycline	SEE doxycycline calcium For suspension, use specially marked measuring spoon or other device to measure each dose	
Minocycline HCl Dynacin Minocin Vectrin	Usually, 200 mg initially followed by 100 mg Q12H, but regimens vary with the type of infection — SEE Prescribing Information (PI)	SEE demeclocycline	SEE doxycycline calcium For suspension, use specially marked measuring spoon or other device to measure each dose	Do not freeze the suspension

Generic Name and Selected Trade Names	Normal Adult Dosage	Major Adverse Effects/Cautions	Key Counseling Points	Miscellaneous Issues
Oxytetra-cycline Terramycin	Usually, 250 to 500 mg Q6H, but regimens vary with the type of infection — SEE Prescribing Information (PI)	SEE demeclocycline	SEE demeclocycline	
Tetracycline HCl Achromycin V	Usually, 1 to 2 G/day divided in 2 or 4 equal doses, but regimens vary with the type of infection — SEE Prescribing Information (PI)	SEE demeclocycline	SEE demeclocycline	

*As a general rule, a medication should not be administered to a patient with a known hypersensitivity to it or a similar agent.
[1]Administration of antimicrobial agents can result in overgrowth of some microorganisms and fungi.
[2]Not recommended for use during pregnancy or breast feeding.

Table 2: Macrolide Antibiotics*,1

Generic Name and Selected Trade Names	Normal Adult Dosage	Major Adverse Effects/Cautions	Key Counseling Points	Miscellaneous Issues
Azithromycin Dihydrate Zithromax	Usually, 250 to 500 mg QD, but regimens vary with the type of infection — SEE Prescribing Information (PI)	Considerations: Serious allergic (including dermal) reactions have occurred; treatment of pneumonia must be done with caution (SEE Prescribing Information); pseudomembranous colitis has occurred; use with caution in patients with liver disease Most common AEs include nausea/vomiting, diarrhea, abdominal pain, rarely angioedema and jaundice Pregnancy category: B	Inform the prescriber if you have liver disease or have had an unusual or allergic reaction to this agent or erythromycin; notify the physician or pharmacist before taking other medications; if symptoms do not improve within a few days, or if they become worse check with the prescriber; seek emergency help if you develop difficulty breathing, fever, joint pain, skin rash, swelling of face, mouth, neck, hands or feet; it is important to take this medication for the full time of treatment even if you are feeling better; take 1 hr before or 2 hrs after meals; if you miss a dose take it as soon as possible, but if it is almost time for the next dose skip the missed dose — do not double doses	

Generic Name and Selected Trade Names	Normal Adult Dosage	Major Adverse Effects/Cautions	Key Counseling Points	Miscellaneous Issues
Clarithromycin Biaxin	Usually, 250 to 500 mg Q12H for 7–14 days, but regimens vary with the type of infection — SEE Prescribing Information (PI) Dosage adjustments may be required in patients with renal impairment — SEE PI	<u>Contraindications</u>: Concomitant administration with cisapride, pimozide, or terfenadine as dangerous arrhythmias may result <u>Considerations</u>: Should not be used in pregnancy unless no other alternative exists; patients presenting with diarrhea should be evaluated for pseudomembranous colitis Most common AEs include diarrhea, nausea, abnormal taste, dyspepsia, abdominal pain, headache, hypersensitivity <u>Pregnancy category</u>: C	Inform the prescriber if you have kidney disease or have had an unusual or allergic reaction to this agent or erythromycin; notify the physician or pharmacist before taking other medications; if symptoms do not improve within a few days, or if they become worse check with the prescriber; contact the prescriber if you develop abdominal tenderness, fever, nausea/vomiting, shortness of breath, skin rash, severe diarrhea; it is important to take this medication for the full time of treatment even if you are feeling better; may be taken without regard to meals;	

Generic Name and Selected Trade Names	Normal Adult Dosage	Major Adverse Effects/Cautions	Key Counseling Points	Miscellaneous Issues
Clarithromycin (continued) Biaxin			If you miss a dose take it as soon as possible, but if it is almost time for the next dose skip the missed dose — do not double doses For oral suspension, use marked measuring spoon or device to measure each dose	

Generic Name and Selected Trade Names	Normal Adult Dosage	Major Adverse Effects/Cautions	Key Counseling Points	Miscellaneous Issues
Erythromycin Base Erythromycin **Delayed-Release erythromycin capsules** ERYC **Delayed-Release erythromycin tablets** E-Mycin Ery-Tab PCE **Erythromycin ophthalmic ointment** Ilotycin	Usual range for tablets and capsules: 250 mg QID, in equally spaced doses or 333 mg Q8H (for Ery-Tab or PCE), or 500 mg Q12H; may be increased to 4 G/day if necessary, but regimens vary with the type of infection — SEE Prescribing Information (PI) Ophthalmic ointment: Apply 1 cm directly to the affected eye up to 6 times per day	Contraindications: Concomitant administration of terfenadine, astemizole, cisapride as dangerous arrhythmias may result Considerations: Hepatic dysfunction has occurred; patients presenting with diarrhea should be evaluated for pseudomembranous colitis Most common AEs include nausea/vomiting, abdominal pain, diarrhea, anorexia, hepatic dysfunction, hypersensitivity reactions Pregnancy category: B	Inform the prescriber if you have heart or liver disease, loss of hearing or have had an unusual or allergic reaction to this agent; notify the physician or pharmacist before taking other medications; if symptoms do not improve within a few days, or if they become worse check with the prescriber; contact the prescriber if you develop fever, skin rash, redness or itching, unusual tiredness, vomiting; it is important to take this medication for the full time of treatment even if you are feeling better;	

Generic Name and Selected Trade Names	Normal Adult Dosage	Major Adverse Effects/Cautions	Key Counseling Points	Miscellaneous Issues
Erythromycin Base (continued) Erythromycin			take with a full glass of water on an empty stomach 1 hr before or 2 hrs after meals, if stomach upset occurs may be taken with food; it is best not to miss any doses and to take the doses at evenly spaced intervals; if you miss a dose take it as soon as possible, but if it is almost time for the next dose skip the missed dose — do not double doses	
Delayed-Release erythromycin capsules ERYC			For delayed release capsules or tablets, swallow whole, do not break, crush, or chew	
Delayed-Release erythromycin tablets E-Mycin Ery-Tab PCE				
Erythromycin ophthalmic ointment Ilotycin			For ointment, make sure patient knows how to instill eye ointments	

Generic Name and Selected Trade Names	Normal Adult Dosage	Major Adverse Effects/Cautions	Key Counseling Points	Miscellaneous Issues
Erythromycin Estolate Ilosone	Usually, 250 mg Q6H, may be increased to 4 G/day if necessary, but regimens vary with the type of infection — SEE Prescribing Information (PI)	SEE erythromycin base; also hepatic dysfunction has occurred	SEE erythromycin base	
Erythromycin Ethylsuccinate EES Ery-Ped	Usually, 400 mg Q6H, increased up to 4 G/day if necessary (may be given Q12H or Q8H), but regimens vary with the type of infection — SEE Prescribing Information (PI) Dosage adjustments in pediatric patients are based upon weight — SEE PI	SEE erythromycin base	SEE erythromycin base	

Generic Name and Selected Trade Names	Normal Adult Dosage	Major Adverse Effects/Cautions	Key Counseling Points	Miscellaneous Issues
Erythromycin Stearate Erythrocin	Usually, 250 mg Q6H or 500 mg Q12H may be increased up to 4 G/day if necessary, but regimens vary with the type of infection — SEE Prescribing Information (PI)	SEE erythromycin base	SEE erythromycin base	

*As a general rule, a medication should not be administered to a patient with a known hypersensitivity to it or a similar agent.
†Administration of antimicrobial agents can result in overgrowth of some microorganisms and fungi.

Table 3: Penicillins*,1

Generic Name and Selected Trade Names	Normal Adult Dosage	Major Adverse Effects/Cautions	Key Counselling Points	Miscellaneous Issues
Amoxicillin Amoxil	Usually, 250 to 500 mg Q8H, but regimens vary with the type of infection — SEE Prescribing Information (PI)	<u>Considerations</u>: Serious and occasionally fatal hypersensitivity reactions have occurred; pseudomembranous colitis has occurred <u>Most common AEs include</u> hypersensitivity, nausea/vomiting, rash, elevation of liver enzymes, blood dyscrasia (rare), agitation, insomnia <u>Pregnancy category</u>: B	Inform the prescriber if you have a history of asthma, hay fever or other allergic conditions, bleeding problems, CHF, hypertension, cystic fibrosis, kidney disease, mononucleosis, stomach or intestinal problems or have had an unusual or allergic reaction to any penicillin or cephalosporin; notify your physician or pharmacist before taking other medications; if symptoms do not improve within a few days, or if they become worse check with the prescriber; if severe diarrhea occurs check with the prescriber;	For liquid dosage forms, may be mixed with formulas, milk, fruit juice, water, ginger ale or other cold drinks

225

Generic Name and Selected Trade Names	Normal Adult Dosage	Major Adverse Effects/Cautions	Key Counselling Points
Amoxicillin (continued) Amoxil			stop taking this medication and seek emergency help if you develop fast, irregular or difficulty breathing, fever, joint pain, lightheadedness or fainting, swelling around the face, red, scaly skin, skin rash, hives or itching; while taking this medication women on oral contraceptives should utilize a different or additional method of birth control; it is important to take this medication for the full time of treatment even if you are feeling better; may be taken without regard to meals; it is best not to miss any doses and to take the doses at evenly spaced intervals; if you miss a dose take it as soon as possible, but if it is almost time for the next dose skip the missed dose — do not double doses For chewable tablets, should be chewed or crushed For oral suspension, use marked measuring spoon or device to measure each dose

Generic Name and Selected Trade Names	Normal Adult Dosage	Major Adverse Effects/Cautions	Key Counseling Points	Miscellaneous Issues
Amoxicillin/ Clavulanate Potassium Augmentin	Usually, 500 mg Q12H or 250 mg Q8H; for severe infections 875 mg Q12H or 500 mg Q8H, but regimens vary with the type of infection — SEE Prescribing Information (PI) Dosage adjustments may be required in patients with renal impairment — SEE PI	SEE amoxicillin	SEE amoxicillin	250 mg tablets and chewable tablets do not contain the same quantity of clavulanic acid and should not be used interchangeably; the 250 and 500 mg tablets contain the same amount of clavulanate and so two 250 mg tablets should not be substituted for one 500 mg tablet

Generic Name and Selected Trade Names	Normal Adult Dosage	Major Adverse Effects/Cautions	Key Counselling Points	Miscellaneous Issues
Ampicillin Omnipen	Usually, 250 to 500 mg Q6H, but regimens vary with the type of infection — SEE Prescribing Information (PI)	<u>Contraindications</u>: Organisms known to produce penicillinase <u>Considerations and most common AEs</u>: SEE amoxicillin <u>Pregnancy category</u>: B	SEE amoxicillin, except take with full glass of water 1 hr before or 2 hrs after meals	
Bacampicillin HCl Spectrobid	Usually, 400 to 800 mg Q12H, but regimens vary with the type of infection — SEE Prescribing Information (PI)	SEE amoxicillin	SEE amoxicillin, except liquid form is best if taken with a full glass of water on an empty stomach, either 1 hr before or 2 hrs after a meal	
Carbenicillin Indanyl Sodium Geocillin	Usually, 1 to 2 tablets QID, but regimens vary with the type of infection — SEE Prescribing Information (PI) Dosage adjustments required in patients with renal impairment — SEE PI	<u>Considerations</u>: SEE amoxicillin <u>Most common AEs</u> include nausea, bad taste, diarrhea, vomiting, flatulence, glossitis, hypersensitivity, rash, elevation of liver enzymes (rare, mild) <u>Pregnancy category</u>: B	SEE amoxicillin, except take with full glass of water 1 hr before or 2 hrs after meals	Use generally restricted to urinary tract infections or prostatitis

Generic Name and Selected Trade Names	Normal Adult Dosage	Major Adverse Effects/Cautions	Key Counseling Points	Miscellaneous Issues
Penicillin V Potassium Beepen-VK Betapen-VK Ledercillin VK PenVee K Veetids	Usually, 125 to 500 mg Q6–8H, but regimens vary with the type of infection — SEE Prescribing Information (PI)	SEE amoxicillin	SEE amoxicillin	Solutions retain potency for 14 days if refrigerated

*As a general rule, a medication should not be administered to a patient with a known hypersensitivity to it or a similar agent.

†Administration of antimicrobial agents can result in overgrowth of some microorganisms and fungi.

Table 4: Cephalosporins and Other Beta-lactam Antibiotics*,1

Generic Name and Selected Trade Names	Normal Adult Dosage	Major Adverse Effects/Cautions	Key Counselling Points	Miscellaneous Issues
Cefaclor Ceclor Ceclor CD	<u>Ceclor</u>: 250 mg Q8H; may increase to 500 mg Q8H for more severe infections <u>Ceclor CD</u>: 375 to 500 mg Q12H Regimens vary with the type of infection — SEE Prescribing Information (PI)	<u>Considerations</u>: Patients with diarrhea should be evaluated for pseudomembranous colitis Most common <u>AEs</u> include hypersensitivity reactions, rhinitis, diarrhea, nausea, vaginitis, abdominal pain <u>Pregnancy category</u>: B	Inform the prescriber if you have kidney disease, stomach or intestinal problems or have had an unusual or allergic reaction to any cephalosporin or penicillin; notify the physician or pharmacist before taking other medication; if symptoms do not improve within a few days, or if they become worse check with the prescriber; check with the prescriber if you develop abdominal pain, fever, or severe diarrhea; it is important to take this medication for the full time of treatment even if you are feeling better;	500 mg BID of CD dosage form is equivalent to 250 mg TID with pulvule, but 500 mg BID of CD is not equivalent to 500 mg TID of other cefaclor formulations, so do not use dosage forms interchangeably; store suspensions in the refrigerator once reconstituted, will retain potency for 14 days, do not freeze; for suspensions, include shake well auxiliary label

Generic Name and Selected Trade Names	Normal Adult Dosage	Major Adverse Effects/Cautions	Key Counseling Points	Miscellaneous Issues
Cefaclor (continued) Ceclor Ceclor CD			may be taken without regard to meals, but if the medication causes stomach upset take with meals; it is best not to miss any doses and to take the doses at even intervals; if you miss a dose take it as soon as possible, but if it is almost time for the next dose skip the missed one — do not double doses For Ceclor CD, administer with food, do not crush or chew; for suspension use marked measuring spoon or device to measure each dose	

Generic Name and Selected Trade Names	Normal Adult Dosage	Major Adverse Effects/Cautions	Key Counseling Points	Miscellaneous Issues
Cefadroxil Monohydrate Duricef Ultracef	Usually, 1 to 2 G either as a single dose or divided BID, but regimens vary with the type of infection — SEE Prescribing Information (PI) Dosage adjustments may be required in patients with renal impairment — SEE PI	<u>Considerations</u>: SEE cefaclor and use with caution in patients with renal impairment <u>Most common AEs</u>: SEE cefaclor <u>Pregnancy category</u>: B	SEE cefaclor	
Cefixime Suprax	Usually, 400 mg daily, either QD or Q12H, but regimens vary with the type of infection — SEE Prescribing Information (PI) Dosage adjustments may be required in patients with renal impairment, or those undergoing peritoneal or hemodialysis — SEE PI	<u>Considerations</u>: SEE cefaclor; also, use with caution in patients with a history of colitis <u>Most common AEs</u>: SEE cefaclor <u>Pregnancy category</u>: B	SEE cefaclor	Suspension does not require refrigeration after reconstitution

Generic Name and Selected Trade Names	Normal Adult Dosage	Major Adverse Effects/Cautions	Key Counseling Points	Miscellaneous Issues
Cefpodoxime Proxetil Vantin	Usually, 100 to 400 mg Q12H, but regimens vary with the type of infection — SEE Prescribing Information (PI) Dosage reduction required in patients with renal impairment — SEE PI	<u>Considerations and most common AEs</u>: SEE cefaclor <u>Pregnancy category</u>: B	SEE cefaclor; also, tablets should be administered with food to increase absorption; suspension may be given without regard to food	
Cefprozil Cefzil	Usually, 250 to 500 mg Q12H or Q24H, but regimens vary with the type of infection — SEE Prescribing Information (PI) Dosage adjustments may be required in patients with renal impairment — SEE PI	<u>Considerations</u>: SEE cefaclor; also, use with caution in patients with GI disorders <u>Most common AEs</u>: SEE cefaclor <u>Pregnancy category</u>: B	SEE cefaclor	Suspension contains phenylalanine

Generic Name and Selected Trade Names	Normal Adult Dosage	Major Adverse Effects/Cautions	Key Counseling Points	Miscellaneous Issues
Ceftibuten Cedax	Usually, 400 mg QD, but regimens vary with the type of infection — SEE Prescribing Information (PI) Dosage adjustments may be required in patients with renal impairment — SEE PI	<u>Considerations</u>: SEE cefaclor <u>Most common AEs</u>: SEE cefaclor <u>Pregnancy category</u>: B	SEE cefaclor and suspension should be taken 2 hrs before a meal or 1 hr after a meal	Suspension contains 1 G sucrose per teaspoonful
Cefuroxime Axetil Ceftin	Tablet: Usually 125 to 500 mg BID Oral suspension for children 3 months to 12 years of age: Usually 20 to 30 mg/kg/day Regimens vary with the type of infection — SEE Prescribing Information (PI)	<u>Considerations and most common AEs</u>: SEE cefaclor <u>Pregnancy category</u>: B	SEE cefaclor, except should be taken with food	Shake suspension well, store in refrigerator or at room temperature after reconstitution; tablets and suspension are not bioequivalent and therefore are not substitutable on a mg/mg basis — SEE Prescribing Information

Generic Name and Selected Trade Names	Normal Adult Dosage	Major Adverse Effects/Cautions	Key Counselling Points	Miscellaneous Issues
Cephalexin Keflex C-Lexin Novo-Lexin Nu-Cephalex	Usually, 1 to 4 G daily in divided doses (Q6–12H), but regimens vary with the type of infection — SEE Prescribing Information (PI) Dosage adjustments may be required in patients with renal impairment — SEE PI	<u>Considerations and most common AEs</u>: SEE cefaclor <u>Pregnancy category</u>: B	SEE cefaclor	
Cephalexin HCl Keftab	SEE cephalexin	SEE cephalexin	SEE cephalexin	

Generic Name and Selected Trade Names	Normal Adult Dosage	Major Adverse Effects/Cautions	Key Counseling Points	Miscellaneous Issues
Loracarbef Lorabid	Usually, 200 to 400 mg Q12H, but regimens vary with the type of infection — SEE Prescribing Information (PI) Dosage adjustments may be required in patients with renal impairment — SEE PI	<u>Considerations</u>: Patients with diarrhea should be evaluated for pseudomembranous colitis Most common AEs include diarrhea, nausea/vomiting abdominal pain, rashes, headache, vaginitis <u>Pregnancy category</u>: B	SEE cefaclor except take at least 1 hr before or 2 hrs after meals	

*As a general rule, a medication should not be administered to a patient with a known hypersensitivity to it or a similar agent.
†Administration of antimicrobial agents can result in overgrowth of some microorganisms and fungi.

Table 5: Quinolone Antibiotics and Related Agents*,1

Generic Name and Selected Trade Names	Normal Adult Dosage	Major Adverse Effects/Cautions	Key Counseling Points	Miscellaneous Issues
Ciprofloxacin HCl Cipro **Ciprofloxacin HCl Ophthalmic Solution** Ciloxan	Oral dosage form, usually 500 mg Q12H; serious infections may be treated with 750 mg Q12H, but regimens vary with the type of infection — SEE Prescribing Information (PI) Dosage adjustments required for patients with renal impairment — SEE PI	Considerations: Safety in children under 18 has not been assessed; CNS stimulation has occurred (tremors, convulsions, hallucinations); patients with diarrhea should be evaluated for pseudomembranous colitis; discontinue in patients that experience pain, inflammation or rupture of a tendon (tendon ruptures have occurred); avoid alkalinization of the urine Most common AEs include nausea/vomiting, diarrhea, abdominal pain, headache, restlessness, rash Pregnancy category: C	Inform the prescriber if you have kidney problems, brain or spinal cord diseases, or had an unusual or allergic reaction to this agent or any other antibiotic; do not take if pregnant or breast feeding; notify the physician or pharmacist before taking other medication; if symptoms do not improve within a few days, or if they become worse check with the prescriber; while on this medication skin may be more sensitive to sunlight, avoid direct sunlight, wear protective clothing and sun block;	

237

Generic Name and Selected Trade Names	Normal Adult Dosage	Major Adverse Effects/Cautions	Key Counseling Points
Ciprofloxacin HCl (continued) Cipro **Ciprofloxacin HCl Ophthalmic Solution** Ciloxan	Ophthalmic solution for bacterial conjunctivitis, usually 1 drop in each eye Q2H, while awake for 2 days, then 1 drop Q4H while awake for 5 days; for corneal ulcers — SEE PI Parenteral form available — SEE PI		may cause some people to become dizzy, lightheaded or drowsy, make sure you know how you react to this medication before you drive a car or operate machinery; check with the prescriber immediately if you develop agitation, confusion, fever, hallucinations, pain in legs or feet, peeling skin, tremors, shortness of breath, rash, itching, redness, swelling; it is important to take this medication for the full time of treatment even if you are feeling better; take with a full glass of water and drink several additional glasses of water each day while on this medication; may be taken without regard to meals; it is best not to miss any doses and to take the doses at evenly spaced intervals; if you miss a dose take it as soon as possible, but if it is almost time for the next dose skip the missed one — do not double doses For ophthalmic form, counsel patient regarding proper use of eye drops

Generic Name and Selected Trade Names	Normal Adult Dosage	Major Adverse Effects/Cautions	Key Counselling Points	Miscellaneous Issues
Enoxacin Penetrex	Usually, 200 to 400 mg Q12H, but regimens vary with the type of infection — SEE Prescribing Information (PI) Dosage adjustments required for patients with renal or liver impairment — SEE PI	<u>Contraindications and considerations</u>: SEE ciprofloxacin <u>Most common AEs</u> include asthenia; also, SEE ciprofloxacin <u>Pregnancy category</u>: C	SEE ciprofloxacin, except take at least 1 hr before or 2 hrs after meals	

Generic Name and Selected Trade Names	Normal Adult Dosage	Major Adverse Effects/Cautions	Key Counselling Points	Miscellaneous Issues
Levofloxacin Levaquin	Usually, 500 mg Q24H, but regimens vary with the type of infection — SEE Prescribing Information (PI) Dosage adjustments required for patients with renal or liver impairment — SEE PI	<u>Contraindications and considerations</u>: SEE ciprofloxacin <u>Most common AEs</u> include vaginitis, flatulence; also, SEE ciprofloxacin <u>Pregnancy category</u>: C	SEE ciprofloxacin	

Generic Name and Selected Trade Names	Normal Adult Dosage	Major Adverse Effects/Cautions	Key Counseling Points	Miscellaneous Issues
Lomefloxacin HCl Maxaquin	Usually, 400 mg Q24H, but regimens vary with the type of infection — SEE Prescribing Information (PI) Dosage adjustments required for patients with renal impairment — SEE PI	<u>Contraindications</u>: SEE ciprofloxacin <u>Considerations</u>: avoid exposure to sunlight (even with sunscreen); also, SEE ciprofloxacin Most common AEs include nausea, headache, photosensitivity, dizziness, diarrhea <u>Pregnancy category</u>: C	SEE ciprofloxacin	

Generic Name and Selected Trade Names	Normal Adult Dosage	Major Adverse Effects/Cautions	Key Counseling Points	Miscellaneous Issues
Norfloxacin Noroxin	Usually, 400 mg Q12H, but regimens vary with the type of infection — SEE Prescribing Information (PI) Dosage adjustments required for patients with renal impairment — SEE PI	<u>Contraindications and considerations</u>: SEE ciprofloxacin <u>Most common AEs</u>: SEE enoxacin <u>Pregnancy category</u>: C	SEE ciprofloxacin, except take at least 1 hr before or 2 hrs after meals	

Generic Name and Selected Trade Names	Normal Adult Dosage	Major Adverse Effects/Cautions	Key Counseling Points	Miscellaneous Issues
Ofloxacin Floxin	Usually, 400 mg Q12H, but regimens vary with the type of infection — SEE Prescribing Information (PI) Dosage adjustments required for patients with renal impairment — SEE PI	<u>Contraindications and considerations</u>: SEE ciprofloxacin Most common AEs include insomnia, vaginitis plus SEE ciprofloxacin <u>Pregnancy category</u>: C	SEE ciprofloxacin, except take at least 1 hr before or 2 hrs after meals	

Generic Name and Selected Trade Names	Normal Adult Dosage	Major Adverse Effects/Cautions	Key Counselling Points	Miscellaneous Issues
Sparfloxacin Zagam	Usually, 400 mg on day one then 200 mg Q24H, but regimens vary with the type of infection — SEE Prescribing Information (PI) Dosage adjustments required for patients with renal impairment — SEE PI	<u>Contraindications</u>: SEE ciprofloxacin, also co-administration with disopyramide and amiodarone or other agents known to prolong the QTc interval or in patients with known QTc prolongation on the ECG <u>Considerations</u>: SEE lomefloxacin Most common AEs include photosensitivity, diarrhea, nausea, headache, dyspepsia, dizziness, insomnia, abdominal pain, pruritus, taste perversion, prolongation of QTc interval <u>Pregnancy category</u>: C	SEE ciprofloxacin	

*As a general rule, a medication should not be administered to a patient with a known hypersensitivity to it or a similar agent.
†Administration of antimicrobial agents can result in overgrowth of some microorganisms and fungi.

244

Table 6: Sulfonamides[*,1]

Generic Name and Selected Trade Names	Normal Adult Dosage	Major Adverse Effects/Cautions	Key Counselling Points	Miscellaneous Issues
Acetyl Sulfisoxazole Gantrisin	For pediatric patient over 2 months of age, 150 mg/kg/24 hrs divided into 4 or 6 doses, initial dose should be one-half the daily maintenance dose. Dosage adjustment required in patient with liver or renal impairment — SEE Prescribing Information (PI)	Contraindications: Infants less than 2 months (except in treatment of congenital toxoplasmosis with pyrimethamine), pregnancy at term, and during nursing. Considerations: Should not be used in group A beta-hemolytic streptococcal infections; severe allergic reactions and blood dyscrasias have occurred; patients with diarrhea should be assessed for pseudomembranous colitis; use caution in patients with glucose-6-phosphate dehydrogenase deficiency or asthma	Inform the prescriber if you have anemia or other blood problems, a glucose-6-phosphate dehydrogenase deficiency, kidney or liver problems, porphyria or have had an unusual or allergic reaction to any sulfa medication; notify the physician or pharmacist before taking other medication; if symptoms do not improve within a few days, or if they become worse check with the prescriber; while on this medication skin may be more sensitive to sunlight, avoid direct sunlight, wear protective clothing and sun block;	Suspension is raspberry flavored

245

Generic Name and Selected Trade Names	Normal Adult Dosage	Major Adverse Effects/Cautions	Key Counseling Points
Acetyl Sulfisoxazole (continued) Gantrisin		Most common AEs include nausea/vomiting, anorexia, diarrhea, headache, allergic reactions, rash Pregnancy category: C	may cause blood problems that can lead to infections, slowed healing and bleeding of the gums, be cautious with dental hygiene; check with the prescriber if you develop itching or a skin rash, a sore throat, fever, pallor, or yellowing of eyes or skin (jaundice) as this could indicate a more serious problem; may cause some people to become dizzy, lightheaded, or drowsy, make sure you know how you react to this medication before driving a car or using machinery; it is important to take this medication for the full time of treatment even if you are feeling better; take with a full glass of water and drink several additional glasses of water each day; may be taken without regard to meals; it is best to not miss any doses and to take the doses at even intervals; if you miss a dose take it as soon as possible, but if it is almost time for the next dose skip the missed dose — do not double doses

Generic Name and Selected Trade Names	Normal Adult Dosage	Major Adverse Effects/Cautions	Key Counseling Points	Miscellaneous Issues
Sulfamethoxazole Gantanol	Usually, 2 G followed by 1 G BID; severe infections may require 1 G TID, but regimens vary with the type of infection — SEE Prescribing Information (PI)	SEE acetyl sulfisoxazole	SEE acetyl sulfisoxazole	

Generic Name and Selected Trade Names	Normal Adult Dosage	Major Adverse Effects/Cautions	Key Counselling Points	Miscellaneous Issues
Sulfasalazine Azulfidine En Tabs	Individualize dosage For ulcerative colitis initial therapy: Usually 3 to 4 G daily in divided doses, may initiate with 1 to 2 G to decrease GI intolerance Maintenance therapy: Usually 2 G QD For rheumatoid arthritis: Usually 2 G daily in divided doses; initiate with 0.5 to 1 G daily to decrease GI intolerance, may titrate by 0.5 G/week up to 4 G/day	Contraindications: Patients under 2 years of age, patients with intestinal or urinary obstruction, or porphyria Considerations: Use with extreme caution in patients with hepatic or renal dysfunction or with blood dyscrasias or glucose-6-phosphate deficiencies; complete blood counts and urinalysis should be conducted periodically; use with caution in patients with asthma Most common AEs include anorexia, headache, nausea, vomiting, gastric distress, reversible oligospermia, and rash (more common in arthritic patients), orange-yellow discoloration of urine or skin Pregnancy category: B	SEE acetyl sulfisoxazole, except this medication should be taken after meals to lessen stomach upset, if stomach upset continues check with prescriber; agent is a chronic medication For suspension, use marked measuring spoon or device to measure each dose For enteric coated tablets, swallow whole, do not break, crush, or chew	

Generic Name and Selected Trade Names	Normal Adult Dosage	Major Adverse Effects/Cautions	Key Counselling Points	Miscellaneous Issues
Trimethoprim and Sulfamethoxazole Bactrim Bactrim DS Septra Septra DS	*For urinary tract infections and shigellosis* Bactrim or Septra: 2 tablets Q12H DS tablets: 1 tablet Q12H Suspension: 4 teaspoonfuls Q12H Regimens vary with the type of infection — SEE Prescribing Information (PI)	<u>Contraindications</u>: Patients with megaloblastic anemia due to folate deficiency; pregnancy or nursing patients; infants under 2 months of age; treatment of streptococcal pharyngitis <u>Considerations</u>: Severe reactions such as Stevens-Johnson syndrome, toxic epidermal necrolysis, fulminant hepatic necrosis, and blood dyscrasias have occurred; use with caution in patients with impaired renal or liver function or those with possible folate deficiencies, patients with asthma or severe allergies, or glucose-6-phosphate deficiency	SEE acetyl sulfisoxazole and not recommended for use during pregnancy or breast feeding For suspension, use marked measuring spoon or device to measure each dose	

Generic Name and Selected Trade Names	Normal Adult Dosage	Major Adverse Effects/Cautions	Key Counseling Points	Miscellaneous Issues
Trimethoprim and Sulfamethoxazole (continued) Bactrim Bactrim DS Septra Septra DS	*For Pneumocystis carinii pneumonia* Administer 15 to 20 mg/kg trimethoprim and 75 to 100 mg/kg sulfamethoxazole Q6H Dosage adjustments may be required in elderly patients — SEE PI	Most common AEs include nausea/vomiting, anorexia, rash, urticaria <u>Pregnancy category</u>: C		

*As a general rule, a medication should not be administered to a patient with a known hypersensitivity to it or a similar agent.
†Administration of antimicrobial agents can result in overgrowth of some microorganisms and fungi.

Table 7: Urinary Antiinfectives*,1

Generic Name and Selected Trade Names	Normal Adult Dosage	Major Adverse Effects/Cautions	Key Counseling Points	Miscellaneous Issues
Fosfomycin Tromethamine Monurol	In women over 18 years of age administer one sachet (3G)	Considerations: More than a single dose for treatment of acute cystitis is not recommended, safety and efficacy in children under 12 years of age has not been adequately evaluated Most common AEs include diarrhea, headache, vaginitis, nausea, rhinitis, back pain, dysmenorrhea Pregnancy category: B	Your symptoms should improve in 2–3 days, if they do not contact the prescriber; can be taken with or without food; pour contents of the sachet into ½ cup of water (do not use hot water) and stir to dissolve and then drink	

Generic Name and Selected Trade Names	Normal Adult Dosage	Major Adverse Effects/Cautions	Key Counseling Points	Miscellaneous Issues
Nalidixic Acid NegGram	Usually, 1 G QID; in long-term therapy (>2 weeks) may be decreased to 2 G (total daily dose) after the initial 2 weeks, but regimens vary with the type of infection — SEE Prescribing Information (PI)	<u>Contraindication</u>: Patients with a history of convulsive disorders <u>Considerations</u>: Use with caution in patients with conditions that may predispose them to seizures; patients who develop diarrhea should be evaluated for pseudomembranous colitis; if therapy persists for more than 2 weeks, conduct blood counts, renal and hepatic testing; use with caution in patients with liver or renal impairment <u>Most common AEs</u> include abdominal pain, nausea/vomiting, diarrhea, rash, drowsiness, weakness, headache, dizziness, vertigo, photosensitivity <u>Pregnancy category</u>: C	Tell the prescriber if you have a convulsive disorder, kidney or liver problem, brain disease, a glucose-6-phosphate dehydrogenase deficiency or have had an unusual or allergic reaction to this agent or any other antibiotic; do not take during pregnancy or breast feeding; notify the physician or pharmacist before taking other medication; if symptoms do not improve within a few days, or if they become worse check with the prescriber; while on this medication skin may be more sensitive to sunlight, avoid direct sunlight, wear protective clothing and sunblock;	Suspension is raspberry flavored

Generic Name and Selected Trade Names	Normal Adult Dosage	Major Adverse Effects/Cautions	Key Counselling Points	Miscellaneous Issues
Nalidixic Acid (continued) NegGram			may cause you to become dizzy, lightheaded or drowsy, make sure you know how you react to this medication before you drive or operate machines; check with the prescriber immediately if you develop any visual problems; it is important to take this medication for the full time even if you are feeling better; take with a full glass of water on an empty stomach; if you miss a dose take it as soon as possible, but if it is almost time for the next dose skip the missed dose — do not double doses	

Generic Name and Selected Trade Names	Normal Adult Dosage	Major Adverse Effects/Cautions	Key Counselling Points	Miscellaneous Issues
Nitrofurantoin Furadantin Macrobid (monohydrate/macrocrystals) Macrodantin (macrocrystals)	Furadantin and Macrodantin: Administer 50 to 100 mg QID Macrobid: 100 mg Q12H Regimens vary with the type of infection — SEE Prescribing Information (PI)	Contraindications: Anuria, oliguria or significant renal impairment (CrCl < 60 mL/min); pregnant patients at term, during labor and delivery, neonates <1 month Considerations: Serious pulmonary toxicities have occurred with long term therapy, monitor patients' respiratory function; hepatic toxicity, optic neuritis, hemolytic anemia, and peripheral neuropathy have occurred; patients presenting with diarrhea should be evaluated for pseudomembranous colitis	Tell the prescriber if you have kidney problems, lung disease, nerve damage or a glucose-6-phosphate dehydrogenase deficiency, or have had an unusual or allergic reaction to any nitrofurantoin; notify the physician or pharmacist before taking other medications; if symptoms do not improve within a few days, or if they become worse check with the prescriber check with the prescriber immediately if you develop chest pain, chills, cough, fever, troubled breathing;	Furandantin Should be dispensed in amber bottles For oral suspension, shake well

Generic Name and Selected Trade Names	Normal Adult Dosage	Major Adverse Effects/Cautions	Key Counseling Points	Miscellaneous Issues
Nitrofurantoin (continued) Furadantin Macrobid (monohydrate/macrocrystals) Macrodantin (macrocrystals)		Most common AEs include pulmonary reactions (manifested as fever, chills, cough, chest pain, dyspnea, pulmonary infiltration, pleural effusion, and eosinophilia), allergic reactions, nausea/vomiting, anorexia, abdominal pain, diarrhea, rash, asthenia, vertigo, nystagmus Pregnancy category: B	It is important to take this medication for the full time even if you are feeling better; take with food or milk; if you miss a dose take it as soon as possible, but if it is almost time for the next dose skip the missed dose — do not double doses For extended-release capsules, swallow whole, do not open, crush, or chew	

*As a general rule, a medication should not be administered to a patient with a known hypersensitivity to it or a similar agent.
†Administration of antimicrobial agents can result in overgrowth of some microorganisms and fungi.

Table 8: Aminoglycosides*,1

Generic Name and Selected Trade Names	Normal Adult Dosage	Major Adverse Effects/Cautions	Key Counseling Points	Miscellaneous Issues
Amikacin Sulfate Amikin	Individualize dosage For patients with normal renal function, 15 mg/kg/day in 2 or 3 equal doses administered in equally divided intervals, IV or IM, but regimens vary with the type of infection — SEE Prescribing Information (PI) Dosage adjustments required in patients with renal impairment and in the elderly — SEE PI	<u>Contraindication</u>: Clinically significant allergy to any aminoglycoside <u>Considerations</u>: Patients should be monitored for renal and ototoxicity; risk of neurotoxicity greater in patients with impaired renal function; avoid use with other neuro- or nephrotoxic agents; use with caution with potent diuretics, neuromuscular blocking agents, anesthetics; use with caution during pregnancy (may cause fetal ototoxicity); if signs of renal toxicity occur hydration should be increased	Tell the prescriber if you have myasthenia gravis, trouble with your hearing and/or balance, kidney or Parkinson's disease; inform the physician or pharmacist if you are receiving any other medications; if you develop any loss of hearing, clumsiness or unsteadiness, dizziness, greatly increased or decreased frequency of urination or amount of urine produced, increased thirst, loss of appetite, nausea or vomiting, muscle twitching or seizures, ringing or buzzing or a feeling of fullness in the ears contact the prescriber immediately;	Incompatible with beta-lactam antibiotics, may occur in vivo as well; serum levels should be monitored during therapy and dosage adjusted, peak measured 30–90 min after injection, trough measured just prior to the next dose

Generic Name and Selected Trade Names	Normal Adult Dosage	Major Adverse Effects/Cautions	Key Counseling Points	Miscellaneous Issues
Amikacin Sulfate (continued) Amikin		Most common AEs include hearing loss, loss of balance, muscular paralysis, renal toxicity, rash, fever, headache, nausea/vomiting, paresthesias, eosinophilia, arthralgia, anemia, and hypotension Pregnancy category: D	it is important that this medication be given for the full treatment even if you begin to feel better; if patient or caregiver is administering the medication ensure he/she is familiar with appropriate aseptic injection technique	

Generic Name and Selected Trade Names	Normal Adult Dosage	Major Adverse Effects/Cautions	Key Counseling Points	Miscellaneous Issues
Gentamicin Sulfate Garamycin	Individualize dosage Parenteral formulation: For patients with normal renal function, 3 mg/kg/day in 3 equal doses Q8H IV or IM, but regimens vary with the type of infection — SEE Prescribing Information (PI) Dosage adjustments required in patients with renal impairment and in the elderly — SEE PI	Contraindications and considerations: SEE amikacin sulfate except, most not applicable for topical forms Most common AEs include renal toxicity, dizziness, vertigo, ataxia, tinnitus, hearing loss, loss of balance, muscular paralysis (including respiratory depression), lethargy confusion, fever, headache, nausea/vomiting; for ointment/cream, main adverse effect is local irritation Pregnancy category: Not specified	SEE amikacin sulfate For ointment/cream, ensure patient knows how to apply it properly	Serum levels should be monitored during therapy and dosage adjusted, peak measured 30–60 min after injection, trough measured just prior to the next dose

Generic Name and Selected Trade Names	Normal Adult Dosage	Major Adverse Effects/Cautions	Key Counseling Points	Miscellaneous Issues
Gentamicin Sulfate (continued) Garamycin	For ointment/cream: Apply a small amount to lesions TID or QID, may cover area with gauze; in impetigo contagiosa, crust should be removed before application For ophthalmic preparations: SEE PI			

Generic Name and Selected Trade Names	Normal Adult Dosage	Major Adverse Effects/Cautions	Key Counselling Points	Miscellaneous Issues
Tobramycin Sulfate Nebcin	Individualize dosage For patients with normal renal function, 3 mg/kg/day in 3 equal doses Q8H IV or IM; may increase to 5 mg/kg/day for serious infections, but regimens vary with the type of infection — SEE Prescribing Information (PI) Dosage adjustments required in patients with renal impairment and in the elderly — SEE PI For ophthalmic preparation: SEE PI	<u>Contraindications and considerations</u>: SEE amikacin sulfate <u>Most common AEs</u>: SEE gentamicin sulfate <u>Pregnancy category</u>: D	SEE amikacin sulfate	Incompatible with beta-lactam antibiotics, may occur in vivo as well; serum levels should be monitored during therapy and dosage adjusted, peak measured 30 min after IV injection (60 min after IM), trough measured just prior to the next dose; contains a bisulfite, which may cause allergic reactions

*As a general rule, a medication should not be administered to a patient with a known hypersensitivity to it or a similar agent.
†Administration of antimicrobial agents can result in overgrowth of some microorganisms and fungi.

Table 9: Antituberculosis Agents* [1,2,3]

Generic Name and Selected Trade Names	Normal Adult Dosage	Major Adverse Effects/Cautions	Key Counseling Points	Miscellaneous Issues
Cycloserine Seromycin	Individualize dosage Initially, 250 mg Q12H for 2 weeks, increased to 500 mg to 1 G daily in divided doses	Contraindications: Patients with epilepsy, depression, psychosis or severe anxiety, severe renal dysfunction; excessive use of alcohol Considerations: Discontinue or decrease dose in patients experiencing allergic dermatitis or CNS toxicity (eg, convulsions, headache, and somnolence); monitor patients for hematologic, renal, and liver function as well as drug levels Most common AEs include convulsions, sedation, headache, tremor, confusion, psychoses, hypersensitivity, rash Pregnancy category: C	Inform the prescriber if you have a history of alcohol abuse, convulsive disorders, kidney disease or mental disorders; notify the physician or pharmacist before taking any other medication; avoid alcoholic beverages while taking this medication; if symptoms do not improve within 2–3 weeks, or if they become worse check with the prescriber; this medication can cause some people to become dizzy or less alert, be sure you know how you react to the agent before driving or operating machines; if you develop any mental changes contact your physician;	

Generic Name and Selected Trade Names	Normal Adult Dosage	Major Adverse Effects/Cautions	Key Counseling Points	Miscellaneous Issues
Cycloserine (continued) Seromycin			it is important that your physician checks your progress at regular visits and that you take this medication as directed for the complete course; may be taken after meals if it causes stomach upset; it is best not to miss any doses and to take the doses at evenly spaced intervals; if you miss a dose take it as soon as possible, but if it is almost time for the next dose skip the missed dose — do not double doses	

Generic Name and Selected Trade Names	Normal Adult Dosage	Major Adverse Effects/Cautions	Key Counselling Points	Miscellaneous Issues
Ethambutol HCl Myambutol	Individualize dosage Initial treatment: 15 mg/kg Q24H Retreatment: 25 mg/kg Q24H, after 60 days decrease dose to 15 mg/kg	Contraindications: Patients with optic neuritis unless clinical judgement determines it can be used Considerations: Not recommended for use in children under 13; lower doses required in patients with renal dysfunction; vision should be assessed periodically Most common AEs include decreased visual acuity, hypersensitivity reactions, dermatitis, joint pain, nausea/vomiting, anorexia, fever, malaise, headache Pregnancy category: Not specified	Inform the prescriber if you have gouty arthritis, kidney disease or eye nerve damage; notify the physician or pharmacist before taking other medication; if your symptoms do not improve within 2–3 weeks, or if they become worse check with the prescriber; this medication can cause some people to become dizzy or less alert, be sure you know how you react to the agent before driving or operating machines; if you develop blurred vision, eye pain, red-green color blindness or loss of vision or chills, pain or swelling in the joints contact the prescriber immediately;	Ethambutol is to be used in combination with other agents

Generic Name and Selected Trade Names	Normal Adult Dosage	Major Adverse Effects/Cautions	Key Counseling Points	Miscellaneous Issues
Ethambutol HCl (continued) Myambutol			It is important that the physician checks your progress at regular visits and that you take this medication as directed for the complete course; may be taken after meals if it causes stomach upset; it is best not to miss any doses and to take the doses at evenly spaced intervals; if you miss a dose take it as soon as possible, but if it is almost time for the next dose skip the missed dose — do not double doses	

Generic Name and Selected Trade Names	Normal Adult Dosage	Major Adverse Effects/Cautions	Key Counseling Points	Miscellaneous Issues
Ethionamide Trecator-SC	Individualize dosage Usually, 0.5 to 1 G daily in divided doses	<u>Contraindications</u>: Severe hepatic dysfunction <u>Considerations</u>: Avoid in pregnancy; liver enzyme levels should be monitored; use with caution in patients with diabetes mellitus Most common AEs include GI intolerance, peripheral neuritis, optic neuritis, psychic disturbances, postural hypotension, rash <u>Pregnancy category</u>: Not specified	Inform the prescriber if you have diabetes mellitus, liver disease or have had an allergic or unusual reaction to any TB medication or niacin; notify the physician or pharmacist before taking any other medication; if symptoms do not improve within 2–3 weeks, or if they become worse check with the prescriber; this medication may cause some blurred vision or loss of vision, be sure you know how you react to the agent before driving or operating machines;	Recommended to be given with pyridoxine

Generic Name and Selected Trade Names	Normal Adult Dosage	Major Adverse Effects/Cautions	Key Counseling Points	Miscellaneous Issues
Ethionamide (continued) Trecator-SC			if you develop unsteadiness, numbness, tingling, burning or pain in the hands or feet contact the prescriber immediately; it is important that the physician checks your progress at regular visits and that this medication is taken as directed for the complete course; the prescriber may want you to take pyridoxine every day to help decrease the adverse effects of this agent; may be taken after meals if it causes stomach upset; it is best not to miss any doses and to take the doses at evenly spaced intervals; if you miss a dose take it as soon as possible, but if it is almost time for the next dose skip the missed dose — do not double doses	

Generic Name and Selected Trade Names	Normal Adult Dosage	Major Adverse Effects/Cautions	Key Counseling Points	Miscellaneous Issues
Isoniazid Laniazid	Individualize dosage For TB prophylaxis: 300 mg QD For TB treatment: Usually, 300 mg QD or 15 mg/kg 2–3 times per week	Contraindications: Previous isoniazid-induced liver damage; previous severe adverse reactions; acute liver dysfunction Considerations: Monitor liver function; if vision changes occur patients should be evaluated for optic neuritis; use with caution in daily users of alcohol, patients with chronic liver disease, or severe renal dysfunction Most common AEs include hepatitis, peripheral neuritis, blood dyscrasias, hypersensitivity, neurotoxicity (seizures, depression), optic neuritis, GI distress Pregnancy category: C	Inform the prescriber if you have a history of alcohol abuse, convulsive disorders, kidney or liver disease or have had an allergic or unusual reaction to any TB medication or niacin; notify the physician or pharmacist before taking other medication; avoid alcoholic beverages while taking this medication; if symptoms do not improve within 2–3 weeks, or if they become worse check with the prescriber; notify the prescriber immediately if you experience fatigue, weakness, malaise, anorexia, nausea/vomiting, blurred vision or loss of vision, or numbness, tingling, burning or pain in the hands or feet;	Recommended to be administered with pyridoxine

Generic Name and Selected Trade Names	Normal Adult Dosage	Major Adverse Effects/Cautions	Key Counselling Points	Miscellaneous Issues
Isoniazid (continued) Laniazid			it is important that the physician checks your progress at regular visits and that this medication is taken as directed for the complete course; the prescriber may want you to take pyridoxine every day to help decrease the adverse effects of this agent; may be taken after meals if it causes stomach upset; it is best not to miss any doses; if you miss a dose take it as soon as possible, but if it is almost time for the next dose skip the missed dose — do not double doses For oral liquid form, use specially marked measuring spoon or other device to measure each dose	

Generic Name and Selected Trade Names	Normal Adult Dosage	Major Adverse Effects/Cautions	Key Counselling Points	Miscellaneous Issues
Pyrazinamide	Individualize dosage Usually, 15 to 30 mg/kg QD, alternatively 50 to 70 mg/kg twice weekly	<u>Contraindications</u>: Severe, hepatic disease, acute gout <u>Considerations</u>: Baseline liver function and uric acid levels should be measured; patients at risk for drug-related hepatitis (preexisting liver disease, alcohol abusers) should be closely monitored; use with caution in patients with a history of diabetes mellitus Most common AEs include hepatotoxicity, gout, porphyria, dysuria, GI disturbances, rash, pruritus <u>Pregnancy category</u>: C	Inform the prescriber if you have gout, liver disease or have had an allergic or unusual reaction to any TB medication or niacin; notify the physician or pharmacist before taking any other medication; if symptoms do not improve within 2–3 weeks, or if they become worse check with the prescriber; if you develop joint pain, fever, loss of appetite, malaise, nausea/vomiting, darkened urine or yellowish discoloration of skin and eyes contact the prescriber immediately;	

Generic Name and Selected Trade Names	Normal Adult Dosage	Major Adverse Effects/Cautions	Key Counseling Points	Miscellaneous Issues
Pyrazinamide (continued)			it is important that the physician checks your progress at regular visits and that this medication is taken as directed for the complete course; it is best not to miss any doses and to take the doses at evenly spaced intervals; if you miss a dose take it as soon as possible, but if it is almost time for the next dose skip the missed dose — do not double doses	

Generic Name and Selected Trade Names	Normal Adult Dosage	Major Adverse Effects/Cautions	Key Counseling Points	Miscellaneous Issues
Rifabutin Mycobutin	Individualize dosage Usually, 300 mg QD for prophylaxis of disseminated mycobacterium avium complex in advanced HIV	<u>Considerations</u>: Not for prophylactic use in patients with active disease; patients who develop signs of TB while on prophylaxis should consult their physician; conduct periodic hematologic monitoring <u>Most common AEs</u> include rash, GI distress, neutropenia, discoloration of bodily fluids <u>Pregnancy category</u>: B	Tell the prescriber if you had an allergic or unusual reaction to this agent or rifampin; notify the physician or pharmacist before taking any other medication; if symptoms do not improve within 2–3 weeks, or if they become worse check with prescriber; your urine, feces, saliva, sputum, perspiration, tears, and skin may be colored brown-orange while on this agent, soft contact lenses may be permanently stained; contact the prescriber if you develop skin rash, changes in taste or vision, fever and sore throat, joint pain, fever, or yellowish discoloration of skin/ eyes;	

Generic Name and Selected Trade Names	Normal Adult Dosage	Major Adverse Effects/Cautions	Key Counseling Points	Miscellaneous Issues
Rifabutin (continued) Mycobutin			it is important that your progress be checked at regular intervals and that this agent be taken as directed for the complete course; may be taken with meals if it produces stomach upset; it is best not to miss any doses and to take the doses at evenly spaced intervals; if you miss a dose take it as soon as possible, but if it is almost time for the next dose skip the missed dose — do not double doses	

Generic Name and Selected Trade Names	Normal Adult Dosage	Major Adverse Effects/Cautions	Key Counseling Points	Miscellaneous Issues
Rifampin Rifadin Rimactane	Individualize dosage For TB: 600 mg Q24H For meningococcal carriers: 600 mg BID for 2 days	Contraindications: Use in the treatment of meningococcal disease Considerations: Use with extreme caution in patients with liver dysfunction; if used patients' liver function should be closely monitored Most common AEs include nausea/vomiting, anorexia, diarrhea, alteration in liver function, headache, fever, rash Pregnancy category: C	Inform the prescriber if you have a history of alcohol abuse or liver disease; notify the physician or pharmacist before taking other medication; avoid alcoholic beverages while taking this medication; oral contraceptives may not work properly while on this medication, a different method of birth control should be used; if symptoms do not improve within 2–3 weeks, or if they become worse check with the prescriber;	Many drug interactions are possible — SEE Prescribing Information (PI); liquid suspension may be prepared from capsules, SEE PI

Generic Name and Selected Trade Names	Normal Adult Dosage	Major Adverse Effects/Cautions	Key Counseling Points
Rifampin (continued) Rifadin Rimactane			your urine, feces, saliva, sputum, perspiration, and tears may be colored a reddish orange to reddish brown while on this agent; soft contact lenses may be permanently stained; if you develop weakness, loss of appetite, nausea/vomiting or any other unusual symptoms contact the prescriber immediately; this agent may produce changes in your blood that make it easier for you to develop an infection or bleeding, be cautious while brushing your teeth; it is important that the physician checks your progress at regular visits and that you take this medication as directed for the complete course; take this medication with a full glass of water on an empty stomach, but may be taken with food if it produces stomach upset; it is best not to miss any doses and to take the doses at evenly spaced intervals; if you miss a dose take it as soon as possible, but if it is almost time for the next dose skip the missed dose — do not double doses

Generic Name and Selected Trade Names	Normal Adult Dosage	Major Adverse Effects/Cautions	Key Counseling Points	Miscellaneous Issues
Streptomycin Sulfate	Individualize dosage For resistant TB in combination with other agents, 15 mg/kg/day (maximum 1 G) OR 25 to 30 mg/kg twice or thrice weekly (maximum 1.5 G) given IM Lower doses required in patients with renal impairment and in the elderly — SEE Prescribing Information (PI)	<u>Contraindications</u>: Clinically significant allergy to any aminoglycoside <u>Considerations</u>: Risk of neurotoxicity greater in patients with impaired renal function, renal function should be monitored; avoid use with other neuro- or nephrotoxic agents; vestibular and ototoxicity can occur, periodic monitoring should be conducted; alkalinization of the urine may decrease nephrotoxicity	Tell the prescriber if you have any kidney, hearing, balance or brain disorder; agent may cause fetal harm, so if you are pregnant or become pregnant contact the prescriber; if you notice any changes in your hearing while on this agent contact the prescriber; if patient or care-giver is administering the agent ensure he/she know proper technique for IM injections	Care should be taken to avoid contact with the skin of the solution; preferred site for IM injection is upper, outer quadrant of buttock or mid-lateral thigh (preferred for children), injection sites should be alternated

Generic Name and Selected Trade Names	Normal Adult Dosage	Major Adverse Effects/Cautions	Key Counseling Points	Miscellaneous Issues
Streptomycin Sulfate (continued)		Most common AEs include nausea/vomiting, vertigo, paresthesias of the face, rash, fever, urticaria, angioneurotic edema, eosinophilia, ototoxicity, dermatitis Pregnancy category: D		

*As a general rule, a medication should not be administered to a patient with a known hypersensitivity to it or a similar agent.

[1]Most tuberculosis patients receive combination therapy, compliance with the regimen is essential, patients should be aware of the importance of full compliance.

[2]Selection of agents for the treatment of tuberculosis is based upon susceptibility and patient factors.

[3]Administration of antimicrobial agents can result in overgrowth of some microorganisms.

Table 10: Antifungal Agents*

Generic Name and Selected Trade Names	Normal Adult Dosage	Major Adverse Effects/Cautions	Key Counseling Points	Miscellaneous Issues
Fluconazole Diflucan	Single dose for vaginal candidiasis: 150 mg Multiple dose for a variety of fungal infections: SEE Prescribing Information (PI) for details; dosage level and duration of therapy is based on infecting organism and patient response to therapy Dosage adjustments required in patients with renal impairment — SEE PI	Contraindication: Concomitant administration with terfenadine Considerations: Hepatic toxicity, anaphylaxis, exfoliative skin disorders have occurred; adverse effects occur more frequently in patients with HIV; drug interactions resulting in torsades de pointes has occurred — SEE Prescribing Information (PI) Most common AEs include headache, nausea, abdominal pain, skin rash, diarrhea Pregnancy category: C	Inform the prescriber if you have too little stomach acid, a history of alcohol abuse, liver or kidney disease, if you are or plan on becoming pregnant while taking this medication; notify the physician or pharmacist before taking other medications; avoid alcoholic beverages and medications such as cough elixirs while receiving this medication; if symptoms do not improve within a few weeks, or if they become worse check with the prescriber; if you develop fever and chills, skin rash or itching contact the prescriber;	For suspension, store between 5 and 30°C; after reconstitution potency remains for 14 days

Generic Name and Selected Trade Names	Normal Adult Dosage	Major Adverse Effects/Cautions	Key Counseling Points	Miscellaneous Issues
Fluconazole (continued) Diflucan			It is important that your doctor checks your progress at regular visits; take with a full glass of water; it is important that you take this medication for the full course even if you begin to feel better; if you miss a dose take it as soon as possible, but if it is almost time for the next dose skip the missed dose — do not double doses For suspension, use specially marked measuring spoon or other device to measure dose	

Generic Name and Selected Trade Names	Normal Adult Dosage	Major Adverse Effects/Cautions	Key Counseling Points	Miscellaneous Issues
Flucytosine Ancobon	Individualize dosage Usually, 50 to 150 mg/kg/ day administered Q6H Dosage adjustments required in patients with renal dysfunction — SEE PI	<u>Considerations</u>: Use with extreme caution in patients with impaired renal or hepatic function; use with caution in patients with bone marrow depression; monitor hematologic, renal and hepatic function; lower doses required in renal patients Most common AEs include nausea/vomiting, diarrhea, rash, photosensitivity, ataxia, hearing loss, headache, hepatic, renal and cardiovascular toxicity has occurred <u>Pregnancy category</u>: C	Inform the prescriber if you have a blood, liver or kidney disease; notify the physician or pharmacist before taking other medications; if symptoms do not improve within a few weeks, or if they become worse check with the prescriber; while on this medication skin may be more sensitive to sunlight, avoid direct sunlight, wear protective clothing and sun block; this agent may cause blood problems which could result in infections, slow healing and bleeding of the gums, use caution with dental hygiene;	

Generic Name and Selected Trade Names	Normal Adult Dosage	Major Adverse Effects/Cautions	Key Counseling Points	Miscellaneous Issues
Flucytosine (continued) Ancobon			if you develop skin rash, redness or itching, sore throat and fever, unusual bleeding or bruising, unusual tiredness or yellow eyes or skin contact the prescriber; it is important that your doctor checks your progress at regular visits; in some patients this agent may cause nausea, so if you are taking more than one capsule, take them over a 15 minute period; it is important that this medication is taken for the full course even if you begin to feel better; if you miss a dose take it as soon as possible, but if it is almost time for the next dose skip the missed dose — do not double doses	

Generic Name and Selected Trade Names	Normal Adult Dosage	Major Adverse Effects/Cautions	Key Counseling Points	Miscellaneous Issues
Griseofulvin Fulvicin P/G Grifulvin V Gris-PEG	Individualize dosage Fulvicin P/G for tinea corporis, tinea cruris, tinea capitis: 330 or 375 mg as a single dose or in divided doses Fulvicin for tinea pedis, tinea unguium: 660 or 750 mg daily in divided doses Grifulvin V for tinea corporis, tinea cruris, tinea capitis: 500 mg/day Grifulvin V for tinea pedis, tinea unguium: 1 G/day	Contraindications: Pregnancy, porphyria, hepatocellular failure Considerations: Safety and efficacy for the prophylaxis of fungal infections has not been proven; periodic monitoring of major organ functioning should be conducted Most common AEs include rashes, urticaria, erythema, oral thrush, nausea/vomiting, epigastric distress, diarrhea, headache, fatigue Pregnancy category: Not specified, but is contraindicated	Inform the prescriber if you have liver disease, lupus, porphyria or have had an unusual or allergic reaction to this agent, a penicillin or penicillamine; not recommended for use during pregnancy; this agent may interfere with certain birth control pills, a different or additional method of birth control should be used while taking this medication and for one month after stopping the medication; notify the physician or pharmacist before taking other medications;	Derived from *penicillium*, cross sensitivity could occur; eradication must be assessed via clinical or laboratory examination

Generic Name and Selected Trade Names	Normal Adult Dosage	Major Adverse Effects/Cautions	Key Counseling Points
Griseofulvin (continued) Fulvicin P/G Grifulvin V Gris-PEG	Gris-PEG for tinea corporis, tinea cruris, tinea capitis: 375 mg QD as a single dose or in divided doses Gris-PEG for tinea pedis, tinea unguium: 750 mg daily in divided doses Duration of therapy: tinea capitis — 4-6 weeks tinea corporis — 2-4 weeks tinea pedis — 4-8 weeks tinea unguium — 4 months (fingernails), 6 months (toenails)		while on this medication skin may be more sensitive to sunlight, avoid direct sunlight, wear protective clothing and sunblock; this agent may potentiate the effects of alcohol, check with the prescriber before consuming alcoholic beverages; this medication can cause some people to become dizzy or less alert, be sure you know how you react to the agent before driving or operating machines; it is important to take appropriate hygienic measures to decrease the incidence of re-infection; if you develop confusion, skin reactions or soreness of mouth or throat, contact the prescriber; it is important to take this medication for the full time of treatment even if you are feeling better; take with or after meals, it is best to take with fatty food, such as ice cream or whole milk; it is best not to miss any doses and to take the doses at evenly spaced intervals; if you miss a dose take it as soon as possible, but if it is almost time for the next dose skip the missed dose — do not double doses

Generic Name and Selected Trade Names	Normal Adult Dosage	Major Adverse Effects/Cautions	Key Counselling Points	Miscellaneous Issues
Itraconazole Sporanox	Individualize dosage <u>Capsules for blastomycosis, histoplasmosis</u>: 200 mg daily, may be increased in 100 mg increments to a maximum of 400 mg if required <u>Capsules for aspergillosis</u>: 200 to 400 mg daily <u>Capsules for fingernail (only) onychomycosis</u>: 200 mg BID for 1 week then 3 weeks later repeat 200 mg BID for 1 week	<u>Contraindications</u>: Pregnancy, co-administration with terfenadine, astemizole, cisapride, midazolam, triazolam, lovastatin and simvastatin <u>Considerations</u>: Capsules and solution should not be used interchangeably; if patient develops signs of hepatic dysfunction the agent should be discontinued Most common AEs include GI distress, rash, pruritus, edema, fatigue, headache, elevated liver enzymes <u>Pregnancy category</u>: C	SEE fluconazole, except take with a meal or snack; also, do not take with astemizole, cisapride, or terfenadine; if taking with antacids or other ulcer medications separate by at least 2 hrs For solution, vigorously swish in mouth for a few seconds and then swallow	Only the solution has been demonstrated to be effective in oral and esophageal candidiasis

Generic Name and Selected Trade Names	Normal Adult Dosage	Major Adverse Effects/Cautions	Key Counselling Points	Miscellaneous Issues
Itraconazole (continued) Sporanox	<u>Capsules for toenail onychomycosis</u>: 200 mg daily for 12 weeks <u>Solution for oropharyngeal candidiasis</u>: 200 mg daily for 1 - 2 weeks <u>Solution for oropharyngeal candidiasis</u>: 100 mg daily for a minimum of 3 weeks, may be increased to 200 mg			

Generic Name and Selected Trade Names	Normal Adult Dosage	Major Adverse Effects/Cautions	Key Counseling Points	Miscellaneous Issues
Ketoconazole Nizoral	Individualize dosage Usually, 200 mg daily; may be increased to 400 mg daily if required	<u>Contraindications:</u> Co-administration with terfenadine, astemizole, cisapride or triazolam <u>Considerations:</u> Liver function should be monitored (severe liver toxicity has occurred); rarely anaphylaxis with the first dose has occurred Most common AEs include hypersensitivity reactions, nausea/vomiting, abdominal pain, pruritus <u>Pregnancy category:</u> C	SEE itraconazole	

285

Generic Name and Selected Trade Names	Normal Adult Dosage	Major Adverse Effects/Cautions	Key Counselling Points	Miscellaneous Issues
Terbinafine HCl Lamisil	Individualize dosage For fingernail onychomycosis: 250 mg daily for 6 weeks For toenail onychomycosis: 250 mg daily for 12 weeks	Considerations: Discontinue if symptoms of hepatobiliary dysfunction occur or if progressive skin rash occurs (Stevens-Johnson syndrome, toxic epidermal necrolysis have occurred) Most common AEs include diarrhea, dyspepsia, abdominal pain, rash, pruritus, urticaria, liver enzyme abnormalities, taste disturbances, visual disturbances Pregnancy category: B	Inform the prescriber if you have a history of alcohol abuse, liver or kidney disease, if you are pregnant or plan on becoming pregnant while taking this medication; notify the physician or pharmacist before taking other medications; avoid alcoholic beverages while taking this medication; if symptoms do not improve within a few weeks, or if they become worse check with the prescriber;	

Generic Name and Selected Trade Names	Normal Adult Dosage	Major Adverse Effects/Cautions	Key Counseling Points	Miscellaneous Issues
Terbinafine HCl (continued) Lamisil			if you develop skin rash or itching contact the prescriber; it is important that your doctor checks your progress at regular visits; may be taken with or without food; it is best not to miss any doses and to take the doses at evenly spaced intervals; if you miss a dose take it as soon as possible, but if it is almost time for the next dose skip the missed dose — do not double doses	

*As a general rule, a medication should not be administered to a patient with a known hypersensitivity to it or a similar agent.

Table 11: AIDS Chemotherapeutic Agents*[1,2]

Generic Name and Selected Trade Names	Normal Adult Dosage	Major Adverse Effects/Cautions	Key Counseling Points	Miscellaneous Issues
Delavirdine Mesylate Rescriptor	Individualize dosage Usually, 400 mg TID in combination regimens	Considerations: Patients with liver impairment may have increased toxicity; resistance develops if given as monotherapy Most common AEs include headache, fatigue, nausea, diarrhea, vomiting, rash, elevation of liver enzymes (AEs are reported from studies with patients on combination therapy) Pregnancy category: C	Inform the prescriber if you have any serious medical conditions; notify the physician or pharmacist before taking any other medication; if you develop a rash contact the prescriber immediately; may be taken with or without food; tablets may be dissolved in at least 3 ounces of water, allow it to sit a few minutes and then stir, drink all 3 ounces, then add more water to ensure all of the powder is consumed; if you have achlorhydria should take this medication with an acidic beverage such as orange juice; if you miss a dose take it as soon as possible, but if it is almost time for the next dose skip the missed one — do not double doses	Many drug interactions are possible — SEE Prescribing Information (PI)

Generic Name and Selected Trade Names	Normal Adult Dosage	Major Adverse Effects/Cautions	Key Counseling Points	Miscellaneous Issues
Didanosine Videx	Individualize dosage Tablets in patients ≥60 kg: 200 mg BID Buffered powder in patients ≥60 kg: 250 mg BID Tablets in patients <60 kg: 125 mg BID Buffered powder in patients <60 kg: 167 mg BID Irrespective of dose, patient must take at least 2 tablets per dose to ensure adequate buffering of gastric acid	Considerations: Use with caution in patients at risk for pancreatitis, if patient develops signs of pancreatitis agent should be discontinued; use with caution in patients with liver disorders; retinal examinations should be performed in children and any patient who experiences changes in vision Most common AEs include pancreatitis, liver failure, retinal changes, peripheral neuropathy, diarrhea Pregnancy category: B	Inform the prescriber if you have liver disease or any other serious medical condition; notify the physician or pharmacist before taking other medications; stop taking the medication and call the physician if you develop severe nausea/vomiting or stomach pain; contact the physician if you develop tingling, burning, numbness, and pain in the hands or feet; it is important that the physician checks your progress at regular visits; take on an empty stomach (ie, 2 hrs before or 2 hrs after eating); take this medication exactly as directed, it is important to try not to miss any doses;	Tablets and solution contain a lot of sodium; tablets contain phenylalanine; specially marked measuring spoon must be used to measure the pediatric suspension accurately

Generic Name and Selected Trade Names	Normal Adult Dosage	Major Adverse Effects/Cautions	Key Counseling Points	Miscellaneous Issues
Didanosine (continued) Videx			If you miss a dose take it as soon as possible, but if it is almost time for the next dose skip the missed dose — do not double doses For tablets, must be chewed or crushed (can be dissolved in water); for oral solution, open foil packet and pour contents into ½ glass of water, stir until dissolved and drink at once	

Generic Name and Selected Trade Names	Normal Adult Dosage	Major Adverse Effects/Cautions	Key Counseling Points	Miscellaneous Issues
Indinavir Sulfate Crixivan	Individualize dosage Usually, 800 mg Q8H; generally used in combination with other agents Dosage adjustments required in patients with liver disease — SEE Prescribing Information (PI)	<u>Considerations</u>: Monitor for signs of nephrolithiasis (flank pain, hematuria) which may warrant suspension of therapy; risk may be lessened if patient maintains adequate hydration Most common AEs include nephrolithiasis, hyper-bilirubinemia, elevation of liver enzymes, rash, upper respiratory infection, dry skin, pharyngitis, taste perversion <u>Pregnancy category</u>: C	Tell the prescriber if you have other medical conditions; contact the prescriber if you have flank pain or notice a change in the color of your urine or blood in your urine; take this medication exactly as directed — do not take more of it; do not stop taking this without discussing it first with the prescriber; take the medication with a full glass of water and at least 1 hour before or 2 hrs after a meal, it is very important that you take this medication every 8 hrs unless otherwise directed and drink plenty of water unless otherwise directed;	

Generic Name and Selected Trade Names	Normal Adult Dosage	Major Adverse Effects/Cautions	Key Counselling Points	Miscellaneous Issues
Indinavir Sulfate (continued) Crixivan			try not to miss any doses, but if you do miss a dose and remember within 2 hrs take it right away, but if you don't remember until later, skip the missed dose and go back to regular dosing schedule — do not double doses	

Generic Name and Selected Trade Names	Normal Adult Dosage	Major Adverse Effects/Cautions	Key Counselling Points	Miscellaneous Issues
Lamivudine Epivir	Individualize dosage Usually, 150 mg BID in combination with zidovudine; dosage adjusted for low weight patients and patients with renal impairment — SEE Prescribing Information (PI)	<u>Considerations</u>: In pediatric patients at risk for pancreatitis the combination of lamivudine and ziduvidine should be used with extreme caution Most common AEs include headache, malaise, nausea, depression, nasal stuffiness, cough, rash, pancreatitis <u>Pregnancy category:</u> C	Inform the prescriber if you have any serious medical condition, especially kidney disease; notify the physician or pharmacist before taking other medications; check with the physician if you develop abdominal or stomach pain, nausea/vomiting, tingling, burning, numbness, or pain in the hands or feet; it is important that the physician checks your progress at regular visits; take this medication exactly as directed; it is important to try and not miss any doses, if you miss a dose take it as soon as possible, but if it is almost time for the next dose skip the missed dose — do not double doses	Specially marked measuring spoon must be used to measure the pediatric suspension accurately

Generic Name and Selected Trade Names	Normal Adult Dosage	Major Adverse Effects/Cautions	Key Counseling Points	Miscellaneous Issues
Nelfinavir Mesylate Viracept	Individualize dosage Usually, 750 mg TID; generally use in combination with nucleoside inhibitors	Considerations: New onset diabetes or aggravation of existing diabetes has occurred with patients on protease inhibitors, use caution in patients with liver disease Most common AEs include diarrhea, flatulence (note: most information is when it is used in combination) Pregnancy category: B	Tell the prescriber if you have diabetes mellitus or a liver disease; if you develop diarrhea do not take any medicine for the diarrhea without first checking with the physician; oral contraceptives (birth control pills) may not work properly — use a different or additional method of birth control; try very hard not to miss any doses; if you miss a dose take it as soon as possible, but if it is almost time for the next dose skip the missed one and return to regular schedule — do not double doses	Powder contains phenylalanine; powder may be mixed with water, milk, or formula and should be consumed within 6 hrs

Generic Name and Selected Trade Names	Normal Adult Dosage	Major Adverse Effects/Cautions	Key Counseling Points	Miscellaneous Issues
Nevirapine Viramune	Individualize dosage Initially, 200 mg daily for 14 days, followed by 200 mg BID; use in combination with nucleoside agents	<u>Considerations</u>: Severe skin reactions have occurred (including Stevens-Johnson syndrome), should be discontinued in patients developing a severe rash or symptoms such as fever, blisters, swelling, muscle or joint pain; incidence of rash is decreased if a lower dose is used initially; liver function test should be performed prior to initiating therapy and during therapy Most common AEs include rash, fever, headache, abnormal liver function tests <u>Pregnancy category</u>: C	Inform the prescriber if you have any serious medical condition, especially kidney disease; notify the physician or pharmacist before taking other medication; stop the medication and check with the physician if you develop a skin rash or a rash accompanied by fever, blistering, oral lesions, conjunctivitis, swelling, muscle or joint pain, or general malaise; it is important that the physician checks your progress at regular visits; take this medication exactly as directed, may be taken with or without food; it is important to try and not miss any doses, if you miss a dose take it as soon as possible, but if it is almost time for the next dose skip the missed dose — do not double doses	

Generic Name and Selected Trade Names	Normal Adult Dosage	Major Adverse Effects/Cautions	Key Counselling Points	Miscellaneous Issues
Ritonavir Norvir	Individualize dosage Usually, 600 mg BID; to decrease the incidence of adverse effects, may be started at 300 mg BID and titrated by 100 mg BID up to 600 mg BID	<u>Contraindications</u>: Many serious drug interactions are possible — SEE Prescribing Information (PI) <u>Considerations</u>: Patient should be monitored for signs of allergic reactions; use with caution in patients with liver disorders Most common AEs include asthenia, nausea/vomiting, anorexia, abdominal pain, taste perversion, paresthesias <u>Pregnancy category</u>: B	SEE indinavir sulfate except take with meals if possible; solution may be mixed with chocolate milk, Ensure or Advera, and consumed within 1 hr	
Saquinavir Mesylate Invirase	Individualize dosage Usually, 600 mg TID in combination with nucleoside inhibitors	<u>Considerations</u>: Safety in children under 16 has not been studied; use with caution in patients with liver disorders Most common AEs include diarrhea, abdominal discomfort, nausea, headache, rash <u>Pregnancy category</u>: B	SEE indinavir sulfate except must be taken within 2 hrs of a full meal	

Generic Name and Selected Trade Names	Normal Adult Dosage	Major Adverse Effects/Cautions	Key Counseling Points	Miscellaneous Issues
Stavudine Zerit	Individualize dosage Patients ≤ 60 kg: 30 mg BID Patients > 60 kg: 40 mg BID Dosage adjustments required in patients with renal impairment — SEE Prescribing Information (PI)	Considerations: Monitor patients for development of peripheral neuropathy; dosage reduced in patients who develop peripheral neuropathy Most common AEs include peripheral neuropathy, elevation of liver enzymes, headache, chills/fever, diarrhea, rash, nausea/vomiting, abdominal pain, myalgia, insomnia Pregnancy category: C	SEE lamivudine and inform the prescriber if you have a history of alcohol abuse, liver disease or peripheral neuropathy	

Generic Name and Selected Trade Names	Normal Adult Dosage	Major Adverse Effects/Cautions	Key Counseling Points	Miscellaneous Issues
Zalcitabine Hivid	Individualize dosage Monotherapy: 0.75 mg Q8H Combination therapy: 0.75 mg with 200 mg zidovudine Q8H Dosage adjustments required in patients with renal impairment — SEE Prescribing Information (PI)	Considerations: Peripheral neuropathy can be severe and irreversible damage can occur if drug is not discontinued; patients at risk for pancreatitis should be carefully monitored; extreme caution should be used in patients with liver disorders Most common AEs include peripheral neuropathy (numbness and burning of distal extremities), pancreatitis, liver damage, oral/esophageal ulcers, cardiomyopathy, allergic reaction Pregnancy category: C	SEE lamivudine; also, inform the prescriber if you have increased blood triglycerides or pancreatitis	

Generic Name and Selected Trade Names	Normal Adult Dosage	Major Adverse Effects/Cautions	Key Counseling Points	Miscellaneous Issues
Zidovudine Retrovir	Individualize dosage Usually, 600 mg/day in divided doses	<u>Considerations</u>: Use with caution in patients with already depressed bone marrow function, and in patients with liver disorders Most common AEs include granulocytopenia, anemia, myopathy, lactic acidosis, liver toxicity, nausea/vomiting <u>Pregnancy category</u>: C	Inform the prescriber if you have anemia or other blood problems, liver disease or low amounts of folic acid or vitamin B_{12} in the blood; notify the physician or pharmacist before taking other medications; may cause blood problems that result in certain infections and slow healing; use caution with dental hygiene; check the prescriber if you develop fever, chills, or sore throat or pale skin or unusual tiredness; it is important that the physician checks your progress at regular visits;	Also used to help prevent pregnant women from passing HIV to their babies — SEE Prescribing Information (PI); specially marked measuring spoon must be used to measure the syrup accurately

Generic Name and Selected Trade Names	Normal Adult Dosage	Major Adverse Effects/Cautions	Key Counseling Points	Miscellaneous Issues
Zidovudine (continued) Retrovir			take this medication exactly as directed, it is important to try not to miss any doses; if you miss a dose take it as soon as possible, but if it is almost time for the next dose skip the missed dose — do not double doses For oral syrup, use marked measuring spoon of device to measure each dose	

*As a general rule, a medication should not be administered to a patient with a known hypersensitivity to it or a similar agent.

[1]Administration of antimicrobial agents can result in overgrowth of some microorganisms and fungi.

[2]Patients should be counseled regarding methods to decrease transmission of the HIV virus and the importance of proper compliance with their entire therapeutic regimen despite the potential for many adverse effects.

Table 12: Antimalarial Agents*[1,2]

Generic Name and Selected Trade Names	Normal Adult Dosage	Major Adverse Effects/Cautions	Key Counselling Points	Miscellaneous Issues
Chloroquine Phosphate Aralen	Individualize dosage. For malaria suppression: 500 mg once per week, on the exact same day. For treatment of an acute attack: 1 G followed by 500 mg after 6–8 hrs and 500 mg daily for the next two days. For extra-intestinal amebiasis: 1 G daily for 2 days followed by 500 mg daily for 2–3 weeks, usually in combination with an intestinal amebicide	<u>Contraindications</u>: Patients with retinal or visual field changes, however, in acute attacks, the risk and benefits of treatment must be weighed. <u>Considerations</u>: Vision should be monitored in chronic therapy; if muscle weakness occurs agent should be discontinued; may precipitate attacks of psoriasis in susceptible patients; may exacerbate porphyria; if a drug-induced blood disorder is suspected the agent should be discontinued; use with caution in patients with liver disease, alcoholics or patients on concomitant agents that produce liver toxicity; use with caution in patients with glucose-6-phosphate dehydrogenase deficiency	Tell the prescriber if you have any serious medical conditions; it is important that the physician checks you at regular intervals if you are taking this agent for a long period of time; if you develop muscle weakness, visual changes, fatigue, lightheadedness, changes in mood, ringing or buzzing in the ears or any change in hearing, sore throat, fever, unusual bleeding, or easy bruising, contact the prescriber; it is important to take this medication for the full course, it works best if you take it on a regular schedule at the same time every day/week;	500 mg chloroquine phosphate is equivalent to 300 mg chloroquine base; low doses can be toxic to children, so keep out of their reach

301

Generic Name and Selected Trade Names	Normal Adult Dosage	Major Adverse Effects/Cautions	Key Counseling Points
Chloroquine Phosphate (continued) Aralen		Most common AEs include irreversible retinal damage, visual disturbances, hearing impairment, skin eruptions, pigment changes, headache, psychic stimulation Pregnancy category: Not specified	if you are taking this medication to prevent malaria you may begin taking it several weeks before travel; take with meals or milk to lessen the chance of stomach upset; if you miss a dose and you are taking one dose per week take the missed one as soon as possible then go back to regular schedule, if you are taking one dose per day take the missed one as soon as possible, but if you remember the next day, skip the missed dose and go back to regular schedule — do not double doses, if you are taking more than one dose per day take the missed one right away if you remember within one hour, but if you remember later, skip the missed one and go back to regular schedule — do not double doses

Generic Name and Selected Trade Names	Normal Adult Dosage	Major Adverse Effects/Cautions	Key Counseling Points	Miscellaneous Issues
Hydroxy-chloroquine Sulfate Plaquenil	Individualize dosage For suppression of malaria: 400 mg once per week on the same day For treatment of an acute attack: 800 mg followed by 400 mg in 6–8 hrs and then 400 mg for 2 days For systemic lupus erythematosus: Initially, 400 mg QD or BID; may be continued for several months, usually prolonged maintenance dose is 200 to 400 mg QD	Contraindications: SEE chloroquine; also, long term therapy in children Considerations: May precipitate an attack of psoriasis in susceptible patients and exacerbate porphyria; use with caution in patients with glucose-6-phosphate dehydrogenase deficiency, patients with liver disease, alcoholics or patients on concomitant agents that produce liver toxicity Most common AEs include headache, dizziness, diarrhea, anorexia, nausea/vomiting, cramps; CNS, muscle, ocular, dermatologic, and hematologic reactions have occurred in patients on long-term therapy Pregnancy category: Not specified	SEE chloroquine; also, for arthritis or lupus, may take several weeks before you begin to feel the agent work and it may take 6 months before you feel the full benefit	For patients unable to swallow whole tablets, may be crushed and place in a capsule, then contents may be mixed with jam, jelly or a gelatin desert; keep out of the reach of children

Generic Name and Selected Trade Names	Normal Adult Dosage	Major Adverse Effects/Cautions	Key Counselling Points	Miscellaneous Issues
Hydroxy-chloroquine Sulfate (continued) Plaquenil	For rheumatoid arthritis: Initially, 400 to 600 mg QD; when a good response is obtained (4–12 weeks) reduce dose by 50% and continue at 200 to 400 mg QD			

Generic Name and Selected Trade Names	Normal Adult Dosage	Major Adverse Effects/Cautions	Key Counseling Points	Miscellaneous Issues
Mefloquine HCl Lariam	For treatment of mild to moderate malaria due to P. vivax or susceptible strains of P. falciparum: 1250 mg as a single dose For malaria prophylaxis: 250 mg once per week, on the same day each week	Considerations: Life-threatening P. falciparum infections should be treated parenterally initially and then continued with oral therapy; caution should be used when driving or operating machinery; discontinue if signs of depression, anxiety, restlessness or confusion are noticed; use with caution in patients with psychiatric conditions; for long-term therapy liver and visual function should be assessed periodically; can affect cardiac rhythm therefore use with caution in patients with cardiac disease Most common AEs include nausea/vomiting, dizziness, syncope, myalgia, fever, headache, chills, diarrhea, rash, fatigue, extrasystoles Pregnancy category: C	SEE chloroquine; also, check with the physician or pharmacist before taking other medications (especially quinidine)	Many drug interactions are possible — SEE Prescribing Information (PI)

Generic Name and Selected Trade Names	Normal Adult Dosage	Major Adverse Effects/Cautions	Key Counselling Points	Miscellaneous Issues
Pyrimethamine Daraprim	<u>For malaria chemoprophylaxis</u>: Usually, 25 mg once per week <u>For treatment of acute attacks</u>: Usually, 25 mg daily for 2 days in combination with other agents in nonimmune persons; if used as monotherapy in semi-immune patients, administer 50 mg for 2 days	<u>Contraindications</u>: Patients with documented megaloblastic anemia due to folate deficiency <u>Considerations</u>: High doses are required to treat toxoplasmosis; patient should be monitored for signs of folate deficiency, if they occur the dose should be lowered or the agent discontinued and folic acid should be administered; small initial doses should be tested in patients with convulsive disorders; use with caution in patients with impaired renal or hepatic dysfunction or in patients with possible folate deficiency	Tell the prescriber if you have anemia or other blood problems, liver disease or a seizure disorder; check with the physician or pharmacist before taking other medications; if you develop a skin rash, stop taking the medication and contact your physician immediately; if you develop sore throat, pallor, purpura, glossitis, unusual bleeding or easy bruising consult your physician as these could be signs of more serious adverse effects;	Keep out of the reach of children

Generic Name and Selected Trade Names	Normal Adult Dosage	Major Adverse Effects/Cautions	Key Counseling Points	Miscellaneous Issues
Pyrimethamine (continued) Daraprim	For toxoplasmosis: Usually, 50 to 75 mg daily (with a sulfapyridine) continued for 1–3 weeks; then decrease to ½ the original dose and continue for 1 month	Most common AEs include hypersensitivity reactions, anorexia, vomiting, blood dyscrasias, hematuria and cardiac rhythm disturbances can occur with higher doses such as those used in the treatment of toxoplasmosis Pregnancy category: C	it is important to take this medication for the full course, it works best if you take it on a regular schedule at the same time every day or week depending on schedule; if you are taking this medication to prevent malaria you may begin taking it several weeks before travel; take with meals or milk to lessen the chance of stomach upset; if you miss a dose take it as soon as possible then go back to your regular schedule, if it is almost time for the next dose skip the dose — do not double doses	

Generic Name and Selected Trade Names	Normal Adult Dosage	Major Adverse Effects/Cautions	Key Counseling Points	Miscellaneous Issues
Quinine Sulfate	Individualize dosage For malaria, 260 to 650 mg TID for 6–12 days Dosage adjustment required in children — SEE Prescribing Information (PI)	Contraindications: Glucose-6-phosphate dehydrogenase deficiency, optic neuritis, tinnitus, history of blackwater fever and thrombocytopenia purpura (associated with previous quinine sulfate therapy), pregnancy Considerations: May produce cinchonism; tinnitus and impaired hearing more likely in sensitive persons; use with caution in patients with cardiac arrhythmias (similar cautions as quinidine — SEE quinidine sulfate)	Tell the prescriber if you have or had any type of a blood disease, are allergic to quinidine or beverages that contain quinine, have a hearing problem, or are or plan to become pregnant while taking this agent; while taking this agent, contact the prescriber if you develop anxiety, back/leg/stomach pains, cold sweats, pale stools, abdominal pain, hives or itching, sore throat and fever, unusual bleeding, easy bruising; take this medicine only as directed, do not take more or less, and take it for the entire course of therapy even if you feel better;	

Generic Name and Selected Trade Names	Normal Adult Dosage	Major Adverse Effects/Cautions	Key Counseling Points	Miscellaneous Issues
Quinine Sulfate (continued)		Most common AEs include visual disturbances, vertigo, restlessness, allergic reactions, anginal symptoms, and GI effects such as nausea, diarrhea and stomach cramps Pregnancy category: X	may cause blurred vision, so know how you react to it before driving or using machinery; you may take this medication with meals to lessen GI upset; if you miss a dose take it as soon as possible, but if it is almost time for the missed dose skip the missed one and return to regular schedule — do not double doses	

*As a general rule, a medication should not be administered to a patient with a known hypersensitivity to it or a similar agent.
[1]Agents are frequently given to patients traveling to prevent malaria, generally therapy begins 2 weeks before travel.
[2]Administration of antimicrobial agents can result in overgrowth of some microorganisms.

Table 13: Miscellaneous Antiinfectives*,1

Generic Name and Selected Trade Names	Normal Adult Dosage	Major Adverse Effects/Cautions	Key Counseling Points	Miscellaneous Issues
Atovaquone Mepron	For *Pneumocystis carinii* pneumonia usually, 750 mg BID with meals for 21 days, but regimens vary with the type of infection — SEE Prescribing Information (PI)	<u>Considerations</u>: Adequate plasma levels may not be achieved in patients with GI disorders; concomitant respiratory infections (bacterial, viral, etc) will require therapy with additional agents <u>Most common AEs</u> include rash, nausea/vomiting, diarrhea, headache, fever, insomnia, asthenia, pruritus, monilia, abdominal pain, constipation, dizziness <u>Pregnancy category</u>: C	Tell the prescriber if you have stomach or intestinal problems; notify the physician or pharmacist before taking other medications; check with the prescriber immediately if you develop fever or skin rash; it is important to take this medication for the full time even if you are feeling better; take with a balanced meal; if you miss a dose take it as soon as possible, but if it is almost time for the next dose skip the missed one — do not double doses For suspension, use marked measuring spoon or device to measure each dose	

Generic Name and Selected Trade Names	Normal Adult Dosage	Major Adverse Effects/Cautions	Key Counseling Points	Miscellaneous Issues
Clindamycin HCl Cleocin HCl Cleocin Cleocin T	Individualize dosage <u>Capsules or oral solution</u>: 150 to 300 mg Q6H; for more severe infections 300 to 450 mg Q6H <u>Vaginal cream</u>: One applicator full intravaginally HS for 7 days <u>Topical solution or gel</u>: Apply a thin film to affected area BID Dosage adjustments may be required for patients with renal or liver impairment — SEE Prescribing Information (PI)	<u>Considerations</u>: Associated with severe colitis, which may be fatal, reserved for serious infections for which less toxic agents are inappropriate; discontinue if significant diarrhea (elderly patients may be more sensitive) occurs; should not be used in the treatment of meningitis (does not penetrate meninges); use with caution in patients with a history of bowel disease; for patients with liver disease, enzyme levels should be monitored; both the vaginal and topical preparations can irritate the eye, so wash hands after handling	Tell the prescriber if you have kidney or liver disease or stomach or intestinal problems; notify the physician or pharmacist before taking other medication; may produce diarrhea, check with the prescriber before taking any antidiarrheal medication; check with the prescriber immediately if you develop severe abdominal pain/cramps, diarrhea, sore throat, fever or skin rash; it is important to take this medication for the full time even if you are feeling better; take the capsules with full glass of water or with meals;	

Generic Name and Selected Trade Names	Normal Adult Dosage	Major Adverse Effects/Cautions	Key Counseling Points
Clindamycin HCl (continued) Cleocin HCl Cleocin Cleocin T		Most common AEs include abdominal pain, esophagitis, nausea/vomiting, diarrhea, rash, urticaria, cervicitis/ vaginitis/irritation (major AE with vaginal cream) Pregnancy category: B	It is best to take this medication at evenly spaced intervals; if you miss a dose take it as soon as possible, but if it is almost time for the next dose skip the missed dose — do not double doses For oral liquid, use marked measuring spoon or device to measure each dose For vaginal cream ensure patient understands proper use of vaginal applicator, best to be used at bedtime, discard each applicator after use For Pledget, remove from foil prior to use and discard each pledget after each use; do not engage in vaginal intercourse during the duration of treatment For topical products, ensure patient knows proper administration technique; if your skin becomes unusually dry, check with the prescriber

Generic Name and Selected Trade Names	Normal Adult Dosage	Major Adverse Effects/Cautions	Key Counseling Points	Miscellaneous Issues
Dapsone	Individualize dosage For dermatitis herpetiformis: Administer 50 to 300 mg QD adjusted according to response For leprosy: Administer 100 mg QD in combination with other agents Regimens vary with the type of infection — SEE Prescribing Information (PI)	Considerations: Severe blood dyscrasias have occurred, therefore complete blood counts should be performed (patients with concomitant disorders or drug therapy that also suppress the bone marrow are at greater risk); severe skin reactions have occurred; blood levels are influenced by acetylation rates Most common AEs include nausea/vomiting, abdominal pain, pancreatitis, vertigo, vision disturbances, peripheral neuropathy, photosensitivity, hemolysis Pregnancy category: C	Tell the prescriber if you have anemia, glucose-6-phosphate dehydrogenase deficiency or methemoglobin reductase deficiency, or liver disease; notify the physician or pharmacist before taking other medication; if your symptoms do not improve within 2–3 months (a few days for dermatitis herpetiform is) or if they become worse notify the prescriber; if you develop back, leg or stomach pains, bluish fingernails, lips or skin, difficult breathing, fever, loss of appetite, pale skin, rash or unusual tiredness or weakness contact the prescriber immediately;	

Generic Name and Selected Trade Names	Normal Adult Dosage	Major Adverse Effects/Cautions	Key Counseling Points	Miscellaneous Issues
Dapsone (continued)			it is important to take this medication for the full time even if you are feeling better; it is best to take this medication at evenly spaced intervals, you may skip a missed dose if it does not make your symptoms come back or get worse, if your symptoms get worse take the missed dose as soon as possible, then return to regular schedule	

Generic Name and Selected Trade Names	Normal Adult Dosage	Major Adverse Effects/Cautions	Key Counseling Points	Miscellaneous Issues
Metronidazole Flagyl	Individualize dosage For trichomoniasis: Administer 375 mg BID for 7 days For amebiasis: Administer 750 mg TID for 5–10 days For anaerobic bacterial infections: Usually, intravenous 7.5 mg/kg Q6H Regimens vary with the type of infection — SEE Prescribing Information (PI) Dosage adjustments required in patients with liver impairment — SEE PI	Contraindications: In patients with trichomoniasis during the first trimester of pregnancy Considerations: Discontinue if abnormal neurological signs occur (seizures and peripheral neuropathy have occurred); use with caution in patients with CNS disorders; candidiasis may present during therapy and will require treatment Most common AEs include nausea/vomiting, headache, diarrhea, anorexia, dizziness, vertigo, ataxia, confusion Pregnancy category: B	Tell the prescriber if you have a blood, brain, heart, or liver disease; notify the physician or pharmacist before taking other medication; if your symptoms do not improve within a few days or if they become worse notify the prescriber; consumption of alcohol may produce side effects, some of which can be severe, so do not drink alcohol or take other alcohol-containing substances while on this medication and for at least 1 day after stopping; may cause dry mouth, metallic taste or a change in taste, may use sugarless candy, gum, ice or saliva substitute if necessary;	

Generic Name and Selected Trade Names	Normal Adult Dosage	Major Adverse Effects/Cautions	Key Counseling Points	Miscellaneous Issues
Metronidazole (continued) Flagyl			may cause some people to become dizzy or lightheaded, make sure you know how you react before driving or using machinery; if you develop numbness, tingling, pain, or weakness in hands or feet contact the prescriber; it is important to take this medication as directed for the entire course even if you begin to feel better; if the medication upsets your stomach it may be taken with meals or a snack; it is best to take at evenly spaced intervals and not miss a dose; if you miss a dose take it as soon as possible, but if it is almost time for the next dose skip the missed one — do not double doses	

Generic Name and Selected Trade Names	Normal Adult Dosage	Major Adverse Effects/Cautions	Key Counselling Points	Miscellaneous Issues
Vancomycin HCl Vancocin HCl	Usually, 500 mg to 2 G in 3–4 divided doses for 7–10 days, but regimens vary with the type of infection — SEE Prescribing Information (PI) Parenteral dosage form available — SEE PI	Considerations: Although the agent is meant for topical treatment of the gut, some patients may experience absorption and therefore systemic adverse effects; not effective via the oral route for uses other than pseudomembranous colitis produced by C. difficile or staphylococcal enterocolitis Most common AEs include nausea, fever, chills, rashes and rarely renal toxicity, ototoxicity Pregnancy category: C	Tell the prescriber if you have kidney disease or any loss of hearing (for parenteral), or any bowel dysfunction (for oral); notify the physician or pharmacist before taking other medication; if your symptoms do not improve within a few days or if they become worse notify the prescriber; if you develop a skin rash check with the physician immediately (others for parenteral, SEE Prescribing Information); it is important to take this medication for the full course even if you are feeling better;	Mix contents of bottle with distilled or deionized water

Generic Name and Selected Trade Names	Normal Adult Dosage	Major Adverse Effects/Cautions	Key Counseling Points	Miscellaneous Issues
Vancomycin HCl (continued) Vancocin HCl			do not take any medications for diarrhea without consulting with the prescriber; if you miss a dose take it as soon as possible, if it is almost time for the next dose, skip the missed one and go back to regular schedule — do not double doses For liquid, use marked measuring spoon or device to measure each dose; may dilute each dose with 1 ounce of fluid; for injection, if patient or caregiver is administering ensure they know the proper technique	

*As a general rule, a medication should not be administered to a patient with a known hypersensitivity to it or a similar agent.
†Administration of antimicrobial agents can result in overgrowth of some microorganisms and fungi.

Antineoplastic Agents

Table: Selected Antineoplastic Agents*[1,2,3]

Generic Name and Selected Trade Names	Normal Adult Dosage	Major Adverse Effects/Cautions	Key Counselling Points	Miscellaneous Issues
Altretamine Hexalen	For palliative treatment in recurrent or persistent ovarian cancer, 260 mg/m²/day for 14 or 21 days in a 28 day cycle, daily doses should be divided into 4 equal doses after meals and at bedtime	Contraindications: Preexisting severe bone marrow depression or severe neurologic toxicity Considerations: Blood counts and neurologic function should be monitored, co-administration with an MAO-inhibitor may result in hypotension Most common AEs include nausea/vomiting, peripheral neuropathy, mood disorders, disorders of consciousness, ataxia, dizziness, mild to moderate myelosuppression Pregnancy category: D	Tell the prescriber if you have chickenpox or shingles (or recent exposure), or any infection, brain, kidney or liver problems, check with the physician or pharmacist before taking any other medication; discuss with your physician if you plan to become pregnant or are pregnant; ensure patient has discussed all the risks and adverse effects associated with this agent; discuss with the physician before having any immunizations;	

Generic Name and Selected Trade Names	Normal Adult Dosage	Major Adverse Effects/Cautions	Key Counseling Points	Miscellaneous Issues
Altretamine (continued) Hexalen			ensure patient knows to avoid infections, bruising, and to report any unusual or severe adverse effects to the physician; it is important that the physician checks your progress regularly, including conducting some blood tests; it is important to take this medication for the full time of treatment even if you experience nausea; if you miss a dose take it as soon as possible, but if it is almost time for the next dose skip the missed dose — do not double doses	

Generic Name and Selected Trade Names	Normal Adult Dosage	Major Adverse Effects/Cautions	Key Counselling Points	Miscellaneous Issues
Anastrozole Arimidex	For advanced breast cancer in post-menopausal women with disease progression following anti-estrogen therapy, usually administer 1 mg QD	<u>Considerations</u>: May cause fetal damage, pregnancy should be ruled out prior to use <u>Most common AEs include</u> diarrhea, asthenia, nausea/vomiting, headache, hot flushes, pain, back pain, cough <u>Pregnancy category</u>: D	Take only as directed — do not take more or less of it or use it for longer than prescribed; try to take the medication even if you become somewhat nauseated; if you miss a dose, skip it and return to regular dose schedule and check with the prescriber — do not double doses	

Generic Name and Selected Trade Names	Normal Adult Dosage	Major Adverse Effects/Cautions	Key Counseling Points	Miscellaneous Issues
Busulfan Myleran	For remission induction, usually administer 4 to 8 mg/day (total daily dose) or by weight 60 mcg/kg or 1.8 mg/m² per day (total daily dose) Frequency and duration of therapy depend upon patient factors including assessment of bone marrow function — SEE Prescribing Information (PI)	<u>Considerations</u>: Bone marrow depression resulting in severe pancytopenia is the most frequent and serious adverse effect; use with extreme caution in patients with comprised bone marrow reserve (eg, prior irradiation, chemotherapy); rarely patients develop bronchopulmonary dysplasia with pulmonary fibrosis which is frequently fatal; patients experiencing any pulmonary symptom should be evaluated as soon as possible; cellular dysplasia in many organs can occur; may produce tumors and/or secondary malignancies; for a more complete list — SEE Prescribing Information (PI)	SEE altretamine and tell the prescriber if you have gout; the physician may want you to drink extra fluids while taking this medication; if you miss a dose skip the missed one — do not double doses	Most bone marrow depression occurs as the result of failure to discontinue dosage in the face of an undetected decrease in leukocyte or platelet counts, leukocyte counts may increase early in therapy, but begin to decrease and continue to decrease following discontinuation of therapy

Generic Name and Selected Trade Names	Normal Adult Dosage	Major Adverse Effects/Cautions	Key Counseling Points	Miscellaneous Issues
Busulfan (continued) Myleran		Most common AEs include leukopenia, thrombocytopenia, anemia, interstitial pulmonary fibrosis, hyperpigmentation, urticaria, alopecia, dry skin, adrenal insufficiency Pregnancy category: D		

Generic Name and Selected Trade Names	Normal Adult Dosage	Major Adverse Effects/Cautions	Key Counselling Points	Miscellaneous Issues
Carboplatin Paraplatin	<u>As monotherapy for ovarian carcinoma</u>: 360 mg/m^2 IV on day 1 every 4 weeks (pending blood counts) <u>Combination therapy with cyclophosphamide for advanced ovarian carcinoma</u>: 300 mg/m^2 IV on day 1 every 4 weeks for 6 cycles Dosage adjustments are required in patients at risk for severe bone marrow depression and in patients with renal dysfunction — SEE Prescribing Information (PI)	<u>Contraindications</u>: Allergy to cisplatin, other platinum-containing compounds or mannitol, not for use in patients with severe bone marrow depression or bleeding <u>Considerations</u>: Dose-dependent bone marrow depression (leukopenia, neutropenia, thrombocytopenia) is the dose-limiting toxicity, incidence is greater in patients who previously received cisplatin or have impaired renal function (lower doses); anemia also occurs; renal toxicity has occurred when combined with aminoglycosides; for a more complete list — SEE Prescribing Information (PI)	SEE altretamine and tell the prescriber if you have any hearing problems; if you are taking other medications in addition, make sure you keep on the prescribed schedule Information on missed dose usually does not apply since the agent is given IV	Blood counts must be monitored during therapy, subsequent doses are generally not advised until blood counts recover; cannot be administered via aluminum containing needles or administration sets, agent will precipitate; administered via infusion over at least 15 minutes, no pre or post hydration necessary

Generic Name and Selected Trade Names	Normal Adult Dosage	Major Adverse Effects/Cautions	Key Counseling Points	Miscellaneous Issues
Carboplatin (continued) Paraplatin		Most common AEs include bone marrow suppression, nausea/vomiting, elevation of liver enzymes, pain, asthenia, alopecia, infections Pregnancy category: D		

Generic Name and Selected Trade Names	Normal Adult Dosage	Major Adverse Effects/Cautions	Key Counselling Points	Miscellaneous Issues
Carmustine BiCNU	As a single agent in previously untreated patient, 150 to 200 mg/m^2 IV every 6 weeks, may be given as a single dose or divided into 2 doses over 2 days Dosage adjustments are required in patients at risk for severe bone marrow depression and when used in combination, subsequent doses are adjusted based upon hematologic response — SEE Prescribing Information (PI)	Considerations: Major toxicity is bone marrow suppression, blood counts should be monitored; pulmonary toxicity is dose-related; secondary malignancies have occurred; monitor liver and renal function Most common AEs include pulmonary fibrosis/ infiltration, delayed myelosuppression, nausea/ vomiting, elevation of liver enzymes, renal abnormalities Pregnancy category: D	SEE altretamine and tell the prescriber if you have lung disease; if you are taking other medications in addition, make sure you keep on the prescribed schedule; if you notice redness, pain or swelling at the injection site, notify the nurse or physician immediately Information on missed dose usually does not apply since the agent is given IV	

Generic Name and Selected Trade Names	Normal Adult Dosage	Major Adverse Effects/Cautions	Key Counseling Points	Miscellaneous Issues
Chlorambucil Leukeran	Usually, 0.1 to 0.2 mg/kg (usually 4–10 mg) QD for 3–6 weeks, dosage must be carefully adjusted according to patient response, must be decreased if there is an abrupt fall in white blood cell count; other regimens have been utilized — SEE Prescribing Information (PI)	Contraindication: Patients whose disease has demonstrated prior resistance to this agent Considerations: Convulsions, infertility, leukemia and secondary malignancies and severe skin reactions (rare) have occurred; lymphopenia and neutropenia generally occur during therapy; should not be given within 4 weeks of radiation or chemotherapy Most common AEs include bone marrow suppression, nausea/vomiting, oral ulceration, diarrhea, tremors, confusion, agitation, ataxia, skin reactions Pregnancy category: D	SEE altretamine and tell the prescriber if you have gout; while taking this medication the physician may want you to drink extra fluid; if you are taking other medications in addition, make sure you keep on the prescribed schedule; for once a day dosing, if you miss a dose take it as soon as possible, but you remember the next day dose skip the missed one — do not double doses; for more than once a day dosing, if you miss a dose take it as soon as possible, but if it is almost time for the next dose skip the missed one — do not double	

Generic Name and Selected Trade Names	Normal Adult Dosage	Major Adverse Effects/Cautions	Key Counseling Points	Miscellaneous Issues
Cisplatin Platinol Platinol-AQ	For metastatic testicular tumors: 20 mg/m² IV daily for 5 days per cycle in combination with other agents For metastatic ovarian tumors: As a single agent, 100 mg/m² IV per cycle every 4 weeks or 75 to 100 mg/m² IV on day 1 per cycle every 4 weeks in combination with cyclophosphamide For advanced bladder cancer: SEE Prescribing Information (PI)	Contraindications: Preexisting renal impairment, myelosuppression or hearing impairment; history of allergy to platinum-containing compounds Considerations: Cumulative nephrotoxicity can be severe so appropriate renal monitoring should be done; other dose-related toxicities include myelosuppression, ototoxicity, nausea/vomiting; severe neuropathies have occurred in patients receiving high doses; routine monitoring includes weekly blood counts, periodic liver function tests and neurologic examinations	SEE altretamine and tell the prescriber if you have any hearing problems or gout; while on this medication the physician may want you to drink extra water; if you are taking other medications in addition, make sure you keep on the prescribed schedule Information on missed dose usually does not apply since the agent is given IV	Cannot be administered via aluminum containing needles or administration sets, medication will precipitate

Generic Name and Selected Trade Names	Normal Adult Dosage	Major Adverse Effects/Cautions	Key Counseling Points	Miscellaneous Issues
Cisplatin (continued) Platinol Platinol-AQ		Most common AEs include nephrotoxicity, ototoxicity, myelosuppression, nausea/vomiting, electrolyte abnormalities, ocular toxicities, allergic reactions Pregnancy category: D		

Generic Name and Selected Trade Names	Normal Adult Dosage	Major Adverse Effects/Cautions	Key Counseling Points	Miscellaneous Issues
Cyclophosphamide Cytoxan	For malignant diseases as a single agent, 40 to 50 mg/kg IV given in divided doses over a period of 2–5 days; oral dosing is usually 1 to 5 mg/kg/day; other regimens have been utilized as well; doses adjusted based upon activity and/or leukopenia; lower doses required in patients on combination therapy — SEE Prescribing Information (PI)	<u>Contraindication</u>: Severely depressed bone marrow function <u>Considerations</u>: Infertility and secondary malignancies have occurred; hemorrhagic cystitis may develop; immune suppression can lead to infections; use with caution in patients with bone marrow suppression, tumor cell infiltration of the bone marrow, previous radiation or cytotoxic therapy, impaired renal or hepatic function Most common AEs include nausea/vomiting, alopecia, leukopenia, cystitis, urinary bladder fibrosis <u>Pregnancy category</u>: D	SEE altretamine and tell the prescriber if you have gout; while on this medication you need to drink extra fluids and empty your bladder frequently, including at least once during the night; if you are taking other medications in addition, it is best to take this medication first thing in the morning; if you miss a dose skip the missed dose — do not double doses	

Generic Name and Selected Trade Names	Normal Adult Dosage	Major Adverse Effects/Cautions	Key Counseling Points	Miscellaneous Issues
Docetaxel Taxotere	For advanced breast cancer, usually 60 to 100 mg/m^2 IV over 1 hr every 3 weeks; dosage adjustments are required based upon patient tolerance and CBC — SEE Prescribing Information (PI)	Contraindications: Hypersensitivity to agents formulated with polysorbate 80; patients with baseline neutropenia of <1,500 WBCs/mm^3 Considerations: Fatalities primarily related to sepsis have occurred and are more frequent in patients with abnormal liver function; avoid in patients with elevated bilirubin or hepatic dysfunction; hypersensitivity reactions and severe fluid retention can occur; bone marrow depression (primarily neutropenia) is the dose-limiting adverse effect; frequent monitoring of blood counts is required; severe neurosensory disturbances can occur and require dose adjustments	SEE altretamine except information on missed dose usually does not apply since the agent is given IV	All patients should be premedicated with corticosteroids to reduce the risk of severe fluid retention

Generic Name and Selected Trade Names	Normal Adult Dosage	Major Adverse Effects/Cautions	Key Counselling Points	Miscellaneous Issues
Docetaxel (continued) Taxotere		Most common AEs include bone marrow suppression, infections, fluid retention, neurosensory disturbances, alopecia, stomatitis, myalgia Pregnancy category: D		

Generic Name and Selected Trade Names	Normal Adult Dosage	Major Adverse Effects/Cautions	Key Counseling Points	Miscellaneous Issues
Doxorubicin HCl Adriamycin RDF Adriamycin PFS	Usually, 60 to 75 mg/m² as a single IV injection every 21 days; indications include a variety of neoplastic diseases — SEE Prescribing Information (PI) Lower dosages required in patients on combination therapy — SEE PI	<u>Contraindications:</u> Patients with marked myelosuppression induced by previous antitumor treatments, patients who have received previous treatment with complete cumulative doses of doxorubicin, daunorubicin, idarubicin, and/or other anthracyclines and anthracenes <u>Considerations:</u> Irreversible dose-related myocardial toxicity is the most severe toxicity, patients at greater risk include prior mediastinal irradiation, concurrent cyclophosphamide therapy, advanced age, and pre-existing heart disease, cardiac function should be monitored during and after therapy;	SEE altretamine and tell the prescriber if you have heart disease or gout; while on this medication you may need to drink extra fluids; will change urine color to red 1–2 days after administration Information on missed dose usually does not apply since the agent is given IV	Extravasation of IV dose can result in severe local tissue reactions; do not administer SC or IM

Generic Name and Selected Trade Names	Normal Adult Dosage	Major Adverse Effects/Cautions	Key Counselling Points	Miscellaneous Issues
Doxorubicin HCl (continued) Adriamycin RDF Adriamycin PFS		bone marrow suppression (primarily leukocytosis) is common, CBC should be monitored; toxicity may be greater in patients with impaired liver function; may enhance toxicity of other cancer chemotherapeutic agents <u>Most common AEs</u> include myelosuppression, cardiotoxicity, alopecia, nausea/vomiting, hypersensitivity reactions <u>Pregnancy category</u>: D		

Generic Name and Selected Trade Names	Normal Adult Dosage	Major Adverse Effects/Cautions	Key Counseling Points	Miscellaneous Issues
Etoposide VePesid	For refractory testicular tumors and small cell lung cancer, regimens vary based upon route of administration and indication — SEE Prescribing Information (PI) Dosage adjustments required in patients with renal dysfunction — SEE PI	Considerations: Dose-limiting myelosuppression is the most important toxicity, CBC must be monitored; severe hypersensitivity reactions have occurred Most common AEs include bone marrow suppression, nausea/vomiting, alopecia Pregnancy category: D	SEE altretamine, except if you miss a dose skip the missed one — do not double doses	

Generic Name and Selected Trade Names	Normal Adult Dosage	Major Adverse Effects/Cautions	Key Counseling Points	Miscellaneous Issues
Fluorouracil Efudex Fluoroplex	For palliative management of carcinoma of the colon, rectum, breast, stomach, and pancreas, usually 12 mg/kg IV QD for 4 successive days; if no toxicity is observed, 6 mg/kg is given on days 6, 8, 10 and 12; courses may be repeated depending upon patient response and tolerance; daily dose should not exceed 800 mg Lower doses may be required in patients at risk for toxicities — SEE Prescribing Information (PI)	Contraindications: Poor nutritional state, depressed bone marrow function, potentially serious infections Considerations: Use with caution in patients with a history of high-dose pelvic irradiation, previous use of alkylating agents, wide-spread involvement of bone marrow by metastatic tumors, and impaired renal or hepatic function; discontinue therapy if stomatitis or esophagopharyngitis, leukopenia, intractable vomiting, diarrhea, GI ulceration or bleeding, thrombocytopenia or hemorrhage occur; associated with hand-foot syndrome (tingling sensation of hands and feet progressing to pain)	SEE altretamine and for topical formulations, after washing the area with soap and water and drying, apply a thin layer of the medication to the skin, may cause redness, soreness, scaling and peeling of the affected skin in 1–2 weeks, skin may continue to be red for several months; avoid sunlight; if you miss a dose apply it as soon as you remember, but if more than a few hours have passed, skip the missed one and go back to regular schedule, if you miss more than one dose check with the prescriber	Recommended for use only under the supervision of a qualified physician with experience with cancer chemotherapy and the use of antimetabolites, initial course should be given in the hospital

Generic Name and Selected Trade Names	Normal Adult Dosage	Major Adverse Effects/Cautions	Key Counselling Points	Miscellaneous Issues
Fluorouracil (continued) Efudex Fluoroplex	Topical preparations available in cream and solution dosage forms — SEE PI	Most common AEs include stomatitis, esopagopharyngitis, diarrhea, anorexia, nausea/vomiting, leukopenia, alopecia, dermatitis Pregnancy category: D		

Generic Name and Selected Trade Names	Normal Adult Dosage	Major Adverse Effects/Cautions	Key Counseling Points	Miscellaneous Issues
Flutamide Eulexin	In combination with LHRH agonists for the Stage B2-C and Stage D2 prostatic cancer, 250 mg Q8H	<u>Considerations</u>: Gynecomastia may occur; may cause fetal harm; alterations in liver function have occurred, monitor liver function tests <u>Most common AEs</u> include loss of libido, diarrhea <u>Pregnancy category</u>: D	Ensure patient has discussed all the risks and adverse effects associated with this agent; report any unusual or severe adverse effects to their physician; it is important that the physician checks your progress regularly; it is important to take this medication for the full time of treatment even if you experience hot flashes, decreased sexual activity or difficulty urinating; usually, you will be taking other medications along with this agent, it is very important that they both be taken as directed; if you miss a dose take it as soon as possible, but if it is almost time for the next dose, skip the missed dose — do not double doses	

Generic Name and Selected Trade Names	Normal Adult Dosage	Major Adverse Effects/Cautions	Key Counselling Points	Miscellaneous Issues
Hydroxyurea Hydrea	For solid tumors, intermittent therapy: 80 mg/kg orally as a single dose every 3rd day For solid tumors or resistant chronic myelocytic leukemia, continuous therapy: 20 to 30 mg/kg orally QD SEE Prescribing Information (PI)	Contraindication: Marked bone marrow suppression Considerations: Bone marrow suppression may occur, usually leukopenia occurs first, which can be followed by thrombocytopenia and anemia; use with caution in patients with renal dysfunction and the elderly; appropriate monitoring of CBC, and liver and renal function should be conducted Most common AEs include bone marrow suppression, stomatitis, anorexia, nausea/vomiting, diarrhea, dermatologic reactions, drowsiness (high doses) Pregnancy category: Not specified	SEE altretamine and tell the prescriber if you have anemia; while receiving this agent the physician may want you to drink extra fluids; if you miss a dose, skip the missed one and return to regular schedule — do not double doses	

Generic Name and Selected Trade Names	Normal Adult Dosage	Major Adverse Effects/Cautions	Key Counseling Points	Miscellaneous Issues
Interferon alfa-2b Intron A	Individualize dosage Regimens vary based upon indication — SEE Prescribing Information (PI)	Considerations: Numerous — SEE Prescribing Information (PI) Most common AEs include flu-like symptoms (fever, headache, chills, myalgia, fatigue), others depend upon dosage and disease being treated; for a more complete list — SEE PI Pregnancy category: C	Tell your physician if you have any serious medical conditions; check with the physician/pharmacist before taking any other medication; ensure patient has discussed all the risks and adverse effects associated with this agent; ensure that the patient has read and understood the patient information sheet, including injection technique; while receiving this agent the physician may want you to drink extra fluids; may produce drowsiness so bedtime dosing may be better tolerated; do not change type of interferon without checking with the prescriber;	

Generic Name and Selected Trade Names	Normal Adult Dosage	Major Adverse Effects/Cautions	Key Counseling Points	Miscellaneous Issues
Interferon alfa-2b (continued) Intron A			may cause some people to become tired or dizzy, make sure you know how you react before driving a car or using machinery; may cause flu-like symptoms, if the prescriber asks you to take acetaminophen, take it as directed; if you experience any unusual or severe adverse effects, check with the physician; if you miss a dose, skip the dose and check with the prescriber — do not double doses	

Generic Name and Selected Trade Names	Normal Adult Dosage	Major Adverse Effects/Cautions	Key Counseling Points	Miscellaneous Issues
Interferon alfa-2a Roferon-A	Individualize dosage Regimens vary for the various indications — SEE Prescribing Information (PI)	Contraindications: Hypersensitivity to alfa interferon, mouse immunoglobulin, or benzyl alcohol Considerations: Numerous, SEE Prescribing Information (PI) Most common AEs include depressive illness, suicidal behavior, flu-like symptoms (fever, headache, chills, myalgia, fatigue), headache, others depend upon dosage and disease being treated; for a more complete list — SEE PI Pregnancy category: C	SEE interferon alfa-2b	

Generic Name and Selected Trade Names	Normal Adult Dosage	Major Adverse Effects/Cautions	Key Counseling Points	Miscellaneous Issues
Lomustine CeeNU	For brain tumors, as a single agent in previously untreated patient, 130 mg/m² as a single oral dose every 6 weeks Dosage adjustments are required in patients at risk for severe bone marrow depression and when used in combination (eg, in Hodgkin's disease); subsequent doses are adjusted based upon hematologic response — SEE Prescribing Information (PI)	SEE carmustine and Prescribing Information (PI)	SEE carmustine, except information regarding injection, this agent is oral	

Generic Name and Selected Trade Names	Normal Adult Dosage	Major Adverse Effects/Cautions	Key Counselling Points	Miscellaneous Issues
Melphalan Alkeran	<u>For multiple melanoma</u>: Usually start with 6 mg QD, dosage is adjusted weekly based upon blood counts; after 2–3 weeks of treatment the agents should be discontinued for up to 4 weeks while blood counts are monitored, when blood counts are rising a maintenance dose of 2 mg/day may be instituted; other dosage regimens have been utilized — SEE Prescribing Information (PI)	<u>Contraindication</u>: Patients whose disease has demonstrated prior resistance to this agent <u>Considerations</u>: Bone marrow suppression is the most common toxicity, appropriate monitoring of blood counts is required; hypersensitivity reactions, infertility, and secondary malignancies have occurred Most common AEs include bone marrow suppression, nausea/vomiting, diarrhea, oral ulceration, pulmonary fibrosis, skin reactions, alopecia <u>Pregnancy category</u>: D	SEE busulfan	

Generic Name and Selected Trade Names	Normal Adult Dosage	Major Adverse Effects/Cautions	Key Counseling Points	Miscellaneous Issues
Melphalan (continued) Alkeran	For epithelial ovarian cancer: One regimen is 0.2 mg/kg/day for 5 days; courses are repeated every 4–5 weeks depending upon hematologic tolerance			

Generic Name and Selected Trade Names	Normal Adult Dosage	Major Adverse Effects/Cautions	Key Counselling Points	Miscellaneous Issues
Mercapto-purine Purinethol	Individualize dosage <u>For induction therapy in acute lymphatic leukemia</u>: 2.5 mg/kg/day; may be increased to 5 mg/kg/day after 4 weeks if needed <u>For maintenance therapy</u>: Usually 1.5 to 2.5 mg/kg/ day, usually in combination with other agents	<u>Contraindications</u>: Patients whose disease has shown resistance to the agent, cross resistance with thioguanine is likely <u>Considerations</u>: Bone marrow suppression (anemia, leukopenia, thrombocytopenia) is the most likely toxicity, agent should be discontinued with any abrupt fall in blood counts, appropriate monitoring should be conducted; hepatic toxicity and immunosuppression may occur Most common AEs include myelosuppression, hyperuricemia, rash, hyperpigmentation, hepatotoxicity <u>Pregnancy category</u>: D	SEE hydroxyurea	Recommended for use only in patients with a diagnosis of acute lymphatic leukemia

Generic Name and Selected Trade Names	Normal Adult Dosage	Major Adverse Effects/Cautions	Key Counseling Points	Miscellaneous Issues
Methotrexate Sodium Immunex Rheumatrex	For neoplastic diseases: 15 to 30 mg/day for a 5 day course usually repeated 3–5 times as required with rest periods of 1 or more weeks For alternative regimens including parenteral administration and use of high dose therapy with leucovorin rescue — SEE Prescribing Information (PI) For psoriasis: 10 to 25 mg once a week given orally, IV, or IM or 2.5 mg Q12H for 3 doses once a week, generally not to exceed 30 mg/week	Contraindications: Pregnancy should be avoided for several months if either partner has received the agent, not to be used in nursing mothers Contraindications for psoriasis or rheumatoid arthritis patients: Pregnancy, alcoholism, chronic liver disease, evidence of immunodeficiency syndromes, blood dyscrasias Considerations: Can produce serious toxicities, if symptoms develop agent should be discontinued and leucovorin calcium therapy should be considered; patients should be carefully monitored; major toxicities include GI distress, anemia, leukopenia, thrombocytopenia, hepatotoxicity, infections, pulmonary toxicity — SEE Prescribing Information (PI)	For cancer SEE mercaptopurine and tell the prescriber if you have any mouth sores or a stomach ulcer; do not drink alcohol while using this medication; do not take medicine for inflammation or pain (eg, aspirin or ibuprofen) unless otherwise directed For noncancerous conditions, tell the prescriber if you have a history of alcohol abuse, chickenpox or shingles (or recent exposure), or any infection, kidney, liver, immune system, intestinal or stomach disease or mouth sores; check with the physician/pharmacist before taking any other medications; do not drink alcohol while taking this agent;	

Generic Name and Selected Trade Names	Normal Adult Dosage	Major Adverse Effects/Cautions	Key Counseling Points	Miscellaneous Issues
Methotrexate Sodium (continued) Immunex Rheumatrex	For rheumatoid arthritis: 7.5 mg once a week or 2.5 mg Q12H for 3 doses once a week; generally do not exceed 20 mg/week	Most common AEs include ulcerative stomatitis, leukopenia, nausea, abdominal distress, malaise, chills and fever, dizziness, for rheumatoid arthritis and psoriasis most common are elevated liver function tests and nausea/vomiting Pregnancy category: X	avoid excess sunlight; it is important that the physician checks your progress regularly; take this medication as directed, it may cause nausea, do not stop taking the agent without consulting with the prescriber; do not take agents for pain or inflammation (aspirin, ibuprofen, etc) while taking this agent; check with the prescriber before receiving any immunizations; if you experience any unusual or severe adverse effects contact the prescriber; try to avoid infections, bruising, injury; if you miss a dose, skip the dose and go back to your regular schedule — do not double doses	

Generic Name and Selected Trade Names	Normal Adult Dosage	Major Adverse Effects/Cautions	Key Counseling Points	Miscellaneous Issues
Mitotane Lysodren	For inoperable adrenal cortical carcinoma, 2 to 6 G/day in divided doses (TID or QID); doses are increased incrementally to 9 to 10 G/day, until a maximum tolerated dose is determined	<u>Considerations</u>: Temporarily discontinue following shock or trauma (patient may require corticosteroids); use with caution in patients with liver dysfunction; long-term treatment for over 2 years has led to neurological or behavioral changes, patients should be monitored; some patients may require corticosteroids due to adrenal suppression <u>Most common AEs</u> include anorexia, nausea/vomiting, diarrhea, lethargy, rash, somnolence, dizziness Pregnancy category: C	Tell the prescriber if you have an infection or liver disease; do not drink alcohol or take other agents that cause drowsiness; some people become dizzy or drowsy while receiving this agent; make sure you know how you react to this agent before driving; if you get an injury, develop an infection or any illness check with the prescriber; take this medication as directed; do not stop taking the agent without consulting with the prescriber; if you miss a dose take it as soon as you remember, if it is almost time for the next dose, skip the missed dose and check with the prescriber — do not double doses	Therapy should be initiated in a hospital setting

Generic Name and Selected Trade Names	Normal Adult Dosage	Major Adverse Effects/Cautions	Key Counseling Points	Miscellaneous Issues
Paclitaxel Taxol	For ovarian cancer in patients previously treated with chemotherapeutic agents: 135 or 175 mg/m² IV over 3 hrs every 3 weeks For carcinoma of the breast: 175 mg/m² IV over 3 hrs every 3 weeks Alternative regimens have been utilized — SEE Prescribing Information (PI)	Contraindications: Hypersensitivity to agents formulated with Cremophor EL; patients with baseline neutropenia of <1,500 WBCs/mm³ Considerations: Severe (sometimes fatal) allergic reactions and severe cardiac conduction abnormalities can occur; bone marrow depression (primarily neutropenia) is the dose-limiting adverse effect, frequent monitoring of CBC is required Most common AEs include bone marrow depression, infections, bleeding, allergic reactions, hypotension, peripheral neuropathy, myalgia/arthralgia, nausea/vomiting, diarrhea, mucositis, alopecia Pregnancy category: D	SEE altretamine and tell the prescriber is you have heart rhythm problems Information on missed dose usually does not apply since the agent is given IV	All patients should be pre-treated with corticosteroids, diphenhydramine, and H₂ antagonists to prevent serious allergic reactions; special instructions for preparation and administration are provided in the Prescribing Information (PI)

Generic Name and Selected Trade Names	Normal Adult Dosage	Major Adverse Effects/Cautions	Key Counselling Points	Miscellaneous Issues
Tamoxifen Citrate Nolvadex	For treatment of breast cancer: Administer 20 to 40 mg/day, doses greater than 20 mg should be given in 2 divided doses For reduction in breast cancer incidence in high risk women: Administer 20 mg daily for 5 years; there are no data to support use for any time period other than 5 years	Considerations: Visual disturbances including corneal changes, cataracts, and retinopathy have occurred; hypercalcemia has been reported in patients with bone metastases; endometrial changes have occurred, so any abnormal vaginal bleeding should be evaluated; increased incidence of uterine cancer is associated with use of this agent; elevation of liver enzymes and bone marrow suppression can occur Most common AEs include hot flashes, nausea/vomiting, vaginal bleeding/discharge, menstrual irregularities, skin rash Pregnancy category: D	Tell the prescriber if you have cataracts or other eye problems or high cholesterol; check with the physician/pharmacist before taking any other medications; for women, it is important to use a method of birth control other than "the pill" while receiving this medication; ensure patient has discussed all the risks and adverse effects associated with this agent; discuss with the physician before having any immunizations; report any unusual or severe adverse effects to the physician, including changes in vision, confusion, shortness of breath, weakness/pain, yellow eyes or skin;	

Generic Name and Selected Trade Names	Normal Adult Dosage	Major Adverse Effects/Cautions	Key Counselling Points	Miscellaneous Issues
Tamoxifen Citrate (continued) Nolvadex			It is important that the physician checks your progress regularly; it is important to take this medication for the full time of treatment even if you experience nausea; if you miss a dose, skip the dose, return to your regular schedule and check with the prescriber — do not double doses For enteric coated, swallow whole, if patient is receiving an antacid it should be separated by 1–2 hrs	

Generic Name and Selected Trade Names	Normal Adult Dosage	Major Adverse Effects/Cautions	Key Counseling Points	Miscellaneous Issues
Vincristine Sulfate Oncovin	For acute leukemia, usually 1.4 mg/m² IV once per week; a 50% reduction in dose recommended for patients with a direct bilirubin more than 3 mg/100 mL	<u>Contraindication</u>: Patients with the demyelinating form of Charcot-Marie-Tooth syndrome <u>Considerations</u>: Acute uric acid nephropathy has occurred; use with caution in patients with leukopenia or an infection; additional agents required to treat CNS leukemia; may potentiate neurotoxicity produced by other agents or in patients with underlying neuromuscular disorders; shortness of breath and bronchospasm have occurred following administration (minutes to weeks); avoid contact with the eye; monitor neurologic function and blood counts	SEE altretamine and tell the prescriber if you have a nerve or muscle disease or gout; while receiving this agent the physician may want you to drink extra fluids or take a laxative to combat constipation, consult with the prescriber; tell the nurse or physician right away if you notice redness, pain or swelling at the injection site Information on missed dose usually does not apply since the agent is given IV	For IV use only, can be fatal if given intrathecally

355

Generic Name and Selected Trade Names	Normal Adult Dosage	Major Adverse Effects/Cautions	Key Counseling Points	Miscellaneous Issues
Vincristine Sulfate (continued) Oncovin		Most common AEs include alopecia, neuromuscular dysfunction, leukopenia, neuritic pain, constipation, nausea/vomiting, for a more complete list — SEE Prescribing Information (PI) <u>Pregnancy category</u>: D		

*As a rule, a medication should not be administered to a patient with a known hypersensitivity to it or a similar agent.
[1]Many cancer chemotherapeutic agents can produce sterility and fetal damage, patients should discuss the issue with their physician.
[2]Since these agents can produce many serious adverse effects, patients should discuss the risks and benefits with the prescriber.
[3]In general, cancer chemotherapy should be under the supervision of a qualified physician experienced in the use of cancer chemotherapeutic agents and when facilities for appropriate patient monitoring and management of complications are available.

Antiarthritic/Antigout Agents

Table 1: Antiarthritic Agents*

Generic Name and Selected Trade Names	Normal Adult Dosage	Major Adverse Effects/Cautions	Key Counseling Points	Miscellaneous Issues
Auranofin Ridaura	Individualize dosage For rheumatoid arthritis, 6 mg daily — either 3 mg BID or 6 mg QD; if response is inadequate after 6 months may increase to 3 mg TID; if response is still inadequate after 3 months agent should be discontinued	Contraindications: Patients with a history of gold-induced anaphylactic reactions, necrotizing enterocolitis, pulmonary fibrosis, exfoliative dermatitis, bone marrow aplasia, or severe hematologic disorders Considerations: Blood counts should be monitored (thrombocytopenia is possible); proteinuria can occur; use with caution in patients with renal, hepatic, inflammatory bowel, or bone marrow dysfunction	Tell the prescriber if you had a reaction to gold therapy previously, and whether you have any serious medical conditions such as blood diseases, colitis, kidney disease, lupus, or skin diseases; while taking this medication, contact the prescriber if you develop a rash or itching, persistent diarrhea, tongue soreness or bloody or cloudy urine; the prescriber will need to check your progress and perform blood and urine tests on a regular basis;	

Generic Name and Selected Trade Names	Normal Adult Dosage	Major Adverse Effects/Cautions	Key Counselling Points	Miscellaneous Issues
Auranofin (continued) Ridaura		Most common AEs include diarrhea, nausea/vomiting, anorexia, abdominal cramps, dermatitis, stomatitis, blood dyscrasias, renal toxicity, rash, pruritus <u>Pregnancy category</u>: C	you may be more sensitive to sunlight when taking this medication, so it is best to avoid direct sunlight, wear protective clothing or use a sun block product (SPF 15 or higher) — do not use a sunlamp or tanning bed; take this medication as prescribed and do not take more than the prescribed amount as this may increase the occurrence of adverse effects; if you miss a dose take the missed dose as soon as possible, but if you do not remember until it is almost time for the next dose, skip the missed one and return to regular dosing schedule — do not double doses	

Generic Name and Selected Trade Names	Normal Adult Dosage	Major Adverse Effects/Cautions	Key Counselling Points	Miscellaneous Issues
Aurothioglucose Solganal	Individualize dosage. For rheumatoid arthritis, first dose is 10 mg, second and third doses 25 mg, fourth and subsequent doses 50 mg, with doses usually separated by 1 week; if patient is improving and no signs of toxicity develop therapy may be continued at 3–4 week intervals but if no improvement after administration of 1 G, therapy should be reconsidered	<u>Contraindications</u>: Uncontrolled diabetes mellitus, severe debilitation, systemic lupus erythematosus, renal disease, hepatic dysfunction, uncontrolled congestive heart failure, marked hypertension, blood dyscrasias, hemorrhagic diathesis, patients who have recently had radiation, concurrent administration of penicillamine or antimalarial agent, pregnancy (usually) <u>Considerations</u>: Blood counts should be monitored (thrombocytopenia is possible); proteinuria can occur; use with caution in patients with renal, hepatic, or bone marrow dysfunction; patients should be checked for sign of allergy before and after each injection	Tell the prescriber if you have lupus erythematosus, a blood disorder, any type of heart, kidney, or liver disease, are pregnant, or ever received radiation therapy; while taking this agent, inform the prescriber if you develop itching, rash, sore mouth, indigestion, or a metallic taste; increased joint pain may occur for a few days following the injection; you may be more sensitive to sunlight when taking this medication, so it is best to avoid direct sunlight, wear protective clothing or use a sunblock product (SPF 15 or higher); if patient or caregiver is administering the medication, ensure he/she understands aseptic administration technique;	

Generic Name and Selected Trade Names	Normal Adult Dosage	Major Adverse Effects/Cautions	Key Counselling Points	Miscellaneous Issues
Aurothio-glucose (continued) Solganal		Most common AEs include dermatitis, pruritus, erythema, stomatitis, allergic reactions <u>Pregnancy category</u>: C	immediately after an injection, you may feel dizzy, flushed, nauseated, etc — if the symptoms do not go away within a few minutes, contact the prescriber immediately	

Generic Name and Selected Trade Names	Normal Adult Dosage	Major Adverse Effects/Cautions	Key Counseling Points	Miscellaneous Issues
Azathioprine Imuran	Individualize dosage For rheumatoid arthritis: Start with 1 mg/kg daily (single dose or divided BID), may be increased after 6–8 weeks if response is inadequate and no serious toxicities have occurred, may titrate in steps at 4 week intervals; dose increments should be 0.5 to 2.5 mg/day For renal homotransplantation: Initially, 3 to 5 mg/kg/day beginning at the time of transplant, dose reduction to 1 to 3 mg/kg/day is usually possible	<u>Contraindications:</u> Pregnancy; patients previously treated with alkylating agents (eg, cyclophosphamide, chlorambucil, melphalan) may be at greater risk for neoplasia <u>Considerations:</u> Severe leukopenia and/or thrombocytopenia, and serious infections can occur; monitor blood counts routinely; patients may be at risk for developing neoplasms Most common AEs include leukopenia, infections, nausea/vomiting, diarrhea, fever, malaise, rash <u>Pregnancy category:</u> D	Tell the prescriber if you are pregnant, or have any medical problem such as recent chicken pox or shingles, gout, infections, kidney or liver disease, or pancreatitis; while taking this agent, contact the prescriber if you develop unusual bleeding, easy bruising, or signs of an infection (eg, fever, malaise); you probably will undergo periodic blood tests while on this agent; this medication may affect your body's ability to fight off infections and form blood clots, so try to avoid getting an infection while receiving this medication — avoid people with infections and maintain good hygiene — and avoid situations such as sports where bruising can occur;	Incidence of adverse effects is greater in patients receiving the agent following organ transplantation as compared with those receiving the agent for arthritis

363

Generic Name and Selected Trade Names	Normal Adult Dosage	Major Adverse Effects/Cautions	Key Counselling Points	Miscellaneous Issues
Azathioprine (continued) Imuran	<u>Dosage adjustments</u>: Lower doses may be required in patients with renal dysfunction — SEE Prescribing Information (PI) Parenteral dosage form available — SEE PI		contact the prescriber if you notice any unusual bleeding; check with the prescriber before considering any immunizations; take this agent after meals or at bedtime to decrease GI upset; if you miss a dose and you are on a once a day schedule do not take the missed dose, instead go back to your original schedule and check with the prescriber, but if you take more than one dose a day take the missed dose as soon as you remember but if it is almost time for your next dose take both doses together, then go back to regular dosing schedule; if you miss more than one dose, check with the prescriber	

Generic Name and Selected Trade Names	Normal Adult Dosage	Major Adverse Effects/Cautions	Key Counselling Points	Miscellaneous Issues
Cyclosporine Neoral Sandimmune	Individualize dosage For rheumatoid arthritis: 2.5 mg/kg/day BID; may be increased after 8 weeks by 0.5 to 0.75 mg/kg/day if tolerated and if a clinical benefit is observed; may increase after 12 weeks to a maximum of 4 mg/kg/day; decrease dose by 25%–50% to control adverse effects For psoriasis: Initially 2.5 mg/kg/day divided BID; if after 4 weeks dosage may be increased at 2 week intervals by 0.5 mg/kg/day up to 4 mg/kg/day	Contraindications: Patients with abnormal renal function, uncontrolled hypertension, or malignancies; for psoriasis patients not to be given with PUVA or UVB therapy or methotrexate, other immunosuppressive agents, coal tar, or radiation Considerations: Can produce renal or hepatic toxicity; renal function should be monitored especially in the elderly Most common AEs include renal dysfunction, tremor, hirsutism, hypertension, gingival hyperplasia, headache, gastrointestinal distress Pregnancy category: C	SEE azathioprine; also, tell the prescriber if you have hypertension or a kidney disorder; if you miss a dose and remember within 12 hrs take the missed dose as soon as you remember but if it is almost time for the next dose go back to your regular dosing schedule — do not double doses For Neoral solution, may be diluted with orange or apple juice that is at room temperature; do not mix with grapefruit juice; dry the dropper used to measure the liquid, but do not rinse with water	Neoral and Sandimmune are not bioequivalent and cannot be interchanged without establishing a new dosage regimen; numerous drug interactions are possible — SEE Prescribing Information (PI)

Generic Name and Selected Trade Names	Normal Adult Dosage	Major Adverse Effects/Cautions	Key Counselling Points	Miscellaneous Issues
Cyclosporine (continued) Neoral Sandimmune	For renal transplant: Dosage regimens are complicated — SEE Prescribing Information (PI)		For Sandimmune, to improve taste, it may be mixed in a glass container with milk, chocolate milk, or orange juice but do not mix with grapefruit juice; dry the dropper used to measure the liquid, but do not rinse with water	

Generic Name and Selected Trade Names	Normal Adult Dosage	Major Adverse Effects/Cautions	Key Counseling Points	Miscellaneous Issues
Gold Sodium Thiomalate Myochrysine	Individualize dosage For active rheumatoid arthritis, inject IM only; usually, the first dose is 10 mg, second dose is 25 mg, third and subsequent doses are 25 to 50 mg, with doses usually separated by 1 week; continue doses until cumulative dose of 1 G or toxicity — SEE Prescribing Information (PI)	<u>Contraindications:</u> Severe toxicity from previous gold or other heavy metal use, severe debilitation, or systemic lupus erythematosus <u>Considerations:</u> Before and throughout therapy, evaluate the patient's hemoglobin, RBCs, WBCs, and differential, platelet counts, and urinalysis; do not use with penicillamine; safety with cytotoxic agents not established; use caution in patients with history of blood dyscrasia caused by drug sensitivity, allergies, skin rash, kidney or liver disease, marked hypertension, compromised cerebral or cardiovascular circulation, diabetes mellitus, CHF; adverse effects most common after a cumulative dose of 400 to 800 mg	SEE aurothioglucose	

Generic Name and Selected Trade Names	Normal Adult Dosage	Major Adverse Effects/Cautions	Key Counselling Points	Miscellaneous Issues
Gold Sodium Thiomalate (continued) Myochrysine		Most common AEs include dermatitis, kidney toxicity such as nephrotic syndrome, allergic reactions — for a more complete list, SEE Product Information (PI) Pregnancy category: C		

Generic Name and Selected Trade Names	Normal Adult Dosage	Major Adverse Effects/Cautions	Key Counseling Points	Miscellaneous Issues
Penicillamine Cuprimine Depen	Individualize dosage For rheumatoid arthritis: Initially, 125 to 250 mg as a single daily dose; increased at 1–3 month intervals by 125 to 250 mg/kg/day as patient response and tolerance indicate; for maintenance doses and management of exacerbations — SEE Prescribing Information (PI) For Wilson's disease: Dosage is based upon measurement of urinary copper excretion and measurement of free copper levels in the serum — SEE PI	Contraindications: Pregnancy (except Wilson's disease) and breast feeding, history of penicillamine-related aplastic anemia or agranulocytosis, patients with renal insufficiency Considerations: Risk of serious hematologic and renal toxicities so renal function and blood counts should be routinely monitored; monitor liver function every 6 months; if drug fever occurs in arthritis patients the agent should be discontinued; skin and mucus membranes should be examined for evidence of allergic reactions Most common AEs include rashes, pemphigus, anorexia, nausea/vomiting, diarrhea, leukopenia, thrombocytopenia, proteinuria, hematuria, tinnitus, optic neuritis, peripheral neuropathies, muscle weakness	Tell the prescriber if you ever had an allergic reaction to penicillin, are pregnant, are breast feeding, or have any type of a blood or kidney disorder; while taking this agent, tell the prescriber if you develop fever, joint pain, rash, hives, itching, swollen/ painful glands, ulcers, sores or white spots on lips or mouth; take this medication exactly as directed and do not stop taking it without first speaking with the prescriber; take on an empty stomach (eg, one hour before or 2 hrs after meals);	In arthritis, response may take 2–3 months to become evident

Generic Name and Selected Trade Names	Normal Adult Dosage	Major Adverse Effects/Cautions	Key Counseling Points	Miscellaneous Issues
Penicillamine (continued) Cuprimine Depen	For cystinuria: Usually, 1 to 4 G/day divided in four equal doses	Pregnancy category: Not specified but is generally contraindicated	if you miss a dose and are taking 1 or 2 doses per day, take the missed dose as soon as possible but if it is almost time for the next dose, skip the missed one and go back to your regular schedule — do not double doses; if you miss a dose and are taking more than 2 doses a day, take the missed dose if you remember within an hour of the missed dose, but if you remember later, skip the missed one and return to regular schedule — do not double doses	

*As a general rule, a medication should not be administered to a patient with a known hypersensitivity to it or a similar agent.

Table 2: Agents for Gouty Arthritis*

Generic Name and Selected Trade Names	Normal Adult Dosage	Major Adverse Effects/Cautions	Key Counseling Points	Miscellaneous Issues
Allopurinol Zyloprim	Individualize dosage For mild gout: On average, administer 200 to 300 mg daily For moderately severe tophaceous gout: On average, administer 400 to 600 mg daily Dosages greater than 300 mg daily should be administered in divided doses To decrease the incidence of flare ups start with 100 mg daily and increase by 100 mg at weekly intervals until serum uric acid levels are below 6 mg/dL, without exceeding maximum dosage	Considerations: Discontinue if any sign of an allergic reaction occurs, including rash; may cause liver toxicity so if patient develops anorexia, weight loss, or pruritus, assess liver function; acute attacks of gouty arthritis may be precipitated early in therapy; use caution in patients with renal disease Most common AEs include increase in acute gout attacks, rash, diarrhea, nausea Pregnancy category: C	Tell the prescriber if you have CHF, diabetes mellitus, hypertension, or kidney disease; while taking this medication, stop therapy and contact the prescriber if you develop a skin rash, painful urination, blood in the urine, irritation of the eyes, or swelling of the lips/mouth; you must drink 10–12 full glasses of fluids each day unless otherwise directed; if you are told to take another medication to make your urine less acidic or to prevent a flare up of your gout during the first few days of therapy please take it; this medication does not work quickly enough to treat an acute attack;	

Generic Name and Selected Trade Names	Normal Adult Dosage	Major Adverse Effects/Cautions	Key Counseling Points	Miscellaneous Issues
Allopurinol (continued) Zyloprim	Dosage adjustment: Patients with renal disease require lower doses than normal — SEE Prescribing Information (PI)		drinking alcoholic beverages can aggravate your condition, so avoid alcohol; this agent may cause drowsiness so be cautious conducting any activity where alertness is required such as driving a car; if you miss a dose, take it as soon as possible but if it is almost time for the next dose, skip the missed one and go back to regular schedule — do not double doses	

Generic Name and Selected Trade Names	Normal Adult Dosage	Major Adverse Effects/Cautions	Key Counseling Points	Miscellaneous Issues
Colchicine	Individualize dosage For prophylactic use in gout: Start with 0.5 to 0.6 mg daily; may be increased to 0.5 to 0.6 mg BID or rarely TID; in mild cases single doses may be administered 1–4 times per week For relief of acute gout attack: Administer 1 to 2 tablets (0.5, 0.6 or 1 mg) initially, then 0.5 to 0.6 mg every 1–2 hrs or 1 to 1.2 mg Q2H until pain is relieved or nausea/vomiting or diarrhea occur, or until 6 mg has been consumed	<u>Contraindications</u>: Hepatic or renal disease <u>Considerations</u>: Use with caution in alcoholic, geriatric, or debilitated patients, and persons with blood dyscrasias, heart disease or a GI disorder; monitoring of complete blood counts required for chronic therapy; excessive dosage is very dangerous — discontinue therapy at first sign of toxicity Most common AEs include diarrhea, nausea/vomiting, stomach pain, loss of appetite, alopecia, bone marrow depression <u>Pregnancy category</u>: D	Tell the prescriber if you have a heart, liver, kidney, or blood disorder; taking too much of this medication can result in serious toxicities so take this medication as directed and do not exceed prescribed dose; drinking alcoholic beverages can aggravate your condition and worsen the stomach upset that can occur with this agent so try to avoid alcohol; for relief of an acute attack, begin to take this medication at the first sign of the attack and stop taking the medication as soon as the pain is relieved or at the first sign of nausea/vomiting, stomach pain, or diarrhea — but, even if none of these symptoms occur do not exceed the amount prescribed;	

Generic Name and Selected Trade Names	Normal Adult Dosage	Major Adverse Effects/Cautions	Key Counselling Points	Miscellaneous Issues
Colchicine (continued)			the first few times you take this medication to treat an acute attack, keep track of how many doses you took before the stomach symptoms occurred and the next time stop taking the medication prior to that dose; after taking the medication to relieve an acute attack do not take it again for 3 days (may be more in elderly)	

Generic Name and Selected Trade Names	Normal Adult Dosage	Major Adverse Effects/Cautions	Key Counseling Points	Miscellaneous Issues
Probenecid Benemid	Individualize dosage For gout: Usually start with 0.25 G BID for one week, followed by 0.5 G BID; may titrate dose by 0.5 G every 4 weeks up to 2 G per day if necessary With penicillin therapy: Usually administer 2 G daily, in divided doses	Contraindications: Children under 2 years of age, patients with known blood dyscrasias or uric acid kidney stones, patients experiencing an acute attack of gouty arthritis, salicylate use Considerations: Exacerbations of gout can occur early in therapy; maintaining adequate urine flow will decrease the formation of uric acid stones; use with caution in patients with peptic ulcer disease Most common AEs include headache, dizziness, nausea/vomiting, anorexia, rash, alopecia, flushing Pregnancy category: Not specified	SEE allopurinol; in addition tell the prescriber if you are being treated for cancer, have stomach ulcers, a blood disorder, or kidney disease/stones, or are taking any other medication; while taking this medication, contact the prescriber if you experience fast/irregular/difficulty in breathing, swelling around the eyes, skin rash, hives or itching; this medication may alter some urine sugar tests in diabetic patients; this medication is not used to treat an acute attack of gout; drinking alcoholic beverages or taking aspirin can aggravate your condition so try to avoid alcohol and aspirin unless otherwise directed;	

Generic Name and Selected Trade Names	Normal Adult Dosage	Major Adverse Effects/Cautions	Key Counseling Points	Miscellaneous Issues
Probenecid (continued) Benemid			if you miss a dose, take it as soon as possible but if it is almost time for the next dose, skip the missed one and go back to regular schedule — do not double doses	

*As a general rule, a medication should not be administered to a patient with a known hypersensitivity to it or a similar agent.

Analgesics

Table 1: Opioid Analgesics*

Generic Name and Selected Trade Names	Normal Adult Dosage	Major Adverse Effects/Cautions	Key Counseling Points	Miscellaneous Issues
Buprenorphine Buprenex	Individualize dosage For pain, 0.3 mg via a deep IM injection (or, may be given IV) Q6H as needed; may repeat once 30 to 60 minutes after the initial dose if needed and risks are considered; high risk patients (eg, elderly, debilitated, those with respiratory disease) should receive one-half the dose; some patients may require 0.6 mg — administer this dose by IM route only	<u>Considerations</u>: Use with caution in patients with impaired respiratory function, elderly, debilitated patients, children, patients with renal or hepatic dysfunction; effects are potentiated in the presence of other CNS and/or respiratory depressants; use with caution in patients with head injuries; may precipitate withdrawal in patients dependent upon narcotics Most common AEs include sedation, nausea/vomiting, dizziness, sweating, headache, hypotension, hypoventilation, miosis <u>Pregnancy category</u>: C	Tell the prescriber if you have a lung, kidney, or liver disorder, or any other serious condition; take this medication as directed by your physician; do not take it for longer than prescribed and do not exceed the recommended dosage — if you feel it is not working properly contact the physician; the medicine could become habit forming; may cause drowsiness/sedation so use caution if performing a task that requires alertness such as driving a car or using machinery; drowsiness may be enhanced by other CNS depressants such as alcohol, antihistamines, and tranquilizers.	Does not substitute for full agonist opioids in dependent individuals

Generic Name and Selected Trade Names	Normal Adult Dosage	Major Adverse Effects/Cautions	Key Counseling Points	Miscellaneous Issues
Buprenorphine (continued) Buprenex			so do not take any other medications without discussing it first with your physician or pharmacist; if you have been taking this medication for several weeks do not suddenly stop, the prescriber may want to decrease the dosage gradually; if patient or caregiver is injecting, ensure that he/she is familiar with proper aseptic injection technique; be sure to store this medication out of the reach of children; if you are taking this medication on a regular schedule and miss a dose take it as soon as you remember but if it is almost time for your next dose skip the missed one and go back to regular dosing schedule — do not double doses	

Generic Name and Selected Trade Names	Normal Adult Dosage	Major Adverse Effects/Cautions	Key Counselling Points	Miscellaneous Issues
Butorphanol Tartrate Stadol Stadol NS	Individualize dosage for pain Injectable: 0.5 to 2 mg Q3–4H as needed IV; 1 to 4 mg IM Q3–4H as needed Nasal spray: 1 mg (1 spray in 1 nostril), repeat in 60 to 90 min if necessary then Q3–4H as needed Dosage adjustment: Lower doses used in elderly patients — SEE Prescribing Information (PI)	Contraindication: Not to be used in patients under 18 Most common AEs include somnolence, dizziness, nausea/vomiting, nasal congestion, irritation, and for spray formulation unpleasant taste Pregnancy category: C	SEE buprenorphine For spray, blow nose gently, remove cover and protective clip from spray, ensure patient knows how to prime the pump and how to use a nasal spray properly	

Generic Name and Selected Trade Names	Normal Adult Dosage	Major Adverse Effects/Cautions	Key Counselling Points	Miscellaneous Issues
Codeine Phosphate	Individualize dosage For pain: Administer 15 to 60 mg Q3–6H as needed For cough: Administer 10 to 20 mg Q 4–6H	Most common AEs include constipation, somnolence, dizziness, nausea/vomiting Pregnancy category: C	SEE buprenorphine	Lower risk of dependency than other opioids For cough: Children under two are more prone to breathing problems — do not use unless directed by physician; although dose of codeine is lower than for analgesia, there is a risk of sedation, mental confusion, etc
Codeine Sulfate	SEE codeine phosphate	SEE codeine phosphate	SEE buprenorphine	SEE codeine phosphate

Generic Name and Selected Trade Names	Normal Adult Dosage	Major Adverse Effects/Cautions	Key Counselling Points	Miscellaneous Issues
Fentanyl Transdermal System Duragesic	Individualize dosage Dosage depends upon the patient's previous opioid therapy (agent and dose), the degree of tolerance, and the general medical status of the patient; dosage range is 25 to 300 mcg/hr; patches generally last 72 hrs — SEE prescribing information (PI)	Contraindications: Management of post-operative pain, mild pain, or doses exceeding 25 mcg/hr when initiating therapy Considerations: Should not be administered to patients under 12 years of age or patients under 18 years of age who weigh <50 kG; doses must be decreased if used in conjunction with other CNS depressants; effects will last for at least 12 hrs following removal of the patch; avoid exposing the patch to heat Most common AEs include headache, abdominal discomfort, sedation, urinary retention, sweating, and pruritus, but most serious are respiratory and cardiovascular depression Pregnancy category: C	Tell the prescriber if you are taking any other pain medication, antihistamines/sleep aids/tranquilizers or any other type of medication that makes you drowsy; ensure patient reviews the patient instructions supplied with the medication; this agent may cause drowsiness and dizziness so use caution if you need to drive a car or use machinery; apply the patch to a non-irritated flat area of the skin, such as chest/back/flank/upper arm, clip (do not shave) hair at the application site, do not put oil/lotion on the skin, apply patch only when skin is dry, do not cut or tear the patch.	

Generic Name and Selected Trade Names	Normal Adult Dosage	Major Adverse Effects/Cautions	Key Counselling Points	Miscellaneous Issues
Fentanyl Transdermal System (continued) Duragesic			each patch should be worn for 72 hrs unless otherwise directed and when you need another remove the first and apply the new patch in a different area; used patches should be flushed down the toilet as soon as removed; keep patches out of the reach of children	
Hydrocodone Bitartrate Opioid in many combination products	Individualize dosage For pain: Usually, 2.5 to 10 mg Q4–6H as needed For cough: Usually, 5 mg Q4–6H as needed	SEE buprenorphine	SEE buprenorphine	For cough, although dose commonly is lower than for analgesia, there is a risk of sedation, mental confusion, etc

Generic Name and Selected Trade Names	Normal Adult Dosage	Major Adverse Effects/Cautions	Key Counseling Points	Miscellaneous Issues
Hydromorphone HCl Dilaudid	Individualize dosage Oral tablets for pain: Usually, 2 to 4 mg Q4–6H Oral liquid for pain: Give 2.5 to 10 mL Q3–6H as directed by the clinical situation Oral liquid for cough: Administer 5 mL (1 mg) of the syrup Q3–4H Rectal for pain: Insert 1 suppository (3 mg) Q6–8H	<u>Contraindications</u>: Patients with depressed respiration or increased intracranial pressure <u>Considerations</u>: Physical and psychic dependence can occur with prolonged use; respiratory depression is dose-related Most common AEs include sedation, dizziness, nausea, vomiting, sweating, and mood changes, but most serious are respiratory and cardiovascular depression <u>Pregnancy category</u>: C	SEE buprenorphine; for suppository, ensure patient is familiar with administration procedure — eg, remove outer wrapper, insert rectally, retain until product dissolves	

Generic Name and Selected Trade Names	Normal Adult Dosage	Major Adverse Effects/Cautions	Key Counselling Points	Miscellaneous Issues
Hydromorphone HCl (continued) Dilaudid	Dosage adjustments: May be required in patients with hepatic, renal, thyroid or urinary disorders, and in the elderly — SEE Prescribing Information (PI) Injectable form available — SEE PI			

Generic Name and Selected Trade Names	Normal Adult Dosage	Major Adverse Effects/Cautions	Key Counseling Points	Miscellaneous Issues
Levomethadyl Acetate HCl Orlaam	Individualize dosage For management of opiate dependence, dosing is generally 3 days per week, but is complex — SEE Prescribing Information (PI) for details	<u>Considerations</u>: Administration of this agent on a daily basis can lead to accumulation of the drug and overdose; use with caution in elderly, debilitated, head injury, respiratory and cardiac patients Most common AEs in patients on stable therapy include asthenia, abdominal pain, insomnia, nervousness, sweating, sexual dysfunction <u>Pregnancy category</u>: C	Ensure patient reviews the patient instructions supplied with the medication; follow the prescribed regimen very carefully as taking this agent more frequently can lead to overdose; it will take a few days for this medication to work — do not take other narcotic agents or alcoholic beverages during this time; before taking any other type of pain killer, contact your physician or pharmacist; inform your family that you are taking this medication and be sure they can inform any emergency personnel in the case of an overdose; also, SEE buprenorphine	Unlike methadone this agent is not taken daily, but rather three times per week

Generic Name and Selected Trade Names	Normal Adult Dosage	Major Adverse Effects/Cautions	Key Counselling Points	Miscellaneous Issues
Levorphanol Tartrate Levo-Dromoran	Individualize dosage For pain, initially 2 mg, repeat in 6–8H as needed, may be increased to 3 mg; assess patient for hypoventilation	Considerations and most common AEs: SEE buprenorphine Pregnancy category: C	SEE buprenorphine	
Meperidine HCl Demerol	Individualize dosage Oral or IM for pain, 50 to 150 mg Q3–4H as needed Dosage adjustments: May be required in patients with hepatic, renal, thyroid, or urinary disorders, and in elderly patients — SEE Prescribing Information (PI)	Contraindications: Patients receiving MAO inhibitors Considerations: Physical and psychic dependence can occur with prolonged use; more likely to cause convulsions than other opioids Most common AEs include dizziness, sedation, nausea/vomiting, sweating, constipation, but most serious are respiratory and cardiovascular depression Pregnancy category: Not specified	Tell the prescriber if you have a liver or kidney disorder; also, SEE buprenorphine For syrup, may be diluted in ½ glass (4 ounces) of water unless otherwise directed	Syrup is non-alcoholic and banana-flavored

Generic Name and Selected Trade Names	Normal Adult Dosage	Major Adverse Effects/Cautions	Key Counseling Points	Miscellaneous Issues
Methadone HCl Dolophine Methadose	Individualize dosage <u>Concentrate and solution for pain</u>: Usually, 5 to 20 mg Q4-8H as needed <u>Tablets for pain</u>: Usually, 2.5 to 10 mg Q3-4H as needed <u>Maintenance programs</u>: Regimens are complicated — SEE Prescribing Information (PI)	<u>Considerations</u>: SEE buprenorphine <u>Most common AEs</u>: SEE meperidine HCl <u>Pregnancy category</u>: Not specified	SEE buprenorphine and levomethadyl acetate	

Generic Name and Selected Trade Names	Normal Adult Dosage	Major Adverse Effects/Cautions	Key Counselling Points	Miscellaneous Issues
Morphine Sulfate MS Contin OraMorph SR Roxanol Roxanol-T Roxanol 100 Kadian (SR) MSIR	Individualize dosage MS Contin, OraMorph SR, Kadian SR for pain: Generally used after a patient has been titrated with immediate release morphine — SEE Prescribing Information (PI) to convert dosage regimen Roxanol for pain: Usually, 10 to 30 mg Q4H MSIR for pain: Usually, 5 to 30 mg Q4H Injectable dosage form available — SEE PI	Considerations — SEE buprenorphine Pregnancy Category: C	SEE buprenorphine For MS Contin, OraMorph SR, Kadian SR, do not break, chew or crush tablets For MSIR capsules, contents may be added to soft food (eg, pudding, applesauce) and swallowed immediately	
Oxycodone HCl OxyContin	Individualize dosage SEE Prescribing Information (PI) for details	SEE buprenorphine	SEE buprenorphine; also, do not break, crush, or chew tablets	Opioid found in many combination products

Generic Name and Selected Trade Names	Normal Adult Dosage	Major Adverse Effects/Cautions	Key Counselling Points	Miscellaneous Issues
Oxymorphone HCl Numorphan	Individualize dosage For pain, 5 mg (1 suppository) Q4–6H as needed	SEE buprenorphine	SEE buprenorphine, also ensure patient knows how to use a suppository properly — eg, remove outer wrapper, insert rectally, retain until product dissolves	Suppositories should be stored in refrigerator, but not frozen
Pentazocine HCl + Naloxone HCl Talwin Nx	Individualize dosage For pain, usually 50 mg Q 3–4H as needed, increased to 100 mg if needed	<u>Considerations</u>: SEE buprenorphine; and intended for oral use only as potentially fatal reactions can occur if injected Most common AEs include hypotension, tachycardia, hallucinations, disorientation, confusion, dizziness, sedation, euphoria, headache, sweating, nausea/vomiting <u>Pregnancy category</u>: C	SEE buprenorphine	May be less habit forming than other opioids

Generic Name and Selected Trade Names	Normal Adult Dosage	Major Adverse Effects/Cautions	Key Counselling Points	Miscellaneous Issues
Propoxyphene Napsylate Darvon-N	Individualize dosage For pain, usually 100 to 600 mg/day divided Q4H as needed Reduced dosage may be required in patients with hepatic or renal impairment	<u>Considerations</u>: Not for use in patients who are suicidal or addiction-prone; use with caution in patients receiving other CNS depressants and in patients with liver or kidney dysfunction; not recommended for use in patients under 12 years of age Most common AEs include dizziness, sedation, nausea/vomiting, constipation, rash, headache, weakness <u>Pregnancy category</u>: C	Tell the prescriber if you have a liver or kidney disorder; may cause drowsiness/sedation so use caution if performing a task that requires alertness such as driving a car or using machinery; drowsiness may be enhanced by other CNS depressants such as alcohol, antihistamines, and tranquilizers, so try not to drink alcoholic beverages and do not take any other medication (eg, tranquilizers, cold remedies, antihistamines, and sleep aids) without discussing it first with your physician or pharmacist;	Component of many combination analgesics

Generic Name and Selected Trade Names	Normal Adult Dosage	Major Adverse Effects/Cautions	Key Counseling Points	Miscellaneous Issues
Propoxyphene Napsylate (continued) Darvon-N			if you are taking this medication on a regular schedule and miss a dose take it as soon as you remember but if it is almost time for your next dose skip the missed one and go back to regular dosing schedule — do not double doses	
Propoxyphene HCl Darvon	Individualize dosage For pain, 65 mg Q4H as needed; maximum recommended dose is 390 mg/day Reduced dosage may be required in patients with hepatic or renal impairment	SEE propoxyphene napsylate	SEE propoxyphene napsylate	SEE propoxyphene napsylate

*As a general rule, a medication should not be administered to a patient with a known hypersensitivity to it or a similar agent.
Note: Many opioids are commonly combined with aspirin or acetaminophen.

Table 2: Non-Steroidal Antiinflammatory Agents and Related Agents*

Generic Name and Selected Trade Names	Normal Adult Dosage	Major Adverse Effects/Cautions	Key Counseling Points	Miscellaneous Issues
Bromfenac Sodium Duract	Individualize dosage For pain, 25 mg Q6–8H as needed, usually for less than 10 days; higher doses may be necessary if taken with a high fat meal	<u>Contraindications</u>: Patients with chronic hepatitis; patients allergic to or who experienced severe adverse reactions due to other NSAIDS <u>Considerations</u>: Elevations of liver enzymes have occurred (incidence higher if therapy longer than 10 days in duration); may cause renal toxicity; use with caution in patients with liver disease, cardiovascular disorders, and ulcer disease; GI distress is possible and can include bleeding (more likely with higher doses, in elderly patients, with certain concomitant agents, smoking, alcohol intake, and if debilitated); avoid in late pregnancy; may prolong bleeding time	Tell the prescriber if you have any type of heart, kidney, liver, or ulcer disorder; do not take more than the prescribed amount; take with a full glass of water and remain upright for 15 to 30 minutes after taking the medication; to lessen stomach upset you may take this medication with food or an antacid; alcoholic beverages may worsen the stomach upset that may occur with this medication, so try to avoid; if stomach upset is bothersome or persistent, check with the physician or pharmacist;	

Generic Name and Selected Trade Names	Normal Adult Dosage	Major Adverse Effects/Cautions	Key Counselling Points	Miscellaneous Issues
Bromfenac Sodium (continued) Duract		Most common AEs include abdominal pain, dyspepsia, nausea, dizziness, somnolence, headache — for more complete list, SEE Prescribing Information (PI) Pregnancy category: C	use with other pain relievers can increase the chance of unwanted effects, so do not take any without discussing it first with the physician or pharmacist; some people taking this may become dizzy or experience visual disturbances, so make sure you know how you react to this medication before you drive a car or operate machinery; if you are taking this medication on a regular schedule and miss a dose take it as soon as you remember but if it is almost time for your next dose skip the missed one and go back to regular dosing schedule	

Generic Name and Selected Trade Names	Normal Adult Dosage	Major Adverse Effects/Cautions	Key Counselling Points	Miscellaneous Issues
Choline Salicylate and Magnesium Salicylate Trilisate	Individualize dosage For rheumatoid arthritis, osteoarthritis, severe arthritides, and acute painful shoulder, start with 1500 mg BID, then titrate based upon patient response Dosage adjustment: Lower doses required in elderly patients — SEE Prescribing Information (PI)	Considerations: Avoid in children with chicken pox, influenza, or flu-like symptoms (Reye's syndrome); use caution in patients with peptic ulcer disease, renal, or liver dysfunction Most common AEs include tinnitus, gastrointestinal distress (nausea/vomiting, heartburn, diarrhea), hearing impairment, headache, dizziness Pregnancy category: C	SEE bromfenac; also, ensure the patient is not receiving any other salicylate containing preparation, including OTCs such as shampoos; for diabetic patients, this agent can affect urine sugar tests For arthritis: This medication must be taken regularly as prescribed; the medication usually begins to work within one week, but may take several weeks before you feel the full effects	

Generic Name and Selected Trade Names	Normal Adult Dosage	Major Adverse Effects/Cautions	Key Counselling Points	Miscellaneous Issues
Diclofenac Potassium Cataflam	Individualize dosage For osteoarthritis: Usually, 100 to 150 mg/day as 50 mg BID or TID For rheumatoid arthritis: Usually 100 to 200 mg/day as 50 mg TID or QID For analgesia and primary dysmenorrhea: Usually, 50 mg TID	Contraindication: Patients allergic to or who experienced severe adverse reactions due to other NSAIDS Considerations and most common AEs: SEE bromfenac Pregnancy category: B	SEE bromfenac For arthritis: This medication must be taken regularly as prescribed; the medication usually begins to work within one week, but may take several weeks before you feel the full effects	

Generic Name and Selected Trade Names	Normal Adult Dosage	Major Adverse Effects/Cautions	Key Counseling Points	Miscellaneous Issues
Diclofenac Sodium Voltaren Voltaren-XR	Individualize dosage <u>Voltaren for osteoarthritis</u>: Usually, 100 to 150 mg/day, as 50 mg BID or TID or 75 mg BID <u>Voltaren for rheumatoid arthritis</u>: Usually, 100 to 200 mg/day, as 50 mg TID or QID or 75 mg BID <u>Voltaren for ankylosing spondylitis</u>: Usually, 100 to 125 mg/day, as 25 mg QID with an extra 25 mg dose at bedtime <u>Voltaren-XR for osteoarthritis and rheumatoid arthritis</u>: 100 to 150 mg QD or in 2 or 3 divided doses	SEE diclofenac potassium	SEE diclofenac potassium	

Generic Name and Selected Trade Names	Normal Adult Dosage	Major Adverse Effects/Cautions	Key Counselling Points	Miscellaneous Issues
Diflunisal Dolobid	Individualize dosage For mild to moderate pain: Start with 1000 mg followed by 500 mg Q12H; some patients may require 500 mg Q8H For osteoarthritis and rheumatoid arthritis: Usually, 500 to 1000 mg daily in two divided doses	<u>Contraindication</u>: SEE diclofenac potassium <u>Considerations and most common AEs</u>: SEE bromfenac <u>Pregnancy category</u>: C	SEE bromfenac and diclofenac potassium; also, tablets must be swallowed whole	

Generic Name and Selected Trade Names	Normal Adult Dosage	Major Adverse Effects/Cautions	Key Counseling Points	Miscellaneous Issues
Etodolac Lodine Lodine XL	Individualize dosage <u>Lodine for pain:</u> Usually, 200 to 400 mg Q6–8H; may be increased to 1000 mg/day <u>Lodine for osteoarthritis and rheumatoid arthritis:</u> Initially, 300 mg BID or TID, or 400 to 500 mg BID; then, titrate dosage based upon patient response <u>Lodine XL for osteoarthritis and rheumatoid arthritis:</u> Usually, 400 to 1000 mg daily	<u>Contraindication</u>: SEE diclofenac potassium <u>Considerations and most common AEs</u>: SEE bromfenac <u>Pregnancy category</u>: C	SEE bromfenac and diclofenac potassium Also for Lodine XL, tablets must be swallowed whole; if you miss a dose, take the missed dose only if you remember within an hour or two after the dose should have been taken, but if you remember later, skip the missed dose and go back to your regular dosing schedule	

Generic Name and Selected Trade Names	Normal Adult Dosage	Major Adverse Effects/Cautions	Key Counseling Points	Miscellaneous Issues
Fenoprofen Calcium Nalfon Nalfon 200	Individualize dosage For pain: Usually, 200 mg Q4–6H as needed For osteoarthritis and rheumatoid arthritis: Usually, 300 to 600 mg TID or QID	Contraindication: SEE diclofenac potassium Considerations and most common AEs: SEE bromfenac; also should not be administered to patients with significant renal impairment Pregnancy category: Not specified	SEE bromfenac and diclofenac potassium	

Generic Name and Selected Trade Names	Normal Adult Dosage	Major Adverse Effects/Cautions	Key Counselling Points	Miscellaneous Issues
Ibuprofen Motrin Rufen Saleto-400 and 800	Individualize dosage For osteoarthritis and rheumatoid arthritis: Usually start with 1200 to 3200 mg daily in 3–4 divided doses; after response achieved, reduce dose to the lowest maintenance dose that controls symptoms For pain, fever or dysmenorrhea: Usually, 200 to 400 mg Q4–6H as needed	<u>Contraindication</u>: SEE diclofenac potassium <u>Considerations and most common AEs</u>: SEE bromfenac <u>Pregnancy category</u>: Not specified	SEE bromfenac and diclofenac potassium	

Generic Name and Selected Trade Names	Normal Adult Dosage	Major Adverse Effects/Cautions	Key Counseling Points	Miscellaneous Issues
Indomethacin Indocin Indocin SR	Individualize dosage Indocin for rheumatoid and osteoarthritis and ankylosing spondylitis: Usually start with 25 mg BID or TID; may titrate dose by 25 to 50 mg at weekly intervals up to a total daily dose of 150 to 200 mg Indocin SR for rheumatoid and osteoarthritis and ankylosing spondylitis: Begin with 75 mg daily; may increase to 75 mg BID if needed and if the patient tolerates the therapy	<u>Contraindications:</u> Suppositories should not be used in patients with a history of proctitis or recent rectal bleeding, patients allergic to or who experienced severe adverse reactions due to other NSAIDS <u>Considerations:</u> SEE bromfenac and not recommended for use in patients under 14 years of age; corneal deposits and retinal lesions have occurred; may aggravate CNS disorders such as epilepsy, psychiatric conditions, and Parkinson's disease; adverse effects increase with higher doses Most common AEs include nausea/vomiting, dyspepsia, diarrhea, abdominal distress, headache, dizziness, vertigo, somnolence, depression, tinnitus <u>Pregnancy category:</u> Not specified, but not recommended	SEE bromfenac and diclofenac potassium For suppositories, not necessary to take with a full glass of water; ensure patient knows how to use a suppository properly — eg, remove outer wrapper, insert rectally, retain until product dissolves Indocin SR, capsules must be swallowed whole; take at the same time every day; if you miss a dose take the missed one only if you remember within an hour or two after the dose should have been taken, but if you remember later skip the missed dose and go back to regular dosing schedule	

Generic Name and Selected Trade Names	Normal Adult Dosage	Major Adverse Effects/Cautions	Key Counseling Points	Miscellaneous Issues
Indomethacin (continued) Indocin Indocin SR	<u>Indocin SR for acute painful shoulder:</u> Initially 75 to 150 mg in 3–4 divided doses, usually for 7–14 days; discontinue when symptoms resolve <u>Indocin SR for acute gouty arthritis:</u> Usually 50 mg TID until pain is tolerable, rapidly reduce when pain subsides			

Generic Name and Selected Trade Names	Normal Adult Dosage	Major Adverse Effects/Cautions	Key Counselling Points	Miscellaneous Issues
Ketoprofen Orudis Oruvail	Individualize dosage Orudis for rheumatoid arthritis and osteoarthritis: Usually, either 75 mg TID or 50 mg QID Orudis for pain and dysmenorrhea: Usually, 25 to 50 mg Q6–8H as needed Oruvail for rheumatoid arthritis and osteoarthritis: Usually, 200 mg QD	<u>Considerations and most common AEs</u>: SEE bromfenac <u>Pregnancy category</u>: B	SEE bromfenac and diclofenac potassium Also, for Oruvail, swallow tablet whole; not necessary to take with food or an antacid; take at the same time every day; also, SEE Indocin SR	

Generic Name and Selected Trade Names	Normal Adult Dosage	Major Adverse Effects/Cautions	Key Counselling Points	Miscellaneous Issues
Ketorolac Tromethamine Toradol	Individualize dosage Indicated for up to 5 days of therapy; oral therapy is only indicated following IV/IM therapy — SEE Prescribing Information (PI)	Contraindications: Patients with peptic ulcer, GI bleeding, advanced renal impairment, during labor and delivery, in nursing mothers, patients at risk for bleeding (eg, pre-operatively, presence of cerebrovascular bleeding), concomitant use with aspirin, NSAIDs or probenecid, not for epidural or intrathecal use Considerations: Use is limited to 5 days (combined parenteral and oral); hypovolemia should be treated before therapy is started; severe GI toxicity can occur; use with caution in patients with renal or hepatic dysfunction; may prolong bleeding time	SEE bromfenac Also for IV/IM, if patient or caregiver is injecting the medication, ensure he/she is familiar with proper aseptic administration technique	

Generic Name and Selected Trade Names	Normal Adult Dosage	Major Adverse Effects/Cautions	Key Counseling Points	Miscellaneous Issues
Ketorolac Tromethamine (continued) Toradol		Most common AEs include nausea, dyspepsia, GI pain, diarrhea, headache, edema, drowsiness, dizziness — for a more complete list, SEE Prescribing Information (PI) Pregnancy category: C		

Generic Name and Selected Trade Names	Normal Adult Dosage	Major Adverse Effects/Cautions	Key Counselling Points	Miscellaneous Issues
Mefenamic Acid Ponstel	Individualize dosage For acute pain: Start with 500 mg followed by 250 mg Q6H as needed but usually not to exceed 1 week For primary dysmenorrhea: Start with 500 mg followed by 250 mg Q6H starting with the onset of bleeding and associated symptoms, usually for 2–3 days	<u>Contraindications</u>: Avoid in patients with renal disease, also SEE diclofenac potassium <u>Considerations</u>: SEE bromfenac; and if diarrhea occurs dosage should be reduced or the agent should be temporarily suspended; if rash occurs discontinue therapy Most common AEs include diarrhea, also SEE bromfenac <u>Pregnancy category</u>: C	SEE bromfenac; also, this medication must be taken with food or an antacid; do not take for more than 7 days unless directed by the prescriber	

Generic Name and Selected Trade Names	Normal Adult Dosage	Major Adverse Effects/Cautions	Key Counseling Points	Miscellaneous Issues
Nabumetone Relafen	Individualize dosage For osteoarthritis and rheumatoid arthritis, start with 1000 mg as a single dose with or without food; may titrate to 1500 to 2000 mg/day if needed	<u>Contraindications</u>: SEE diclofenac potassium <u>Considerations and most common AEs</u>: SEE bromfenac <u>Pregnancy category</u>: C	SEE bromfenac and diclofenac potassium	

Generic Name and Selected Trade Names	Normal Adult Dosage	Major Adverse Effects/Cautions	Key Counselling Points	Miscellaneous Issues
Naproxen Sodium Anaprox Anaprox DS **Naproxen** Naprosyn Naprosyn Suspension EC-Naprosyn	Individualize dosage Naprosyn (tablets or suspension) for osteoarthritis, rheumatoid arthritis, and ankylosing spondylitis: Usually, 250, 375 or 500 mg BID Naprosyn for acute gout: Start with 750 mg followed by 250 mg Q8H until attack subsides EC-Naprosyn for osteoarthritis, rheumatoid arthritis, and ankylosing spondylitis: Usually, 375 or 500 mg BID	Contraindications: SEE diclofenac potassium Consideration and most common AEs: Different formulations and salts should not be used concurrently; also, SEE bromfenac Pregnancy category: B	SEE bromfenac and diclofenac potassium; also for enteric coated and long-acting products do not break, crush, or chew For EC-Naproysn, it may not be necessary to take with food or antacid	

410

Generic Name and Selected Trade Names	Normal Adult Dosage	Key Counselling Points	Miscellaneous Issues
Naproxen Sodium (continued) Anaprox Anaprox DS **Naproxen** Naprosyn Naprosyn Suspension EC-Naprosyn	<u>Anaprox for osteoarthritis, rheumatoid arthritis, and ankylosing spondylitis</u>: Usually, 275 mg BID <u>Anaprox for pain, primary dysmenorrhea, and acute tendinitis or bursitis</u>: Start with 550 mg then 550 mg Q12H or 275 mg Q6-8H as needed <u>Anaprox for acute gout</u>: Start with 825 mg, then 275 mg Q8H <u>Anaprox DS for osteoarthritis, rheumatoid arthritis, and ankylosing spondylitis</u>: Usually, 550 mg BID <u>For pain, primary dysmenorrhea, and acute tendinitis or bursitis</u>: Start with 550 mg, then 550 mg Q12H or 275 mg Q6-8H as needed		

Generic Name and Selected Trade Names	Normal Adult Dosage	Major Adverse Effects/Cautions	Key Counselling Points	Miscellaneous Issues
Oxaprozin Daypro	Individualize dosage For rheumatoid arthritis and osteoarthritis, usually 1200 mg QD although some patients (eg, low-weight persons with osteoarthritis) may require less — SEE Prescribing Information (PI)	<u>Contraindications</u>: SEE diclofenac potassium <u>Considerations</u>: SEE bromfenac; also photosensitivity has occurred <u>Most common AEs</u> include rash; also SEE bromfenac <u>Pregnancy category</u>: C	SEE bromfenac, diclofenac potassium, and Indocin SR	
Piroxicam Feldene	Individualize dosage For rheumatoid arthritis and osteoarthritis, 20 mg QD	<u>Contraindications</u>: SEE diclofenac potassium <u>Considerations and most common AEs</u>: SEE bromfenac <u>Pregnancy category</u>: Not specified, but is not recommended	SEE bromfenac, diclofenac potassium, and Indocin SR	

Generic Name and Selected Trade Names	Normal Adult Dosage	Major Adverse Effects/Cautions	Key Counselling Points	Miscellaneous Issues
Salsalate Disalcid Salflex Mono-gesic	Individualize dosage For rheumatoid arthritis and osteoarthritis, usually 3000 mg/day in divided doses	<u>Considerations</u>: Avoid in children with chicken pox, influenza, or flu-like symptoms (Reye's syndrome) <u>Most common AEs</u> include tinnitus, nausea, hearing impairment, rash, and vertigo <u>Pregnancy category</u>: C	SEE choline salicylate and magnesium salicylate	
Sulindac Clinoril	Individualize dosage For rheumatoid arthritis, osteoarthritis, and ankylosing spondylitis: Start with 150 mg BID; may titrate to a maximum of 400 mg/day For acute painful shoulder or acute gouty arthritis: Usually, 200 mg BID, then reduce according to response	<u>Contraindication</u>: SEE diclofenac potassium <u>Considerations</u>: SEE bromfenac <u>Most common AEs</u> include rash; also SEE bromfenac <u>Pregnancy category</u>: Not specified	SEE bromfenac, diclofenac potassium, and Indocin SR	

Generic Name and Selected Trade Names	Normal Adult Dosage	Major Adverse Effects/Cautions	Key Counselling Points	Miscellaneous Issues
Tolmetin Sodium Tolectin 200 Tolectin 600 Tolectin DS	Individualize dosage For rheumatoid arthritis and osteoarthritis, start with 400 mg TID; may titrate after 1–2 weeks up to 600 to 1800 mg daily	<u>Contraindication</u>: SEE diclofenac potassium <u>Considerations</u>: SEE bromfenac Most common AEs include asthenia (weakness), weight gain or loss, increased blood pressure, edema; also SEE bromfenac <u>Pregnancy category</u>: C	SEE bromfenac and diclofenac potassium	

*As a general rule, a medication should not be administered to a patient with a known hypersensitivity to it or a similar agent.

Psychotherapeutic Agents

Table 1: Antianxiety Agents*

Generic Name and Selected Trade Names	Normal Adult Dosage	Major Adverse Effects/Cautions	Key Counseling Points	Miscellaneous Issues
Alprazolam Xanax	Individualize dosage For anxiety disorders and transient symptoms of anxiety: 0.25 to 0.5 mg TID; may be increased every 3–4 days to a maximum of 4 mg/day For panic disorder: Usually, 1 to 10 mg daily; initiate at 0.5 mg TID; increase every 3–4 days by increments of 1 mg if necessary	Contraindications: Acute narrow angle glaucoma; use with ketoconazole or itraconazole Considerations: Risk of dependence and withdrawal reactions, agent should not be discontinued abruptly; use with caution with other psychotropic agents and in patients with impaired renal, hepatic, or respiratory function Most common AEs include drowsiness, impaired coordination, dysarthria, constipation Pregnancy category: D	Tell the prescriber if you have any serious medical conditions such as glaucoma, respiratory, liver, or kidney disease; do not use if pregnant or breast feeding without speaking first with the prescriber; notify the physician or pharmacist before taking any other medication; avoid alcohol or other agents that may make you drowsy, such as antihistamines or pain killers; this agent may cause some people to become drowsy, dizzy, lightheaded, clumsy or unsteady, so make sure you know how you react before driving a car or using machinery;	

Generic Name and Selected Trade Names	Normal Adult Dosage	Major Adverse Effects/Cautions	Key Counselling Points	Miscellaneous Issues
Alprazolam (continued) Xanax			if you feel this medication is not working properly, do not take more, contact prescriber; take this medication only as directed; do not take more and do not stop taking it without consulting the prescriber; it may be habit forming; if you develop any unusual symptoms while on this medication contact the prescriber; if you are taking this medication regularly and you miss a dose and you remember within 1 hour, take it right away, if you do not remember until later skip the missed one — do not double doses	

Generic Name and Selected Trade Names	Normal Adult Dosage	Major Adverse Effects/Cautions	Key Counseling Points	Miscellaneous Issues
Buspirone HCl Buspar	Individualize dosage For anxiety start with 7.5 mg BID; may increase by 5 mg/day at 2–3 day intervals; not to exceed 60 mg/day	Considerations: Not for use in lieu of appropriate antipsychotics; will not inhibit withdrawal symptoms from benzodiazepines Most common AEs include dizziness, nausea, headache, nervousness, lightheadedness, excitement Pregnancy category: B	Tell the prescriber if you have a history of drug abuse/dependence or kidney or liver disease; notify the physician or pharmacist before taking other medication; avoid alcohol or other agents that may make you drowsy, such as antihistamines or pain killers; this agent may cause some people to become drowsy, dizzy, lightheaded, make sure you know how you react before driving a car or using machinery; it may take several weeks before you feel the full effects of this medication; take this medication only as directed do not take more;	Less sedating than many other anxiolytics

Generic Name and Selected Trade Names	Normal Adult Dosage	Major Adverse Effects/Cautions	Key Counselling Points	Miscellaneous Issues
Buspirone HCl (continued) Buspar			if you develop chest pain, confusion, mental depression, racing heartbeat, or any unusual symptoms while on this medication contact the prescriber; if you are taking this medication regularly and you miss a dose take as soon as possible, but if it is almost time for the next dose, skip the missed one — do not double doses	

Generic Name and Selected Trade Names	Normal Adult Dosage	Major Adverse Effects/Cautions	Key Counseling Points	Miscellaneous Issues
Chlordiazepoxide HCl Librium	Individualize dosage For mild and moderate anxiety disorders and symptoms of anxiety: Usually, 5 or 10 mg TID or QID For severe anxiety disorders and symptoms of anxiety: Usually, 20 or 25 mg TID or QID Dosage adjustments required in elderly and debilitated patients — SEE Prescribing Information (PI) Parenteral dosage form available — SEE PI	Considerations: Not recommended for use during pregnancy; use with caution with other psychotropic agents; paradoxical excitement can occur in some patients Most common AEs include drowsiness, ataxia, confusion, skin eruptions, edema, minor menstrual irregularities, nausea, constipation, extrapyramidal symptoms, changes in libido Pregnancy category: Not specified	SEE alprazolam	

Generic Name and Selected Trade Names	Normal Adult Dosage	Major Adverse Effects/Cautions	Key Counseling Points	Miscellaneous Issues
Clorazepate Dipotassium Tranxene T-Tab Tranxene SD Tranxene SD Half Strength	Individualize dosage For symptomatic relief of acute anxiety: *Tranxene T-Tab* Usually, 15 to 60 mg in divided doses; adjust the dose slowly based upon patient response; alternatively administer a single 15 mg dose at bedtime *Tranxene-SD or Tranxene-SD Half Strength* Usually, 1 tablet (22.5 mg or 11.25 mg) daily For symptomatic relief of acute alcohol withdrawal: Day 1 give 30 mg;	Contraindications: Acute narrow angle glaucoma Considerations: Not recommended for use in patients with a primary depressive disorder or psychosis; withdrawal symptoms have occurred following abrupt withdrawal, after continuous therapy agent should be tapered, addiction-prone patients should be carefully monitored; in patients with depression accompanied by anxiety the possibility of suicide should be considered; use with caution in patients with impaired liver or renal function, or in elderly or debilitated patients; not recommended for use in patients under 9 years of age; not recommended for use in pregnancy or lactation	SEE alprazolam	

Generic Name and Selected Trade Names	Normal Adult Dosage	Major Adverse Effects/Cautions	Key Counselling Points	Miscellaneous Issues
Clorazepate Dipotassium (continued) Tranxene T-Tab Tranxene SD Tranxene SD Half Strength	followed by 30 to 60 mg in divided doses; day 2 give 45 to 90 mg in divided doses; day 3 give 22.5 to 45 mg in divided doses; day 4 give 15 to 30 mg in divided doses, then gradually reduce daily dose to 7.5 to 15 mg; discontinue when patient stable For adjunct treatment of epilepsy: Start with 7.5 mg TID; increase by no more than 7.5 mg every week; do not exceed 90 mg/day Dosage adjustments required in elderly and debilitated patients — SEE Prescribing Information (PI)	Most common AEs include drowsiness, dizziness, GI complaints, nervousness, blurred vision, dry mouth, headache, confusion Pregnancy category: Not specified, but not recommended		

423

Generic Name and Selected Trade Names	Normal Adult Dosage	Major Adverse Effects/Cautions	Key Counseling Points	Miscellaneous Issues
Diazepam Valium	Individualize dosage For anxiety: Usually, 2 to 10 mg BID to QID For symptomatic relief of acute alcohol withdrawal: Usually, 10 mg TID or QID during the first 24 hrs; reduce to 5 mg TID or QID as needed For adjunct therapy of muscle spasm: Usually, 2 to 10 mg TID or QID For adjunct treatment of epilepsy: Usually, 2 to 10 mg BID to QID Dosage adjustments required in elderly and debilitated patients — SEE Prescribing Information (PI)	Contraindications: Acute narrow angle glaucoma; patients under 6 months of age Considerations: Not recommended for use in patients with psychosis; withdrawal symptoms have occurred following abrupt withdrawal, after continuous therapy agent should be tapered; use with caution in patients with impaired liver or renal function, or in elderly or debilitated patients; not recommended for use in pregnancy Most common AEs include drowsiness, fatigue, ataxia, confusion, constipation Pregnancy category: Not specified, but not recommended	SEE alprazolam	

Generic Name and Selected Trade Names	Normal Adult Dosage	Major Adverse Effects/Cautions	Key Counselling Points	Miscellaneous Issues
Diazepam (continued) Valium	Parenteral dosage form available — SEE PI			
Hydroxyzine HCl[1] Atarax Axanil				
Hydroxyzine Pamoate[1] Vistaril				

Generic Name and Selected Trade Names	Normal Adult Dosage	Major Adverse Effects/Cautions	Key Counselling Points	Miscellaneous Issues
Lorazepam Ativan	Individualize dosage <u>For anxiety</u>: Initially, 2 to 3 mg/day given BID or TID; usual maintenance dosage is 2 to 6 mg/day in divided doses; may vary from 1 to 10 mg/day <u>For insomnia due to anxiety of transient situational stress</u>: Usually, 2 to 4 mg at bedtime Dosage adjustments required in elderly and debilitated patients — SEE Prescribing Information (PI) Parenteral dosage form available — SEE PI	<u>Contraindications and considerations</u>: SEE clorazepate dipotassium Most common AEs include sedation, dizziness, weakness, unsteadiness <u>Pregnancy category</u>: SEE clorazepate dipotassium	SEE alprazolam For oral solution, may be diluted with water or soda or semisolid foods	

Generic Name and Selected Trade Names	Normal Adult Dosage	Major Adverse Effects/Cautions	Key Counseling Points	Miscellaneous Issues
Oxazepam Serax	Individualize dosage. For mild to moderate anxiety: Usually, 10 to 15 mg TID or QID. Severe anxiety: Usually, 15 to 30 mg TID or QID. Alcoholics with acute inebriation, tremulousness, or anxiety on withdrawal: Usually, 15 to 30 mg TID or QID. Dosage adjustments required in elderly and debilitated patients — SEE Prescribing Information (PI)	<u>Contraindications</u>: Psychoses; patients under 6 years of age. <u>Considerations</u>: SEE clorazepate dipotassium, also use with caution in patients for which hypotension would be problematic; paradoxical excitement has occurred in psychiatric patients. Most common AEs include headache, vertigo, also SEE lorazepam. <u>Pregnancy category</u>: Not specified	SEE alprazolam	15 mg tablets contain tartrazine

*As a general rule, a medication should not be administered to a patient with a known hypersensitivity to it or a similar agent.
†SEE antihistamines.

427

Table 2: Antidepressants and Agents for Obsessive Compulsive Disorder*,1

Generic Name and Selected Trade Names	Normal Adult Dosage	Major Adverse Effects/Cautions	Key Counselling Points	Miscellaneous Issues
Amitriptyline HCl Elavil	For depression, start with 75 mg/day in divided doses; may increase to 150 mg/day if necessary (usually increase the bedtime dose due to sedative effects); alternative regimens are available — SEE Prescribing Information (PI) Dosage adjustment required in elderly patients — SEE PI Parenteral dosage form available — SEE PI	<u>Contraindications:</u> Co-administration with MAO inhibitors (within 14 days); during the acute recovery phase following a myocardial infarction <u>Considerations:</u> Use with caution in patients with a history of seizures, urinary retention, angle-closure glaucoma, increased intraocular pressure, cardiovascular disorders, thyroid disorders, or impaired liver function; use with caution with other CNS depressants including alcohol	Tell the prescriber if you have any serious medical conditions; do not use if pregnant or breast feeding without speaking first with the prescriber; notify the physician or pharmacist before taking any other medication; avoid alcohol and other agents that may make you drowsy, such as antihistamines or pain killers; this agent may cause some people to become drowsy, dizzy, lightheaded, clumsy or unsteady, make sure you know how you react before driving a car or using machinery; you may experience dry mouth, try sugarless gum or candy or ice chips, if it persists	

Generic Name and Selected Trade Names	Normal Adult Dosage	Major Adverse Effects/Cautions	Key Counseling Points
Amitriptyline HCl (continued) Elavil		Most common AEs include hypotension, syncope, arrhythmias, GI symptoms, anticholinergic effects, sexual dysfunction, increases or decreases in glucose levels, fatigue, headache, insomnia, for a more complete list — SEE Prescribing Information (PI) Pregnancy category: Not specified, but not recommended	check with the prescriber; your skin may be more sensitive to sunlight, avoid the sun and wear protective clothing and sunblock; if you develop convulsions, difficult or rapid breathing, fever with increased sweating, changes in blood pressure, loss of bladder control, severe muscle stiffness, pale skin, or unusual weakness or tiredness contact the prescriber; it may take several weeks before you begin to feel better; it is important that the prescriber checks your progress regularly; take this medication only as directed; do not take more or do not stop taking without consulting the prescriber; may be taken with food; if you are taking only a bedtime dose and you miss a dose, don't take the dose in the morning, instead consult the prescriber; if you are taking more than one dose per day and you miss a dose take it as soon as possible, but if it is almost time for the next dose, skip the missed one — do not double doses

Generic Name and Selected Trade Names	Normal Adult Dosage	Major Adverse Effects/Cautions	Key Counseling Points	Miscellaneous Issues
Bupropion HCl Wellbutrin Wellbutrin SR Zyban	Individualize dosage <u>Wellbutrin for depression</u>: Start with 100 mg BID; if necessary increase to 100 mg TID after at least 3 days of therapy; may increase to a maximum of 450 mg/day, no single dose should exceed 150 mg; dose escalation must be done with caution to avoid adverse effects (eg, seizures) — SEE Prescribing Information (PI)	<u>Contraindications</u>: Seizure disorders, bulimia or anorexia nervosa (higher incidence of seizures), co-administration with a MAO inhibitor <u>Considerations</u>: Use with caution in any patient at risk for seizures (eg, head trauma, CNS tumor); some patients may develop neuropsychiatric signs and symptoms; use with caution in patients with cardiovascular disease; use with caution in patients with pre-existing weight loss Most common AEs include restlessness, anxiety, insomnia, weight loss, dry mouth, headache, nausea/vomiting, constipation, tremor <u>Pregnancy category</u>: B	Tell the prescriber if you have epilepsy, a nervous, mental or emotional condition, or any other medical condition; notify the physician or pharmacist before taking any other medication; avoid alcohol; this agent may cause some people to become drowsy or dizzy, so make sure you know how you react before driving a car or using machinery; if you develop agitation, excitement, anxiety, confusion, fast or irregular heart rate, or trouble sleeping contact the prescriber; it may take several weeks before you begin to feel better; it is important that the prescriber checks your progress regularly;	

Generic Name and Selected Trade Names	Normal Adult Dosage	Major Adverse Effects/Cautions	Key Counseling Points	Miscellaneous Issues
Bupropion HCl (continued) Wellbutrin Wellbutrin SR Zyban	Wellbutrin SR for depression: Start with 150 mg QAM; if necessary increase to 150 mg BID after at least 4 days of therapy, may increase to a maximum of 400 mg/day; dose escalation must be done with caution to avoid adverse effects (eg. seizures) — SEE PI Dosage adjustments required in patients with liver or renal impairment — SEE PI Zyban for smoking cessation: Usually, 150 mg QAM for 3 days; on day four begin 150 mg BID		take this agent only as directed, do not take more and do not stop taking it without consulting the prescriber; may be taken with food if you experience stomach upset; if you miss a dose take it as soon as possible, but if it is within 4 hrs of the net dose skip the missed one and go back to regular schedule — do not double doses	

Generic Name and Selected Trade Names	Normal Adult Dosage	Major Adverse Effects/Cautions	Key Counselling Points	Miscellaneous Issues
Clomipramine HCl Anafranil	For obsessive compulsive disorder, start with 25 mg QD; may increase gradually during the first 2 weeks to 100 mg/day; should be given in divided doses initially; then may increase gradually to a maximum of 250 mg/day and after titration the total dose may be given at bedtime	<u>Contraindications and considerations</u>: SEE amitriptyline HCl Most common AEs include dry mouth, constipation, nausea, anorexia, somnolence, tremor, dizziness, nervousness, myoclonus, sexual dysfunction, sweating, increased appetite, weight gain, visual changes <u>Pregnancy category</u>: C	SEE amitriptyline HCl	

Generic Name and Selected Trade Names	Normal Adult Dosage	Major Adverse Effects/Cautions	Key Counselling Points	Miscellaneous Issues
Desipramine HCl Norpramin	Individualize dosage For depression, start with 100 to 200 mg/day; may increase to 300 mg/day if necessary	SEE amitriptyline HCl	SEE amitriptyline HCl	
Doxepin HCl Sinequan	Individualize dosage For depression, start with 75 mg/day; may be slowly increased up to 300 mg/day if necessary; may be given QD or in divided doses, however, no more than 150 mg should be given as a QD dose; some patients with mild depression respond to 25 to 50 mg/day	Contraindications: SEE amitriptyline HCl, also patients with glaucoma or urinary retention Considerations: Not recommended for use in children under 12; use with caution in elderly patients Most common AEs: SEE amitriptyline HCl Pregnancy category: Not specified	SEE amitriptyline HCl	150 mg tablet is meant for maintenance therapy only and not for the initiation of therapy

Generic Name and Selected Trade Names	Normal Adult Dosage	Major Adverse Effects/Cautions	Key Counselling Points	Miscellaneous Issues
Fluoxetine HCl Prozac	Individualize dosage For depression or obsessive compulsive disorder: Start with 20 mg QAM; may increase after several weeks up to 80 mg/day (QAM or BID) For bulimia nervosa: Start with 60 mg QAM; may be advisable to titrate the dose up to 60 mg over several days Dosage adjustments required in elderly and in patients with liver impairment — SEE Prescribing Information (PI)	Contraindications: Co-administration with an MAO inhibitor (within 14 days) Considerations: Discontinue if rash or other signs of allergy not attributable to another cause occur; use with caution in patients with seizure disorders, with conditions that could affect hemodynamics and metabolism Most common AEs include asthenia, nausea, diarrhea, anorexia, dry mouth, anxiety, insomnia Pregnancy category: C	Tell the prescriber if you have diabetes, kidney or liver disease, or a seizure disorder; notify the physician or pharmacist before taking any other medication; avoid alcohol; this agent may cause some people to become drowsy, so make sure you know how you react before driving a car or using machinery; you may experience dry mouth, try sugarless gum or candy, or ice chips, if it persists check with the prescriber; if you develop skin rash, hives, chills or fever, joint or muscle pain, or trouble breathing contact the prescriber immediately; it may take several weeks before you begin to feel better;	Many drug interactions

Generic Name and Selected Trade Names	Normal Adult Dosage	Major Adverse Effects/Cautions	Key Counselling Points	Miscellaneous Issues
Fluoxetine HCl (continued) Prozac			it is important that the prescriber checks your progress regularly; take this medication only as directed do not take more or do not stop taking without consulting the prescriber; may be taken with food if you experience stomach upset; if you miss a dose skip the missed one and go back to regular schedule — do not double doses	

Generic Name and Selected Trade Names	Normal Adult Dosage	Major Adverse Effects/Cautions	Key Counseling Points	Miscellaneous Issues
Fluvoxamine Maleate Luvox	Individualize dosage For obsessive compulsive disorder, start with 50 mg HS; may increase in 50 mg increments every 4–7 days as tolerated until a maximum therapeutic benefit is achieved, but not to exceed 300 mg/day; total daily doses of greater than 100 mg should be administered BID either as equal doses or the larger dose at bedtime Dosage adjustments required in elderly, debilitated patients, and patients with liver impairment — SEE Prescribing Information (PI)	<u>Contraindications</u>: Co-administration with terfenadine, astemizole, or cisapride <u>Considerations</u>: Avoid in patients receiving (within 14 days) MAO inhibitors; use with caution in patients with seizure disorders; use with caution in patients with conditions that could affect hemodynamics and metabolism Most common AEs include headache, asthenia, abdominal pain, nausea/vomiting, diarrhea, anorexia, somnolence, dizziness, insomnia, tremor, nervousness, dry mouth <u>Pregnancy category</u>: C	SEE fluoxetine HCl	Many drug interactions

Generic Name and Selected Trade Names	Normal Adult Dosage	Major Adverse Effects/Cautions	Key Counseling Points	Miscellaneous Issues
Imipramine HCl Tofranil	Individualize dosage For depression, 25 to 50 mg TID or QID; dosage adjusted based upon patient response; in hospitalized patients 300 mg/day may be required	SEE amitriptyline HCl	SEE amitriptyline HCl	

Generic Name and Selected Trade Names	Normal Adult Dosage	Major Adverse Effects/Cautions	Key Counseling Points	Miscellaneous Issues
Imipramine Pamoate Tofranil-PM	Individualize dosage. For depression, 75 mg/day in divided doses (or HS); may increase to 150 mg/day or 200 mg/day; in hospitalized patients usually start with 100 to 150 mg/day; may increase in a few days to 200 mg/day and then up to 300 mg/day depending upon patient response	SEE amitriptyline HCl	SEE amitriptyline HCl	

Generic Name and Selected Trade Names	Normal Adult Dosage	Major Adverse Effects/Cautions	Key Counseling Points	Miscellaneous Issues
Mirtazapine Remeron	Individualize dosage For depression, start with 15 mg/day as a single dose; may increase dose up to 45 mg/day in 1–2 week intervals Dosage adjustments may be required in elderly and patients with liver or renal impairment — SEE Prescribing Information (PI)	<u>Considerations</u>: Rarely, agranulocytosis has occurred; patients should be monitored for signs of infection (eg, sore throat, fever); do not use within 14 days of receiving an MAO inhibitor; elevations in cholesterol and triglyceride levels have occurred; elevation of liver enzymes have occurred Most common AEs include somnolence, dizziness, increased appetite, weight gain, nausea, asthenia, dry mouth <u>Pregnancy category</u>: C	Tell the prescriber if you are taking an MAO inhibitor or were taking 1 during the last 2 weeks; do not take any other medication without first discussing it with your physician or pharmacist; take this medication only as directed, do not take any more and do not stop without first discussing it with the prescriber; it is important that the prescriber checks your progress regularly; avoid alcohol; this agent may cause some people to become drowsy or dizzy, so make sure you know how you react before driving a car or using machinery;	

Generic Name and Selected Trade Names	Normal Adult Dosage	Major Adverse Effects/Cautions	Key Counselling Points	Miscellaneous Issues
Mirtazapine (continued) Remeron			you may experience dry mouth, try sugarless gum or candy or ice chips, if it persists check with the prescriber; may be taken with or without food; if you miss a dose take it as soon as possible, but if it is almost time for the next dose, skip the missed one — do not double doses	

Generic Name and Selected Trade Names	Normal Adult Dosage	Major Adverse Effects/Cautions	Key Counseling Points	Miscellaneous Issues
Nefazodone HCl Serzone	Individualize dosage For depression, usually start with 200 mg/day in divided doses (BID); may increase dose by 100 to 200 mg/day at intervals of at least 1 week, up to 600 mg/day Dosage adjustments required in elderly or debilitated patients — SEE Prescribing Information (PI)	<u>Contraindications:</u> Co-administration with terfenadine, astemizole, or cisapride <u>Considerations:</u> Avoid co-administration with triazolam or MAO inhibitors; use with caution in patients with cardiovascular or cerebrovascular disorders that could be aggravated by hypotension; priapism has occurred, patients with prolonged or inappropriate erections should seek medical attention Most common AEs include postural hypotension, nausea, dizziness, insomnia, asthenia, agitation, dry mouth, constipation, blurred vision, confusion <u>Pregnancy category:</u> C	SEE mirtazapine	

441

Generic Name and Selected Trade Names	Normal Adult Dosage	Major Adverse Effects/Cautions	Key Counselling Points	Miscellaneous Issues
Nortriptyline HCl Pamelor	Individualize dosage. For depression, usually start with 25 mg TID – QID; should be initiated at low levels and gradually increased; for doses above 100 mg/day plasma levels should be monitored	<u>Contraindications</u>: SEE amitriptyline HCl <u>Considerations</u>: SEE amitriptyline HCl, also not recommended for use in children <u>Most common AEs</u>: SEE amitriptyline HCl <u>Pregnancy category</u>: Not specified	SEE amitriptyline HCl	Many drug interactions are possible — SEE Prescribing Information (PI)

Generic Name and Selected Trade Names	Normal Adult Dosage	Major Adverse Effects/Cautions	Key Counseling Points	Miscellaneous Issues
Paroxetine HCl Paxil	Individualize dosage For depression: Start with 20 mg QAM; may increase in 10 mg/day increments in at least one week intervals up to 50 mg/day For obsessive compulsive disorder: Start with 20 mg QAM; may increase in 10 mg/day increments in at least one week intervals up to 60 mg/day For panic disorder: Start with 10 mg QAM; may increase in 10 mg/day increments in at least one week intervals up to 60 mg/day	Contraindications: SEE fluoxetine HCl Considerations: Use with caution in patients with seizure disorders and use with caution in patients with conditions that could affect hemodynamics and metabolism; hyponatremia has occurred Most common AEs include asthenia, sweating, anorexia, somnolence, dizziness, insomnia, tremor, nervousness, sexual dysfunction, dry mouth, nausea, constipation Pregnancy category: C	Tell the prescriber if you have a history of drug abuse, kidney or liver disease, or a seizure disorder; notify the physician or pharmacist before taking any other medication; avoid alcohol; this agent may cause some people to become drowsy or have blurred vision, so make sure you know how you react before driving a car or using machinery; you may experience dry mouth, try sugarless gum or candy, or ice chips, if it persists check with the prescriber; if you develop skin rash, agitation, lightheadedness or fainting, or muscle pain or weakness contact the prescriber immediately; it may take several weeks before you begin to feel better;	

Generic Name and Selected Trade Names	Normal Adult Dosage	Major Adverse Effects/Cautions	Key Counselling Points	Miscellaneous Issues
Paroxetine HCl (continued) Paxil	Dosage adjustments required in elderly, debilitated patients, and patients with liver or renal dysfunction		it is important that the prescriber checks your progress regularly; take this agent only as directed; do not take more and do not stop taking it without consulting the prescriber; may be taken with or without food; if you miss a dose take it as soon as possible, but if it is almost time for the next dose, skip the missed one and go back to regular schedule — do not double doses	

Generic Name and Selected Trade Names	Normal Adult Dosage	Major Adverse Effects/Cautions	Key Counselling Points	Miscellaneous Issues
Phenelzine Sulfate Nardil	Individualize dosage For depression, initially 15 mg TID; increase to 90 mg/day based upon patient tolerance; after maximum benefit is achieved, dosage should be reduced slowly over several weeks; maintenance dose may be as low as 15 mg QD or QOD	Contraindications: Pheochromocytoma, CHF, history of liver disease or abnormal liver function tests; concomitant use with sympathomimetics (eg, amphetamine, cocaine, epinephrine, L-dopa), meperidine, alcohol, antidepressants, general anesthetics (no elective surgery) Considerations: Blood pressure should be monitored as hypertensive crisis has occurred; use with caution with any antihypertensive medication Most common AEs include dizziness, headache, sleep disturbances, constipation, dry mouth, GI disturbances, weight gain, postural hypotension, edema, sexual disturbances Pregnancy category: Not specified, but not recommended	Tell the prescriber if you have any other medical conditions, it is very important to check with the physician or pharmacist before taking any other medication; certain foods cannot be eaten while receiving this medication, consult the physician or pharmacist; not recommended for use during pregnancy; avoid alcohol; this agent may cause some people to become drowsy or have blurred vision, so make sure you know how you react before driving a car or using machinery; if you develop severe headache, stiff neck, chest pains, fast heartbeat or nausea and vomiting contact the prescriber immediately; it may take several weeks before you begin to feel better;	Many food and drug interactions which can result in fatal reactions are possible — SEE Prescribing Information (PI)

Generic Name and Selected Trade Names	Normal Adult Dosage	Major Adverse Effects/Cautions	Key Counselling Points	Miscellaneous Issues
Phenelzine Sulfate (continued) Nardil			it is important that the prescriber checks your progress regularly; take this medication only as directed do not take more or do not stop taking without consulting the prescriber; may be taken with or without food; if you miss a dose take it as soon as possible, but if it is within 2 hrs of the next dose skip the missed one, return to regular schedule — do not double doses	

Generic Name and Selected Trade Names	Normal Adult Dosage	Major Adverse Effects/Cautions	Key Counseling Points	Miscellaneous Issues
Protriptyline HCl Vivactil	Individualize dosage For depression, start with 15 to 40 mg/day divided into 3–4 doses; may increase to 60 mg/day if necessary	SEE amitriptyline HCl	SEE amitriptyline HCl	
Sertraline Zoloft	Individualize dosage For depression or obsessive compulsive disorder: Usually, 50 mg QD For panic disorder: Start with 25 mg QD; increase after 1 week to 50 mg QD; may increase up to 200 mg/day at 1 week intervals if necessary	Contraindications: SEE fluoxetine HCl Considerations and most common AEs: SEE paroxetine HCl Pregnancy category: C	SEE paroxetine HCl, except consult the prescriber about any missed doses	

Generic Name and Selected Trade Names	Normal Adult Dosage	Major Adverse Effects/Cautions	Key Counselling Points	Miscellaneous Issues
Tranylcypromine Sulfate Parnate	Individualize dosage For depression, start with 30 mg/day in divided doses; if no improvement is seen in 2 weeks may increase in 10 mg/day increments at intervals of 1–3 weeks up to a maximum of 60 mg/day	<u>Contraindications and considerations</u>: SEE phenelzine sulfate <u>Most common AEs</u> include restlessness, insomnia, weakness, drowsiness, dizziness, dry mouth, nausea, diarrhea, abdominal pain, constipation <u>Pregnancy category</u>: Not specified, but not recommended	SEE phenelzine sulfate	SEE phenelzine sulfate

Generic Name and Selected Trade Names	Normal Adult Dosage	Major Adverse Effects/Cautions	Key Counselling Points	Miscellaneous Issues
Trazodone HCl Desyrel	Individualize dosage For depression, start with 150 mg/day in divided doses; may increase by 50 mg/day every 3–4 days; usually not to exceed 400 mg/day for outpatients and 600 mg/day for inpatients	<u>Considerations</u>: Priapism has occurred, male patients with prolonged or inappropriate erections should seek medical attention; not recommended for use in patients recovering from an MI; use with caution in patients with cardiac disease, as hypotension has occurred, antihypertensive medications may require adjustment Most common AEs include blurred vision, constipation, dry mouth, hypotension, syncope, dizziness, fatigue, nervousness, pruritus/rash <u>Pregnancy category</u>: C	Tell the prescriber if you have a history of alcohol abuse, heart, liver or kidney disease; check with the physician or pharmacist before taking any other medication; avoid alcohol; this agent may cause some people to become drowsy, so make sure you know how you react before driving a car or using machinery; you may experience dry mouth, try sugarless gum or candy or ice chips, if it persists check with the prescriber; if you develop confusion or muscle tremors contact the prescriber; for men this agent can cause a prolonged or inappropriate erection of the penis, if this occurs contact the prescriber;	

Generic Name and Selected Trade Names	Normal Adult Dosage	Major Adverse Effects/Cautions	Key Counselling Points	Miscellaneous Issues
Trazodone HCl (continued) Desyrel			it may take several weeks before you begin to feel better; it is important that the prescriber checks your progress regularly; take this medication only as directed; do not take more or do not stop taking without consulting the prescriber; may be taken with food to lessen stomach upset and dizziness; if you miss a dose take it as soon as possible, but if it is within 4 hrs of the next dose, skip the missed one, return to regular schedule — do not double doses	

Generic Name and Selected Trade Names	Normal Adult Dosage	Major Adverse Effects/Cautions	Key Counseling Points	Miscellaneous Issues
Trimipramine Maleate Surmontil	Individualize dosage. For depression, usually start with 75 mg/day in divided doses (or HS); may increase to 150 mg/day; in hospitalized patients usually start with 100 mg/day, may increase in a few days to 200 mg/day, and then up to 300 mg/day depending upon patient response	<u>Contraindications, considerations, and most common AEs:</u> SEE amitriptyline HCl <u>Pregnancy category:</u> C	SEE amitriptyline HCl	

Generic Name and Selected Trade Names	Normal Adult Dosage	Major Adverse Effects/Cautions	Key Counseling Points	Miscellaneous Issues
Venlafaxine HCl Effexor	Individualize dosage For depression, start with 75 mg/day in 2–3 divided doses; may increase to 150 mg/day after at least 4 days if needed; then may further increase to 225 mg/day, severely depressed patients may require up to 375 mg/day Dosage adjustments required in patients with liver or renal dysfunction — SEE Prescribing Information (PI)	<u>Contraindication</u>: Concomitant use with MAO inhibitors (not to begin within 14 days of receiving an MAO inhibitor) <u>Considerations</u>: Blood pressure monitoring is recommended due to increases in blood pressure that have occurred; seizures have occurred (more frequent in patients with seizure disorders); if the agent must be discontinued taper over at least 2 weeks <u>Most common AEs</u> include nausea, anxiety, nervousness, insomnia, anorexia, asthenia, sweating, constipation, somnolence <u>Pregnancy category</u>: C	Tell the prescriber if you have a seizure disorder, hypertension or hypotension, severe liver disease, a history of drug abuse or dependence, or if you are taking an MAO inhibitor or took one within the past 2 weeks; take only as directed, do not take more or stop without first discussing it with the prescriber; do not take any other medication without first discussing it with the physician or pharmacist; avoid alcohol; this medication may cause some people to become drowsy or dizzy, so make sure you know how you react before driving a car or using machinery;	

Generic Name and Selected Trade Names	Normal Adult Dosage	Major Adverse Effects/Cautions	Key Counseling Points	Miscellaneous Issues
Venlafaxine Hcl (continued) Effexor			you may experience dry mouth, try sugarless gum or candy or ice chips; you may need to take this agent for up to 4 weeks before you feel better; take with food unless otherwise directed; if you miss a dose take is as soon as possible, but if it is within 2 hrs of the next dose skip the missed one and go back to regular dosing schedule — do not double doses	

*As a general rule, a medication should not be administered to a patient with a known hypersensitivity to it or a similar agent.
†All patients with depression should be monitored for suicidal tendencies during initiation of therapy.

Table 3: Anti-Manic and Anti-Panic Agents*

Generic Name and Selected Trade Names	Normal Adult Dosage	Major Adverse Effects/Cautions	Key Counselling Points	Miscellaneous Issues
Alprazolam[1] Xanax				
Divalproex Sodium[2] Depakote				

Generic Name and Selected Trade Names	Normal Adult Dosage	Major Adverse Effects/Cautions	Key Counseling Points	Miscellaneous Issues
Clonazepam Klonopin	Individualize dosage For panic disorders: Start with 0.25 mg BID; may increase to 1 mg/day after 3 days; some patients may require higher doses — SEE Prescribing Information (PI) For seizure disorders: Initial dose should not exceed 1.5 mg/day divided into 3 doses; increase in increments of 0.5 to 1 mg every 3 days until seizures are adequately controlled or until adverse effects preclude higher doses; maximum recommended dose is 20 mg/day	Contraindications: Significant liver disease; acute narrow angle glaucoma Considerations: May precipitate seizures in patients with several types of seizure disorders or status epilepticus which also can be precipitated if the agent is abruptly withdrawn; use with caution in patients with renal dysfunction; may produce excess salivation, use with caution in patients with swallowing difficulties; may cause respiratory depression, use with caution in patients with depressed respiration Most common AEs include somnolence, ataxia, behavioral problems, depression, abnormal coordination Pregnancy category: D	Tell the prescriber if you have any serious medical conditions; do not use if pregnant or breast feeding without speaking first with prescriber; notify the physician or pharmacist before taking other medication; avoid alcohol or other agents that may make you drowsy, such as antihistamines or pain killers; this agent may cause some people to become drowsy, dizzy, lightheaded, clumsy or unsteady, so make sure you know how you react before driving a car or using machinery; if you feel this medication is not working properly, do not take more, contact prescriber;	

Generic Name and Selected Trade Names	Normal Adult Dosage	Major Adverse Effects/Cautions	Key Counseling Points	Miscellaneous Issues
Clonazepam (continued) Klonopin			take this medication only as directed do not take more or do not stop taking it without consulting the prescriber, may be habit forming; if you develop any unusual symptoms while on this medication contact the prescriber; if you are taking this medication regularly and miss a dose take it right away if you remember within 1 hr, but if you do not remember until later skip the missed dose and return to regular dosing schedule — do not double doses	

Generic Name and Selected Trade Names	Normal Adult Dosage	Major Adverse Effects/Cautions	Key Counselling Points	Miscellaneous Issues
Lithium Carbonate Eskalith Eskalith CR Lithobid Lithonate Lithotabs	Individualize dosage according to serum levels and individual response For acute control of mania, usually 1800 mg/day in divided doses; usual maintenance dose is 900 to 1200 mg per day in divided doses — SEE Prescribing Information (PI) Immediate release products are generally given TID or QID and controlled release products are given BID	Considerations: Use with caution in patients with cardiovascular or renal disease, or patients with severe debilitation, dehydration or sodium depletion; chronic therapy may decrease renal concentrating ability and patients may occasionally present with nephrogenic diabetes insipidus; renal function and lithium levels should be monitored during therapy; co-administration with neuroleptics has resulted in an encephalopathic syndrome; use with caution in patients receiving diuretics Most common AEs include fine hand tremor, polyuria, mild thirst, diarrhea, vomiting, drowsiness, muscular weakness, lack of coordination Pregnancy category: Not specified	Tell the prescriber if you have any medical conditions; check with the physician or pharmacist before taking any other medication; may cause some people to become dizzy or drowsy, so make sure you know how you react before driving a car or using machinery; contact the prescriber if you develop diarrhea, vomiting, tremor, mild ataxia, drowsiness or muscular weakness; be cautious in hot weather, as excess fluid and salt loss can lead to serious adverse effects; do not go on a diet or make any changes to your diet without consulting with the prescriber; it is important that the prescriber checks your progress regularly, take as directed;	Many drug interactions are possible — SEE Prescribing Information (PI); to switch patients between immediate and controlled release preparations — SEE PI

Generic Name and Selected Trade Names	Normal Adult Dosage	Major Adverse Effects/Cautions	Key Counseling Points	Miscellaneous Issues
Lithium Carbonate (continued) Eskalith Eskalith CR Lithobid Lithonate Lithotabs			may take several weeks before you begin to feel better; may be taken after a meal or snack; drink 2 or 3 quarts of water or other fluids (not caffeinated beverages) every day and use a normal amount of salt in your food unless otherwise directed by the prescriber; if you miss a dose take it as soon as possible, but if it is within 4 hrs (6 hrs for extended release products) of the next dose, skip the missed one, return to regular schedule — do not double doses For slow release dosage forms, swallow whole, do not break, crush, or chew; for syrup dilute in fruit juice or another flavored beverage	

Generic Name and Selected Trade Names	Normal Adult Dosage	Major Adverse Effects/Cautions	Key Counseling Points	Miscellaneous Issues
Paroxetine HCl[3] Paxil				
Sertraline[3] Zoloft				

*As a general rule, a medication should not be administered to a patient with a known hypersensitivity to it or a similar agent.

[1]SEE antianxiety agents.
[2]SEE antiepileptics.
[3]SEE antidepressants.

Table 4: Antipsychotics*

Generic Name and Selected Trade Names	Normal Adult Dosage	Major Adverse Effects/Cautions	Key Counseling Points	Miscellaneous Issues
Chlorpromazine Thorazine	Individualize dosage <u>For psychotic disorders:</u> Dosage is increased gradually until symptoms are controlled; optimal dosage is continued for 2 weeks, then gradually reduce to the lowest effective maintenance level; dosages of 200 to 800 mg/day are not unusual <u>Intramuscular for acutely disturbed patients:</u> 25 mg; if necessary give 25 to 50 mg in 1 hr, doses may be increased over the next several days — SEE Prescribing Information (PI)	<u>Contraindications:</u> Severe CNS depression or comatose patients <u>Considerations:</u> Avoid in children and adolescents whose signs and symptoms suggest Reye's syndrome; tardive dyskinesia can occur with chronic therapy; neuroleptic malignant syndrome (hyperpyrexia, rigidity, catonia) can occur and has been fatal; use with caution in patients at risk for seizures; elevations in prolactin levels can occur; can inhibit the vomiting reflex which can mask drug overdoses, other disorders, and adverse effects of agents such as chemotherapeutics; use with caution in patients with cardiovascular, liver or renal disease	Tell the prescriber if you have any medical conditions; check with the physician or pharmacist before taking any other medication; avoid alcohol or other agents that may make you drowsy such as antihistamines or pain killers; this agent may cause some people to become drowsy, so make sure you know how you react before driving a car or using machinery; your skin may be more sensitive to sunlight while receiving this medication, so avoid sunlight and wear protective clothing and sunblock, also wear sunglasses to protect your eyes; you may experience dry mouth, try sugarless gum or candy, or ice chips.	

Generic Name and Selected Trade Names	Normal Adult Dosage	Major Adverse Effects/Cautions	Key Counselling Points	Miscellaneous Issues
Chlorpromazine (continued) Thorazine	Oral for nausea/vomiting: 10 to 25 mg Q4–6H as needed Intramuscular for nausea/vomiting: 25 mg; if no hypotension occurs, 25 to 50 mg Q3–4H may be given until vomiting stops; then switch to oral dosage form Suppositories for nausea/vomiting: 100 mg Q6–8H as needed; some patients may require less Oral for intractable hiccups: 25 to 50 mg TID or QID; if symptoms persist IM or IV therapy may be warranted — SEE PI	Most common AEs include drowsiness, jaundice, hematologic disorders, postural hypotension, tachycardia, ECG changes, extrapyramidal symptoms (Parkinson's-like syndrome, dystonias, akathisia), behavioral changes, urticaria and photo-sensitivity, for a more complete list — SEE Prescribing Information (PI) Pregnancy category: Not specified	if it persists check with the prescriber; be careful not to become overheated, as this agent my impair your ability to sweat; take this medication only as directed; do not take more or do not stop taking it without consulting the prescriber; if you develop any unusual symptoms such as lip smacking or puckering of the lips or uncontrolled movements while on this medication contact the prescriber; it is important for the prescriber to check your progress regularly; may be taken with food or a full glass of water or milk; if you miss a dose and you are taking one dose a day, take the missed dose as soon as possible, but if you do not remember until the next day skip the missed one,	

Generic Name and Selected Trade Names	Normal Adult Dosage	Major Adverse Effects/Cautions	Key Counseling Points	Miscellaneous Issues
Chlorpro-mazine (continued) Thorazine	Oral for acute intermittent porphyria: 25 to 50 mg TID or QID Intramuscular for acute intermittent porphyria: 25 mg TID or QID until patient can take oral Intramuscular for tetanus: 25 to 50 mg TID or QID in conjunction with barbiturates; dose determined by patient's response		if you are taking more than one dose a day and you remember within an hour or so take the missed dose but if you do not remember until later skip the missed dose and return to regular schedule — do not double doses For extended release capsules, swallow whole do not break, crush, or chew; for suppositories ensure patient knows proper administration technique (eg, remove foil, moisten suppository with cold water, lie on side, insert, retain until medication dissolves); for IM dosage form, if patient or caregiver is administering, ensure he/she is familiar with proper aseptic injection technique	

Generic Name and Selected Trade Names	Normal Adult Dosage	Major Adverse Effects/Cautions	Key Counselling Points	Miscellaneous Issues
Clozapine Clozaril	Individualize dosage according to individual response; monitoring of CBCs is required. For psychosis, start with 12.5 mg QD or BID; may increase daily in increments of 25 to 50 mg/day if well tolerated to a target dose of 300 to 450 mg/day by the end of 2 weeks; subsequent increases should be made 1-2 times per week in increments of no more than 100 mg	Contraindications: Myeloproliferative disorders, uncontrolled epilepsy, history of clozapine-induced agranulocytosis, severe CNS depression or comatose patients; co-administration with other myelosuppressive agents. Considerations: Due to the potential for life-threatening bone marrow suppression, this agent is reserved for use in patients unresponsive to or unable to tolerate other agents; patients must have blood counts monitored before and throughout therapy; serious adverse reactions such as bone marrow suppression seizures, hyperglycemia, and orthostatic hypotension have occurred; for a more complete list — SEE Prescribing Information (PI)	Tell the prescriber if the patient has any of the conditions listed under "contraindications"; ensure patient has read the patient information leaflet supplied by the manufacturer and is aware of the importance of regular monitoring of CBC	Available only through a distribution system that ensures adequate monitoring of the patient

463

Generic Name and Selected Trade Names	Normal Adult Dosage	Major Adverse Effects/Cautions	Key Counselling Points	Miscellaneous Issues
Clozapine (continued) Clozaril		Most common AEs include sedation, dizziness, tachycardia, hypotension, nausea/vomiting, fever, hematologic changes <u>Pregnancy category</u>: B		

Generic Name and Selected Trade Names	Normal Adult Dosage	Major Adverse Effects/Cautions	Key Counseling Points	Miscellaneous Issues
Haloperidol Haldol	Individualize dosage For psychosis, usual range 0.5 to 5.0 mg BID or TID, depending upon the severity of symptoms; IM administration may be utilized for acute management — SEE Prescribing Information (PI)	<u>Contraindications</u>: Parkinson's disease or patients with severe CNS depression or those in a coma <u>Considerations</u>: Tardive dyskinesia may occur with chronic therapy; neuroleptic malignant syndrome (hyperpyrexia, rigidity, catonia) may occur and has been fatal; bronchopneumonia has occurred; use with caution in patients with cardiovascular disorders, patients receiving anticonvulsant or anticoagulant; prolactin levels will increase so use caution in patients with a history or breast cancer Most common AEs include extrapyramidal syndrome (Parkinson's-like syndrome, dystonias, akathisia), insomnia, restlessness, anorexia, constipation <u>Pregnancy category</u>: C	SEE chlorpromazine except for missed dose take as soon as possible then take any remaining doses for that day at regularly spaced intervals — do not double doses For depot injection, effects last up to 6 weeks, so the considerations noted apply during this entire time	For liquid, should be mixed with water, juice, or cola, but do not mix with tea or coffee

Generic Name and Selected Trade Names	Normal Adult Dosage	Major Adverse Effects/Cautions	Key Counselling Points	Miscellaneous Issues
Mesoridazine Besylate Serentil	Individualize dosage For schizophrenia: Start with 50 mg TID; usual optimal dose is 100 to 400 mg/day For behavioral problems in mental deficiency and chronic brain syndrome: Start with 25 mg TID; usual optimal dose is 75 to 300 mg/day For alcoholism: Start with 25 mg BID; usual optimal dose is 50 to 200 mg/day For psychoneurotic manifestations: Start with 10 mg TID; usual optimal dose is 30 to 150 mg/day	<u>Contraindications</u>: Patients in a comatose state or in the presence of large amounts of CNS depressants <u>Considerations</u>: Tardive dyskinesia may occur with chronic therapy; neuroleptic malignant syndrome (hyperpyrexia, rigidity, catonia) may occur and has been fatal; use with caution in patients at risk for seizures; elevations in prolactin levels may occur Most common AEs include drowsiness, hypotension, tachycardia, extrapyramidal symptoms (eg, Parkinson's-like syndrome, dystonias, akathisia), dry mouth, impotence, dizziness, rash <u>Pregnancy category</u>: Not specified	SEE chlorpromazine	

Generic Name and Selected Trade Names	Normal Adult Dosage	Major Adverse Effects/Cautions	Key Counselling Points	Miscellaneous Issues
Mesoridazine Besylate (continued) Serentil	Parenteral dosage form available — SEE Prescribing Information (PI)			

Generic Name and Selected Trade Names	Normal Adult Dosage	Major Adverse Effects/Cautions	Key Counselling Points	Miscellaneous Issues
Olanzapine Zyprexa	Individualize dosage For psychosis, start with 5 to 10 mg QD; titrate to target dose of 10 mg within several days; may increase or decrease by 5 mg QD if necessary at 1 week intervals	<u>Considerations:</u> Tardive dyskinesia may occur with chronic therapy; neuroleptic malignant syndrome (eg, hyperpyrexia, rigidity, catonia); orthostatic hypotension may be lessened by initiating therapy with lower doses (consider in elderly, debilitated, renal, hepatic or cardiovascular patients); use with caution in patients with a history of seizures; elevations in prolactin levels may occur; use with caution in patients with diseases that affect hemodynamics or metabolism <u>Most common AEs include</u> constipation, weight gain, dizziness, behavioral changes, asthenia, dry mouth, sedation, tremor, extrapyramidal symptoms <u>Pregnancy category:</u> C	Tell the prescriber if you have kidney, liver or cardiovascular disease or a history of seizures; check with the physician or pharmacist before taking any other medication; avoid alcohol or other agents that may make you drowsy such as antihistamines or pain killers; this agent may cause some people to become drowsy, so make sure you know how you react before driving a car or using machinery; be careful not to become overheated, as this agent my impair your ability to sweat; take this medication only as directed; do not take more or do not stop taking it without consulting the prescriber; may be given without regard to meals;	

Generic Name and Selected Trade Names	Normal Adult Dosage	Major Adverse Effects/Cautions	Key Counseling Points	Miscellaneous Issues
Olanzapine (continued) Zyprexa			if you miss a dose take it as soon as possible, but if it is almost time for the next dose, skip the missed one — do not double doses	

Generic Name and Selected Trade Names	Normal Adult Dosage	Major Adverse Effects/Cautions	Key Counseling Points	Miscellaneous Issues
Perphenazine Trilafon	Individualize dosage For moderately disturbed non-hospitalized psychotic patients: Start with 4 to 8 mg TID; reduce to minimum effective dose as soon as possible For hospitalized psychotic patients: 8 to 16 mg BID – QID; avoid daily doses over 64 mg For severe nausea/vomiting: 8 to 16 mg daily in divided doses Parenteral dosage form available for acute situations — SEE Prescribing Information (PI)	Contraindications: SEE chlorpromazine and presence of existing blood dyscrasias, bone marrow depression, or liver damage, patients with subcortical brain damage Considerations: SEE mesoridazine besylate and not recommended for use in children under 12 years of age; liver damage, corneal and lenticular deposits have occurred; photosensitivity may occur Most common AEs: SEE chlorpromazine Pregnancy category: Not specified	SEE chlorpromazine, except information regarding suppositories and extended release preparations does not apply	Injectable form contains sodium bisulfite, which may cause an allergic reaction in some patients Liquid concentrate dosage form should be diluted with water, saline, Seven-Up, homogenized milk, carbonated orange drink, pineapple, apricot, prune, orange, V-8, tomato or grapefruit juices, use 2 ounces for every teaspoonful of concentrate

Generic Name and Selected Trade Names	Normal Adult Dosage	Major Adverse Effects/Cautions	Key Counseling Points	Miscellaneous Issues
Pimozide Orap	Individualize dosage For control of tics in Tourette's syndrome, start with 1 to 2 mg per day in divided doses; may increase every other day up to 0.2 mg/kg/day or 10 mg/day whichever is less; periodic attempts at dosage reduction should be made	Contraindications: Treatment of simple tics or tics other than those associated with Tourette's syndrome; co-administration with agents that produce motor and phonic tics (eg, pemoline, methylphenidate); congenital QT prolongation; patients with a history of arrhythmias or on other agents that prolong QT interval; patients with severe CNS depression or in a coma; co-administration with macrolide antibiotics Considerations: Tardive dyskinesia can occur with chronic therapy; neuroleptic malignant syndrome (hyperpyrexia, rigidity, catonia) may occur and has been fatal; use with caution in patients at risk for seizures; ECG should be performed prior to initiation and during therapy; use with caution in patients with liver or kidney dysfunction	Tell the prescriber if patient has any of the conditions listed under contraindications or a history of breast cancer; check with the physician or pharmacist before taking any other medication; avoid alcohol or other agents that may make you drowsy such as antihistamines or pain killers; this agent may cause some people to become drowsy, so make sure you know how you react before driving a car or operating machinery; you may experience dry mouth, try sugarless gum or candy or ice chips, if it persists check with the prescriber; if you develop convulsions, difficult or fast breathing, fast or irregular heartbeat, fever, change in blood pressure, increased sweating.	

Generic Name and Selected Trade Names	Normal Adult Dosage	Major Adverse Effects/Cautions	Key Counseling Points	Miscellaneous Issues
Pimozide (continued) Orap		Most common AEs include extrapyramidal syndrome, ECG changes, dry mouth, sedation, behavioral changes, visual disturbances, impotence, asthenia, headache Pregnancy category: C	loss of bladder control, muscle stiffness, tiredness or weakness, or unusually pale skin contact the prescriber; take as directed, do not take it more often or stop taking it without consulting the prescriber; the prescriber must check your progress, as the amount of medication that controls your condition may change; if you miss a dose take it as soon as possible then take any remaining doses for that day at regularly spaced intervals — do not double doses	

Generic Name and Selected Trade Names	Normal Adult Dosage	Major Adverse Effects/Cautions	Key Counseling Points	Miscellaneous Issues
Prochlorperazine Compazine	Individualize dosage Tablets for severe nausea/vomiting: 5 or 10 mg TID to QID Spansules for severe nausea/vomiting: 15 mg on arising or 10 mg Q12H Suppositories for severe nausea/vomiting: 25 mg BID Intramuscular for severe nausea/vomiting: Start with 5 to 10 mg injected deeply into upper outer quadrant of the buttock; if necessary repeat Q3–4H; total should not exceed 40 mg/day	Contraindications: Patients in a comatose state or in the presence of large amounts of CNS depressants, pediatric surgery, patients under 2 years of age or 20 pounds, children for conditions in which dosages have not been established Considerations: Avoid in children and adolescents whose signs and symptoms suggest Reye's syndrome; tardive dyskinesia may occur with chronic therapy; a neuroleptic malignant syndrome (hyperpyrexia, rigidity, catonia) may occur and has been fatal; use with caution in patients at risk for seizures; elevations in prolactin levels may occur; can inhibit the vomiting reflex which can mask drug overdoses, other disorders, and adverse effects of agents such as chemotherapeutics	SEE chlorpromazine	Subcutaneous administration is not advised due to local irritation

Generic Name and Selected Trade Names	Normal Adult Dosage	Major Adverse Effects/Cautions	Miscellaneous Issues
Prochlorperazine (continued) Compazine	Tablets for non-psychotic anxiety: 5 mg TID or QID; do not administer in doses of more than 20 mg/day for longer than 12 weeks Spansules for non-psychotic anxiety: 15 mg on arising or 10 mg Q12H; do not administer in doses of more than 20 mg/day for longer than 12 weeks For mild psychotic disorders: 5 or 10 mg TID or QID For moderate to severe psychotic disorders: Start with 10 mg TID or QID; may increase gradually every 2–3 days to limit adverse effects up to 50 to 75 mg/day; some patients may require 100 to 150 mg/day Intramuscular for immediate control of severely disturbed patients: 10 to 20 mg injected deeply into the upper outer quadrant of the buttock; may be repeated every 2–4 hrs if necessary	Most common AEs include drowsiness, amenorrhea, blurred vision, skin reactions, hypotension, cholestatic jaundice, leukopenia and agranulocytosis, extra-pyramidal symptoms (eg, Parkinson's-like syndrome, dystonias, akathisia), for a more complete list — SEE Prescribing Information (PI) Pregnancy category: Not specified	

Generic Name and Selected Trade Names	Normal Adult Dosage	Major Adverse Effects/Cautions	Key Counselling Points	Miscellaneous Issues
Risperidone Risperdal	Individualize dosage For psychosis, initial dose should be 1 mg BID; may increase in increments of 1 mg BID on the 2nd and 3rd day as tolerated, to a target dose of 3 mg BID by the 3rd day; further adjustments of 1 mg BID may be made at 1 week intervals; usual maintenance dosage is 4 to 16 mg/day; for patients at risk for orthostatic hypotension begin with 0.5 mg BID — SEE Prescribing Information (PI)	Considerations: Tardive dyskinesia may occur with chronic therapy; a neuroleptic malignant syndrome (hyperpyrexia, rigidity, catonia) may occur and has been fatal; may prolong the QT interval; orthostatic hypotension may be lessened by initiating with lower doses (consider in elderly, debilitated, renal, hepatic or cardiovascular patients), use with caution in patients with a history of seizures and in patients with diseases that affect hemodynamics or metabolism; elevations in prolactin levels may occur Most common AEs include dyspepsia, rhinitis, rash, extrapyramidal symptoms Pregnancy category: C	Tell the prescriber if you have any other medical conditions; check with the physician or pharmacist before taking any other medication; avoid alcohol or other agents that may make you drowsy such as antihistamines or pain killers; this agent may cause some people to become drowsy, so make sure you know how you react before driving a car or using machinery; your skin may be more sensitive to sunlight while receiving this medication, so avoid sunlight and wear protective clothing and sunblock, also wear sunglasses to protect your eyes; you may experience dry mouth, try sugarless gum or candy or ice chips, if it persists check with the prescriber;	

Generic Name and Selected Trade Names	Normal Adult Dosage	Major Adverse Effects/Cautions	Key Counselling Points
Risperidone (continued) Risperdal			be careful not to become overheated, as this agent my impair your ability to sweat; if you develop convulsions, difficult or fast breathing, fast or irregular heartbeat, fever, change in blood pressure, increased sweating, loss of bladder control, muscle stiffness, tiredness or weakness, or unusually pale skin contact the prescriber; if you develop any unusual symptoms such as lip smacking or puckering of the lips or uncontrolled movements while on this medication contact the prescriber; take this medication only as directed; it is important for the prescriber to check your progress regularly; do not stop taking this medication without first speaking with the prescriber; if you miss a dose take it as soon as possible, but if it is almost time for the next dose, skip the missed one and return to regular schedule — do not double doses

Generic Name and Selected Trade Names	Normal Adult Dosage	Major Adverse Effects/Cautions	Key Counselling Points	Miscellaneous Issues
Thiothixene Navane	Individualize dosage. For psychosis, start with 2 mg TID in mild conditions and 5 mg BID in more severe conditions; may increase to 15 to 60 mg/day depending upon the patient's condition and response	<u>Contraindications</u>: Patients with CNS depression, a blood dyscrasia, circulatory collapse or in a coma; children under 12 years of age <u>Considerations</u>: Tardive dyskinesia may occur with chronic therapy; a neuroleptic malignant syndrome (eg, hyperpyrexia, rigidity, catonia) may occur and has been fatal; use with caution in patients at risk for seizures; pigmentary retinopathy, lenticular pigmentation, blood dyscrasias and liver toxicity have occurred	SEE chlorpromazine except for missed dose take as soon as possible, but if it is within 2 hrs of the next dose, skip the missed dose, return to regular schedule — do not double doses and information regarding suppositories does not apply	For oral solution, may be diluted in water, milk, tomato or fruit juice, soup, or carbonated beverages

Generic Name and Selected Trade Names	Normal Adult Dosage	Major Adverse Effects/Cautions	Key Counseling Points	Miscellaneous Issues
Thiothixene (continued) Navane		Most common AEs include tachycardia, hypotension, dizziness, drowsiness, restlessness, extrapyramidal symptoms, rash, pruritus, dry mouth, blurred vision, nasal congestion, constipation, anorexia, nausea/vomiting <u>Pregnancy category</u>: Not specified		

Generic Name and Selected Trade Names	Normal Adult Dosage	Major Adverse Effects/Cautions	Key Counselling Points	Miscellaneous Issues
Trifluoperazine HCl Stelazine	Individualize dosage For non-psychotic anxiety: Usually, 1 to 2 mg BID; do not administer doses of more than 6 mg/day or for longer than 12 weeks For psychotic disorders: Start with 2 to 5 mg BID; usual optimal dosage is 15 to 20 mg/day; some patients may require 40 mg/day Intramuscular for prompt control: 1 to 2 mg by deep injection Q4–6H as needed	<u>Contraindications</u>: Comatose patients; patients with CNS depression, blood dyscrasias, bone marrow depression, or pre-existing liver damage <u>Considerations</u>: SEE mesoridazine besylate Most common AEs include drowsiness, dizziness, skin reactions, rash, dry mouth, insomnia, amenorrhea, fatigue, muscular weakness, anorexia, lactation, blurred vision, extrapyramidal reactions <u>Pregnancy category</u>: Not specified	SEE chlorpromazine; information regarding suppositories does not apply	For liquid concentrate dosage form dilute in 60 ml tomato or fruit juice, milk, simple syrup, orange syrup, carbonated beverages, coffee, tea or water, or semisolid foods, and then drink immediately

*As a general rule, a medication should not be administered to a patient with a known hypersensitivity to it or a similar agent.

Table 5: Sedative Hypnotics*

Generic Name and Selected Trade Names	Normal Adult Dosage	Major Adverse Effects/Cautions	Key Counselling Points	Miscellaneous Issues
Estazolam Prosom	For insomnia, start with 1 mg at bedtime; some patients may require 2 mg, while others (eg, elderly/debilitated) may respond to 0.5 mg. Dosage adjustments may be required; limit dosage in elderly and debilitated patients — SEE Prescribing Information (PI)	<u>Contraindication</u>: Pregnancy <u>Considerations</u>: Risk of dependence and withdrawal reactions, agent should not be discontinued abruptly; use caution with other CNS depressants, in patients with impaired renal, hepatic or respiratory function; use with caution in depressed patients or patients at risk for suicide; not recommended for use in patients under 18 years of age. Most common AEs include dizziness, drowsiness, impaired coordination. <u>Pregnancy category</u>: X	Tell the prescriber if you have any serious medical conditions; do not use if pregnant or breast feeding; notify the physician or pharmacist before taking other medication; avoid alcohol or other agents that may make you drowsy, such as antihistamines or pain killers; this agent may cause some people to become drowsy, dizzy, lightheaded, clumsy or unsteady, so make sure you know how you react before driving a car or operating machinery; if you feel this medication is not working properly, do not take more, contact prescriber; take this medication only as directed;	

Generic Name and Selected Trade Names	Normal Adult Dosage	Major Adverse Effects/Cautions	Key Counseling Points	Miscellaneous Issues
Estazolam (continued) Prosom			it may be habit forming; if you develop any unusual symptoms while on this medication contact the prescriber; should be taken prior to bedtime	
Flurazepam HCl Dalmane	Individualize dosage For sedation, usually 30 mg at bedtime; 15 mg may suffice in some patients Dosage adjustments required in elderly and debilitated patients — SEE Prescribing Information (PI)	<u>Contraindication</u>: Pregnancy <u>Considerations</u>: SEE estazolam and not recommended for use in children under 15 years of age Most common AEs include dizziness, drowsiness, impaired coordination, headache, heartburn, nausea/vomiting, diarrhea, constipation <u>Pregnancy category</u>: Not specified	SEE estazolam	

Generic Name and Selected Trade Names	Normal Adult Dosage	Major Adverse Effects/Cautions	Key Counseling Points	Miscellaneous Issues
Lorazepam[1] Ativan				
Phenobarbital[2]				

Generic Name and Selected Trade Names	Normal Adult Dosage	Major Adverse Effects/Cautions	Key Counseling Points	Miscellaneous Issues
Promethazine HCl Phenergan	Individualize dosage For sedation: Administer 25 to 50 mg at bedtime For allergy: Usual oral dose is 25 mg taken at bedtime; 12.5 mg may be taken before meals and at bedtime if necessary; suppositories may be used if the oral route is not feasible For motion sickness: Start with 25 mg taken 30–60 min before travel and repeated 8–12 hrs later if necessary; on succeeding days of travel 25 mg can be taken on arising and before the evening meal	Contraindications: Not for treatment of lower respiratory tract symptoms including asthma Considerations: Additive CNS depression may occur if combined with alcohol or other agents; use with caution in patients with seizure disorders or in combination with other agents that lower seizure threshold, patients with narrow-angle glaucoma, stenosing peptic ulcer, pyloroduodenal obstruction, prostatic hypertrophy, cardiovascular diseases or liver dysfunction; has produced cholestatic jaundice; may produce photosensitivity and involuntary movements; avoid in patients with a history of sleep apnea	Tell the prescriber if you have any other medical conditions; check with the physician or pharmacist before taking any other medication; avoid alcohol or other agents that may make you drowsy; this agent may cause some people to become drowsy, so make sure you know how you react before driving a car or using machinery; you may experience dry mouth, try sugarless gum or candy or ice chips; take this medication only as directed; if you develop a sore throat and fever, unusual bleeding or easy bruising, or unusual tiredness or weakness while on this medication contact the prescriber;	

483

Generic Name and Selected Trade Names	Normal Adult Dosage	Major Adverse Effects/Cautions	Key Counseling Points	Miscellaneous Issues
Promethazine HCl (continued) Phenergan	For nausea/vomiting: Usual dose is 25 mg, 12.5 to 25 mg may be repeated as necessary every 4–6 hrs; if oral cannot be tolerated parenteral or rectal routes may be used Parenteral dosage form available — SEE Prescribing Information (PI)	Most common AEs include sedation, blurred vision, dry mouth, dizziness, changes in blood pressure, rash, nausea/vomiting <u>Pregnancy category</u>: C	If you are taking this medication regularly and you miss a dose, take it as soon as possible, if it is almost time for the next dose, skip the missed one, return to regular schedule — do not double doses For suppositories, ensure patient knows proper administration technique (eg, remove foil, moisten suppository with cold water, lie on side, and insert)	

Generic Name and Selected Trade Names	Normal Adult Dosage	Major Adverse Effects/Cautions	Key Counseling Points	Miscellaneous Issues
Quazepam Doral	Individualize dosage For insomnia, start with 15 mg until individual response is determined; some patients may respond to 7.5 mg	<u>Contraindications</u>: SEE flurazepam HCl <u>Considerations</u>: SEE flurazepam HCl, except not recommended for use in patients under 18 years of age Most common AEs include drowsiness, headache, dizziness <u>Pregnancy category</u>: X	SEE estazolam	

Generic Name and Selected Trade Names	Normal Adult Dosage	Major Adverse Effects/Cautions	Key Counseling Points	Miscellaneous Issues
Secobarbital Sodium Seconal	Individualize dosage For sedation, usually 100 mg at bedtime Dosage adjustments required in elderly, debilitated patients, and patients with impaired renal or liver function — SEE Prescribing Information (PI)	<u>Contraindications</u>: Porphyria, marked respiratory depression or liver impairment <u>Considerations</u>: Tolerance, psychological, and physical dependence may occur; paradoxical excitement can occur in patients with pain; potentially hazardous to fetal development <u>Most common AEs</u> include drowsiness, lethargy, vertigo, altered behavior, enhanced sensitivity to pain, nausea/vomiting, constipation <u>Pregnancy category</u>: D	Tell the prescriber if you have any other medical problems; check with the physician or pharmacist before taking any other medication; if you are pregnant or plan on becoming pregnant, discuss this with your physician; this agent may cause drowsiness, vision problems or dizziness, so be cautious when driving or using machinery; may be habit forming; if you develop sores on the lips or mouth, chest pain, fever, muscle or joint pain, changes in your skin including rash, sore throat, fever, swelling of eyelids, face, or lips, difficulty breathing contact the prescriber; take the medication as directed at bedtime	

Generic Name and Selected Trade Names	Normal Adult Dosage	Major Adverse Effects/Cautions	Key Counseling Points	Miscellaneous Issues
Temazepam Restoril	Individualize dosage For insomnia, most patients respond to 15 mg at bedtime; some patients may require 30 mg, while others may respond to 7.5 mg Dosage adjustments required in elderly and debilitated patients — SEE Prescribing Information (PI)	<u>Contraindications</u>: SEE estazolam <u>Considerations</u>: Treatment of sleep disturbances must be done cautiously as they can be manifestation of a physical or psychiatric disorder; if increased daytime anxiety occurs (may be interdose withdrawal) agent should be discontinued; abnormal thinking and behavior have occurred; amnesia may occur if an adequate amount of sleep time is not allowed; use caution in patients with depression <u>Most common AEs</u> include drowsiness, dizziness <u>Pregnancy category</u>: X	SEE estazolam	

Generic Name and Selected Trade Names	Normal Adult Dosage	Major Adverse Effects/Cautions	Key Counselling Points	Miscellaneous Issues
Triazolam Halcion	Individualize dosage For insomnia, usually 0.25 mg at bedtime; some patients may respond to 0.125 mg; rarely patients may require 0.5 mg, but this has been associated with an increased incidence of adverse effects and therefore should be done with caution	Contraindications: SEE flurazepam and co-administration with ketoconazole, itraconazole, and nefazodone, agents that impair metabolism via the cytochrome P450 3A system Considerations: SEE temazepam Most common AEs include drowsiness, dizziness, ataxia, nausea/vomiting Pregnancy category: X	SEE estazolam	Many drug interactions are possible — SEE Prescribing Information (PI)

Generic Name and Selected Trade Names	Normal Adult Dosage	Major Adverse Effects/Cautions	Key Counseling Points	Miscellaneous Issues
Zolpidem Tartrate Ambien	Individualize dosage For insomnia, 10 mg immediately at bedtime Dosage adjustments may be required in elderly patients — SEE Prescribing Information (PI)	Considerations: Treatment of sleep disturbances must be done cautiously as they can be manifestation of a physical or psychiatric disorder; abnormal thinking and behaviors should be evaluated; due to rapid onset of action agent should be ingested only immediately prior to bedtime; use with caution in depressed patients, with other CNS depressants, and in patients with diseases that affect hemodynamics or metabolism Most common AEs include drowsiness, dizziness, headache, nausea/vomiting, amnesia Pregnancy category: B	Tell the prescriber if you have a history of alcohol or drug abuse or dependence, sleep apnea, mental depression, or respiratory, kidney, or liver disease; check with the physician or pharmacist before taking any other medication; do not use if pregnant without first discussing with prescriber; this agent may cause drowsiness, vision problems or dizziness, so be cautious when driving or using machinery; if you develop clumsiness or confusion contact the prescriber;	

489

Generic Name and Selected Trade Names	Normal Adult Dosage	Major Adverse Effects/Cautions	Key Counselling Points	Miscellaneous Issues
Zolpidem Tartrate (continued) Ambien			take this medication just before going to bed as it works very quickly; do not take this medication unless your schedule allows for a full night's sleep; may be taken with or without food	

*As a general rule, a medication should not be administered to a patient with a known hypersensitivity to it or a similar agent.
[1]SEE antianxiety agents.
[2]SEE antiepileptics.

Antiparkinsonian Agents

Table: Antiparkinsonian Agents*

Generic Name and Selected Trade Names	Normal Adult Dosage	Major Adverse Effects/Cautions	Key Counseling Points	Miscellaneous Issues
Amantadine HCl Symadine Symmetrel	Individualize dosage For Parkinson's disease: Usually, 100 mg BID; in patients receiving high doses of other antiparkinsonian agents or with other serious medical conditions, 100 mg daily may be sufficient For drug-induced EPS: 100 mg BID For influenza treatment or prophylaxis: 200 mg QD or 100 mg BID Dosage may need to be adjusted in persons with renal impairment — SEE Prescribing Information (PI)	Considerations: Can exacerbate mental problems and suicide attempts have occurred; use with caution in patients with epilepsy, CHF, edema, or renal impairment; geriatric patients may be sensitive to the anticholinergic effects Most common AEs include nausea, dizziness, insomnia, impaired concentration, depression, anxiety, dry mouth, constipation Pregnancy category: C	Tell the prescriber if you have a history of a mental disorder, a seizure disorder, CHF, or impaired kidney function; contact the prescriber if you develop purplish red, blotchy spots on the skin; alcohol may increase risk of adverse effects such as dizziness, so do not drink alcoholic beverages or take other medicines with alcohol while taking this agent; some people may become dizzy or lightheaded, so know how you react to this medicine before you drive or use machinery; when getting up from a lying or seated position, do so slowly to avoid getting dizzy;	Abrupt withdrawal of medication has resulted in worsening of symptoms

Generic Name and Selected Trade Names	Normal Adult Dosage	Major Adverse Effects/Cautions	Key Counseling Points	Miscellaneous Issues
Amantadine HCl (continued) Symadine Symmetrel			if you develop a dry mouth and it bothers you use ice chips, sugarless gum or candy, or a saliva substitute; if you miss a dose take it as soon as you remember but if it is almost time for the next dose, skip the missed one and return to regular dosing schedule — do not double doses Flu use: If your symptoms do not improve within a few days or get worse, contact the prescriber; speak with your physician about the need for a flu shot; try to space the doses evenly	

Generic Name and Selected Trade Names	Normal Adult Dosage	Major Adverse Effects/Cautions	Key Counselling Points	Miscellaneous Issues
Benztropine Mesylate Cogentin	Individualize dosage For postencephalitic and idiopathic Parkinson's disease: Initiate with 0.5 to 1 mg HS, increase to 4–6 mg based upon patient's response For drug-induced EPS: 1 to 4 mg QD or BID	Contraindication: Patients under 3 years of age Considerations: Caution during hot weather or when administered with other agents with atropine-like actions Most common AEs include dry mouth, urinary retention, constipation, blurred vision, confusion, nervousness, depression Pregnancy category: C	Tell the prescriber if you have glaucoma (narrow angle), a prostate problem, history of depression, or suffer from urinary retention or constipation; do not stop taking this agent without discussing it first with the prescriber; may cause drowsiness and blurred vision, so do not drive or use machinery until you know how you react to the agent; may cause dryness of the mouth, try ice chips, sugarless gum/candy, or saliva substitutes, but if the problem persists contact the prescriber; this medication may decrease your ability to perspire, so use caution and avoid getting overheated if you are exercising or in a warm place;	

Generic Name and Selected Trade Names	Normal Adult Dosage	Major Adverse Effects/Cautions	Key Counseling Points	Miscellaneous Issues
Benztropine Mesylate (continued) Cogentin			if you develop eye pain, urinary retention, or constipation contact the prescriber; the medicine may add to the effects of alcohol and other CNS depressants such as antihistamines, tranquilizers, and barbiturates — contact your physician or pharmacist before taking any other agent; if you miss a dose, take it as soon as you remember but if it is within 2 hrs of the next dose skip the missed one and return to regular dosing schedule — do not double doses	

Generic Name and Selected Trade Names	Normal Adult Dosage	Major Adverse Effects/Cautions	Key Counseling Points	Miscellaneous Issues
Biperiden HCl Akineton	Individualize dosage For Parkinson's disease: 2 mg TID or QID; may titrate up to a maximum of 16 mg per day For drug-induced EPS: 2 mg QD to TID	Contraindications: Narrow angle glaucoma, bowel obstruction, megacolon Considerations: Avoid using other agents with anticholinergic effects (eg, antipsychotics, antidepressants, antihistamines); use cautiously in patients with glaucoma, prostatism, epilepsy, or arrhythmias Most common AEs include dry mouth, blurred vision, drowsiness, euphoria/agitation, urinary retention, postural hypotension, disturbed behavior, constipation Pregnancy category: C	SEE benztropine mesylate	

Generic Name and Selected Trade Names	Normal Adult Dosage	Major Adverse Effects/Cautions	Key Counseling Points	Miscellaneous Issues
Bromocriptine Mesylate Parlodel Parlodel Snap Tabs	Individualize dosage For Parkinson's disease, usually administer 1.25 mg BID with meals; may increase dosage every 14–28 days in 2.5 mg/day increments, if necessary Used for other conditions as well — SEE chapter on "Fertility Agents" and Prescribing Information (PI)	<u>Contraindications:</u> Uncontrolled hypertension, pregnancy <u>Considerations:</u> Increases and decreases in blood pressure may occur so monitor blood pressure during the initiation of therapy Most common AEs include nausea, hypotension, abnormal movements, hallucinations, confusion, "on-off" phenomenon, dizziness, drowsiness <u>Pregnancy category:</u> B	SEE bromocriptine mesylate in chapter on "Fertility Agents"	

Generic Name and Selected Trade Names	Normal Adult Dosage	Major Adverse Effects/Cautions	Key Counseling Points	Miscellaneous Issues
Carbidopa + Levodopa Atamet Sinemet Sinemet CR	Individualize dosage For Sinemet 25–100 or Atamet 25–100: 1 tablet TID; may increase by 1 tablet every day or every other day as needed up to 8 tablets/day For Sinemet 10–100 or Atamet 10–100: 1 tablet TID or QID, increase by 1 tablet every day or every other day as needed until a dosage of 8 tablets/day (given 2 tabs QID) For Sinemet CR: For new patients, 1 tablet Sinemet CR 50 to 200 BID	<u>Contraindications:</u> Concurrent use of MAO-inhibitors, patients with undiagnosed skin lesions or a history of melanoma <u>Considerations:</u> Patients previously on levodopa must discontinue levodopa for at least 12 hrs prior to initiating the combination; CNS adverse effects may occur at lower doses with the combination; use caution in patients with asthma, severe cardiovascular diseases, renal, hepatic, or endocrine disorders; rare cases of a neuroleptic malignant-like syndrome have occurred when patients abruptly stop therapy <u>Most common AEs</u> include dyskinesias (abnormal movement disorders), nausea, mental changes, rash, hypotension, GI bleeding <u>Pregnancy category:</u> C	Tell the prescriber if you are taking a MAO inhibitor, or have diabetes mellitus, a lung disease such as asthma, or a cardiovascular, renal, or liver disorder; take only as directed — do not take more than prescribed; you may need to take this for several weeks or months before you see full benefit; avoid a high protein diet as this may decrease the effect of this medication; this medication should be taken at regular intervals as directed by the prescriber; may cause drowsiness, so do not drive or use machinery until you know how you react to it; when getting up from a lying or seated position, do so slowly to avoid getting dizzy;	

Generic Name and Selected Trade Names	Normal Adult Dosage	Major Adverse Effects/Cautions	Key Counselling Points	Miscellaneous Issues
Carbidopa + Levodopa (continued) Atamet Sinemet Sinemet CR	For guidelines for converting patients from levodopa to carbidopa + levodopa — SEE Prescribing Information (PI)		if you miss a dose take it as soon as possible, but if you remember within 2 hrs of the next dose skip the missed one and return to regular dosing schedule — do not double doses CR dosage form: Tablets may be broken in half, but not crushed	

Generic Name and Selected Trade Names	Normal Adult Dosage	Major Adverse Effects/Cautions	Key Counseling Points	Miscellaneous Issues
Levodopa Dopar Larodopa	Individualize dosage For Parkinson's disease, start with 0.5 to 1 G daily, divided into 2 or more doses taken with food; may titrate dose gradually in increments of no more than 0.75 G every 3–7 days, up to 8 G/day	<u>Contraindications</u>: Concurrent use with MAO inhibitors, narrow angle glaucoma, undiagnosed skin lesions, or a history of melanoma <u>Considerations</u>: Use with caution in patients with severe cardiovascular, pulmonary, renal, hepatic, or endocrine disorders; monitor patients for depression Most common AEs include dyskinesias, cardiac irregularities, nausea, mental changes, hypotension <u>Pregnancy category</u>: C	Do not take vitamin B_6 (pyridoxine) supplements and avoid foods rich in vitamin B_6 such as avocado, bacon, and sweet potato; also, SEE carbidopa + levodopa	

Generic Name and Selected Trade Names	Normal Adult Dosage	Major Adverse Effects/Cautions	Key Counseling Points	Miscellaneous Issues
Pergolide Mesylate Permax	Individualize dosage For Parkinson's disease, initiate with 0.05 mg/day for 2 days, increase by 0.1 to 0.15 mg/day every third day over the next 12 days, then increase by 0.25 mg/day every third day until optimal effect is achieved; usually administered in 3 divided doses/day	<u>Contraindication</u>: Hypersensitivity to any ergot derivative <u>Considerations</u>: Symptomatic hypotension frequently occurs during the initiation of therapy Most common AEs include dyskinesias, hallucinations, somnolence, insomnia, nausea, constipation, diarrhea, rhinitis, hypotension <u>Pregnancy category</u>: B	Tell the prescriber if you had an allergic reaction to any ergot product such as ergotamine; dizziness, fainting, or lightheadedness may occur, whenever you get up from a lying or seated position (especially after the first dose of this medication) so get up slowly to avoid getting dizzy; may cause drowsiness or lightheadedness, so do not drive or use machinery until you know how you react to the medication; you may need to take this agent for several weeks before you see full benefit; may cause dryness of the mouth, try ice chips, sugarless gum or candy, or saliva substitutes, but if the problem persists contact the prescriber;	

Generic Name and Selected Trade Names	Normal Adult Dosage	Major Adverse Effects/Cautions	Key Counseling Points	Miscellaneous Issues
Pergolide Mesylate (continued) Permax			if you miss a dose take it as soon as you remember but if it is almost time for the next dose, skip the missed one and go back to regular dosing schedule — do not double doses	

Generic Name and Selected Trade Names	Normal Adult Dosage	Major Adverse Effects/Cautions	Key Counseling Points	Miscellaneous Issues
Procyclidine HCl Kemadrin	Individualize dosage For Parkinson's disease: 2.5 mg TID after meals; may gradually titrate dosage to 5 mg TID; lower doses required when used in combination with levodopa For drug-induced Parkinson's disease: Initiate with 2.5 mg TID; may increase by 2.5 mg daily until relief of symptoms — usually 10–20 mg/day Dosage adjustment: Elderly patients often require lower doses — SEE Prescribing Information (PI)	<u>Contraindication</u>: Narrow angle glaucoma <u>Considerations</u>: Avoid using other agents with anticholinergic effects (eg, antipsychotics, antidepressants, antihistamines). <u>Most common AEs</u> include dry mouth, blurred vision, dizziness, nausea, nervousness, nausea, constipation, drowsiness <u>Pregnancy category</u>: C	SEE benztropine mesylate	

Generic Name and Selected Trade Names	Normal Adult Dosage	Major Adverse Effects/Cautions	Key Counseling Points	Miscellaneous Issues
Selegiline HCl Atapryl Eldepryl	For Parkinson's disease, 10 mg/day divided between breakfast and lunch	<u>Contraindication</u>: Concurrent use with meperidine <u>Considerations</u>: Do not exceed 10 mg/day dosage due to risks associated with non-selective inhibition of MAO; may exacerbate levodopa's adverse effects Most common AEs include nausea, dizziness, abdominal pain, confusion, dry mouth, hallucinations, vivid dreams, dyskinesias, headache <u>Pregnancy category</u>: C	Take only as directed — do not take more than prescribed; do not take late in the day unless otherwise directed; whenever you get up from a lying or seated position, do so slowly to avoid getting dizzy; may cause dryness of the mouth, try ice chips, sugarless gum or candy, or saliva substitutes, but if the problem persists contact the prescriber; check with your physician or a hospital emergency room if you suddenly develop a severe headache, stiff neck, chest pains, fast heartbeat, or nausea; if you miss a dose take it as soon as possible, but if you do not remember until late afternoon or evening, skip the missed one and go back to regular dosing schedule — do not double doses	Generally administered with carbidopa + levodopa; usually after 2–3 days of therapy the carbidopa + levodopa dose may be decreased 10%–30%; if patient is taking more than 10 mg/day, consider risk of non-selective MAO inhibitor drug-drug and drug-food interactions such as foods with high tyramine content

Generic Name and Selected Trade Names	Normal Adult Dosage	Major Adverse Effects/Cautions	Key Counseling Points	Miscellaneous Issues
Tolcapone Tasmar	Individualize dosage As an adjunct to carbidopa + levodopa for Parkinson's disease, start with 100 or 200 mg TID; may titrate up to 600 mg/day Dosage may need to be reduced in patients with renal or hepatic impairment — SEE Prescribing Information (PI)	Considerations: Usually avoid non-selective MAO inhibitor; may increase liver enzymes so monitor monthly for 3 months then every 6 weeks for 3 months; may cause hypotension, diarrhea, hallucinations, dyskinesias Most common AEs include diarrhea, nausea, muscle cramps, and CNS effects such as sleep disorders and dyskinesias Pregnancy category: C	Tell the prescriber if you have a liver disorder or are taking a MAO inhibitor; dizziness, fainting, or lightheadedness may occur especially when getting up from a seated or lying position so get up slowly; do not drive a car, operate machines, or do any dangerous/difficult tasks until you see how this medication affects you; if you miss a dose take it as soon as you remember but if it is almost time for the next dose, skip the missed one and go back to regular dosing schedule — do not double doses	Levodopa dosage may need to be decreased by about 30%

Generic Name and Selected Trade Names	Normal Adult Dosage	Major Adverse Effects/Cautions	Key Counseling Points	Miscellaneous Issues
Trihexyphenidyl HCl Artane	Individualize dosage For Parkinson's disease: Usually start with 1 mg day 1 then increase by 2 mg every 3–5 days, up to a maximum of 6 to 10 mg/day; lower doses required when used in combination with levodopa For drug-induced Parkinson's disease: Initiate with 1 mg QD then adjust dosage based on the patient's response; generally patients respond at 5 to 15 mg per day	Considerations: Avoid using other agents with anticholinergic effects (eg, antipsychotics, antidepressants, antihistamines); avoid in patients with glaucoma, GI or urinary obstruction, or BPH; elderly patients often require lower doses Most common AEs include dry mouth, blurred vision, dizziness, nervousness, drowsiness, nausea, constipation Pregnancy category: C	SEE benztropine mesylate	

*As a general rule, a medication should not be administered to a patient with a known hypersensitivity to it or a similar agent.

Antiepileptics

Table: Antiepileptics*[1,2]

Generic Name and Selected Trade Names	Normal Adult Dosage	Major Adverse Effects/Cautions	Key Counseling Points	Miscellaneous Issues
Carbamazepine Tegretol Tegretol-XR	Individualize dosage For epilepsy: Start with 200 mg BID (tablets and XR tablets) or 1 teaspoonful QID (suspension); may increase at weekly intervals adding 200 mg/day until optimal response is obtained; long-term XR is given BID; tablets and suspension given TID or QID; usual maintenance dose is 800 to 1200 mg/day	Contraindications: Patients with a history of previous bone marrow depression, in combination with MAO inhibitors Considerations: Aplastic anemia and agranulocytosis have occurred, but are rare; any patient with a history of adverse hematologic reactions to other medications should be monitored carefully; elevations of intraocular pressure have occurred, monitor patients with concurrent elevations Most common AEs include dizziness, drowsiness, unsteadiness, nausea/vomiting, blurred or double vision, nystagmus Pregnancy category: C	Tell the prescriber if you have any other health problems such as heart or blood vessel disease, glaucoma, anemia, diabetes mellitus, kidney or liver disease, problems with urination, history of alcohol abuse or behavioral problems; check with the physician or pharmacist before taking any other medication; if you are pregnant or plan on becoming pregnant, discuss this with the physician; medication may alter the effectiveness of oral contraceptives, so an additional or different method of birth control is recommended;	Do not crush, break, or chew the XR tablets; coating is excreted in the feces; many drug interactions are possible — SEE Prescribing Information (PI)

Generic Name and Selected Trade Names	Normal Adult Dosage	Major Adverse Effects/Cautions	Key Counseling Points
Carbamazepine (continued) Tegretol Tegretol-XR	For trigeminal neuralgia: Start with 100 mg BID for tablets or XR tablets or ½ teaspoonful QID for suspension; increase by up to 200 mg/day using 100 mg increments Q12H for tablets and XR tablets and 50 mg QID for suspension; usual maintenance dose is 400 to 800 mg/day		this agent may cause drowsiness, vision problems or dizziness early in therapy so be cautious when driving a car or using machinery; if you experience fever, sore throat, rash, ulcers in the mouth or easy bruising contact the prescriber; generally you should have frequent blood tests while on this agent; this agent may make you more sensitive to sunlight so avoid direct sunlight and wear protective clothing and sunblock; it is important that the physician monitors your progress on a regular basis; it is important that you take this medication as directed; take with meals; if you miss a dose take it as soon as you remember but if it is almost time for your next dose, skip the missed dose and return to regular schedule — do not double doses For suspension, shake well, do not take with any other liquids For sustained release, swallow whole, do not break, crush, or chew

Generic Name and Selected Trade Names	Normal Adult Dosage	Major Adverse Effects/Cautions	Key Counselling Points	Miscellaneous Issues
Divalproex Sodium Depakote Depakote Sprinkle	Individualize dosage Regimens depend upon disease state, concomitant therapies, and monitoring of blood levels For epilepsy: Generally therapy is initiated with 10 to 15 mg/kg/day; increased by 5 to 10 mg/kg/week until optimal effect is achieved; maximum dose is 60 mg/kg/day For mania: Initially 750 mg daily in divided doses; increased until desired effect achieved; maximum dose is 60 mg/kg/day	Contraindications: Patients with hepatic disease or significant hepatic dysfunction Considerations: Liver function should be monitored; thrombocytopenia and alterations in clotting have occurred; may cause birth defects Most common AEs include GI distress, weight gain or loss, headache, sedation, tremor, hallucinations, altered bleeding time Pregnancy Category: D	Tell the prescriber if you have a blood, brain, kidney, or liver disease; check with the physician or pharmacist before taking any other medication; if you are pregnant or plan on becoming pregnant, discuss this with the physician; may cause drowsiness, so make sure you know how you react before driving a car or operating machinery; it is important that the prescriber checks your progress regularly; take this agent as directed, the prescriber may increase your dose gradually to decrease the occurrence of side effects; do not stop taking the medication without first discussing it with the prescriber; may be taken with meals or snacks;	Coated particles from the sprinkles have appeared in the feces; many drug interactions are possible — SEE Prescribing Information (PI)

Generic Name and Selected Trade Names	Normal Adult Dosage	Major Adverse Effects/Cautions	Key Counseling Points	Miscellaneous Issues
Divalproex Sodium (continued) Depakote Depakote Sprinkle	For migraine: Start with 250 mg BID; may increase up to 1000 mg/day Dosage adjustments may be required in elderly patients — SEE Prescribing Information (PI)		If you miss a dose and you are taking the medication once a day, take the missed dose as soon as you remember, if you do not remember until the next day, skip the dose and return to regular schedule — do not double doses; if you take two or more doses a day and you remember within 6 hrs of the missed dose, take it right away, then take the rest of the doses for the day at equally spaced intervals — do not double doses For tablets, swallow whole, do not break, chew, or crush For sprinkle capsules, may be swallowed whole or opened and the contents sprinkled on a small amount of soft food (eg. applesauce) and then swallowed without chewing	

Generic Name and Selected Trade Names	Normal Adult Dosage	Major Adverse Effects/Cautions	Key Counseling Points	Miscellaneous Issues
Ethosuximide Zarontin	Individualize dosage For epilepsy in patients over 6 years of age, start with 500 mg per day (usually 250 mg BID); may increase daily dose by 250 mg every 4–7 days until optimal response is achieved with minimal adverse effects	<u>Considerations</u>: Blood dyscrasias have occurred so CBC should be monitored; use extreme caution in patients with liver or renal disease; lupus erythematosus has occurred <u>Most common AEs include</u> anorexia, nausea/vomiting, drowsiness, headache, dizziness, dermatologic reactions, myopia <u>Pregnancy category</u>: Not specified	Tell the prescriber if you have any other health problems such as blood, kidney, or liver disease, or porphyria; check with the physician or pharmacist before taking any other medication; this agent may cause drowsiness, vision problems or dizziness early in therapy so be cautious when driving or using machinery; call the physician if you develop a sore throat or fever, muscle pain, rash and itching, or swollen glands; it is important that the prescriber checks your progress at regular visits; take this medication as directed;	For syrup, do not refrigerate

Generic Name and Selected Trade Names	Normal Adult Dosage	Major Adverse Effects/Cautions	Key Counselling Points	Miscellaneous Issues
Ethosuximide (continued) Zarontin			if you experience stomach upset you may take this medication with food; if you miss a dose take it as soon as possible but if it is within 4 hrs of the next dose, skip the missed dose and go back to your regular schedule — do not double doses	

Generic Name and Selected Trade Names	Normal Adult Dosage	Major Adverse Effects/Cautions	Key Counseling Points	Miscellaneous Issues
Gabapentin Neurontin	Individualize dosage For add-on therapy in epilepsy, 300 mg on day 1, 300 mg BID on day 2, 300 mg TID on day 3; may gradually increase to 900 to 1800 mg/day; doses up to 3600 mg/day have been well tolerated Dosage adjustment required for patients with renal impairment — SEE Prescribing Information (PI)	Most common AEs include sedation, dizziness, ataxia, nystagmus Pregnancy category: C	Tell the prescriber if you have kidney disease; may cause blurred vision, unsteadiness, dizziness, drowsiness, or trouble thinking, so make sure you know how you react to this medication before driving or using machinery; if you develop clumsiness or unsteadiness, or continuous rolling eye movements contact the physician; it is important that the prescriber check your progress regularly; initial dose should be taken at bedtime to decrease the occurrence of sedation; take as directed and do not stop taking without first discussing this with the prescriber; may be taken with or without food;	Dose is usually titrated up over several days to minimize AEs

Generic Name and Selected Trade Names	Normal Adult Dosage	Major Adverse Effects/Cautions	Key Counselling Points	Miscellaneous Issues
Gabapentin (continued) Neurontin			if you miss a dose take it as soon as possible, if it is less than 2 hrs until your next dose, take the missed dose right away, take the next dose 1–2 hrs later, then return to regular schedule— do not double doses	
Clonazepam[1] Klonopin				

Generic Name and Selected Trade Names	Normal Adult Dosage	Major Adverse Effects/Cautions	Key Counselling Points	Miscellaneous Issues
Lamotrigine Lamictal	Individualize dosage Dosage for epilepsy depends upon concomitant therapies — SEE Prescribing Information (PI) Dosage adjustment may be required for patients with renal impairment — SEE PI	<u>Considerations</u>: Severe dermatologic reactions (eg, rash, Stevens-Johnson syndrome, toxic epidermal necrolysis) have occurred Most common AEs include dizziness, diplopia, nausea, headache, ataxia somnolence, rash <u>Pregnancy Category</u>: C	Tell the prescriber if you have heart, kidney, or liver disease or anemia; check with the physician or pharmacist before taking any other medication; may cause dizziness or sedation, so do not drive a car or use machinery until you know how this agent affects you; if you develop a rash or symptoms of allergy (eg, swelling, difficulty breathing, fever, swollen lymph nodes) or if your seizures become worse contact the physician immediately; it is important that the prescriber checks your progress regularly;	

Generic Name and Selected Trade Names	Normal Adult Dosage	Major Adverse Effects/Cautions	Key Counseling Points	Miscellaneous Issues
Lamotrigine (continued) Lamictal			take as directed and do not stop taking this medication without talking to the prescriber; may be taken with or without food; if you miss a dose take it as soon as possible but if it is almost time for your next dose skip the missed one and go back to your regular schedule — do not double doses	

Generic Name and Selected Trade Names	Normal Adult Dosage	Major Adverse Effects/Cautions	Key Counseling Points	Miscellaneous Issues
Phenobarbital	Individualize dosage For epilepsy: Usually 60 to 200 mg/day as a single dose or in divided doses For sedation: Usually 30 to 120 mg as needed based upon the patient's response Dosage adjustments required in elderly patients and patients with impaired renal or liver function — SEE Prescribing Information (PI) Injectable form available — SEE PI	Contraindications: Porphyria, marked respiratory depression or liver impairment Considerations: Tolerance, psychological and physical dependence can occur; paradoxical excitement can occur in patients in pain; potentially hazardous to fetal development; reported to be associated with cognitive deficits in children receiving it for complicated febrile seizures Most common AEs include drowsiness, lethargy, vertigo, altered behavior, enhanced sensitivity to pain Pregnancy category: D	Tell the prescriber if you have any other medical problems; check with the physician or pharmacist before taking any other medication; if you are pregnant or plan on becoming pregnant, discuss this with the physician; may alter the effectiveness of oral contraceptives, so an additional or different method of birth control is recommended; this agent may cause drowsiness, vision problems, or dizziness early in therapy so be cautious when driving or using machinery;	Elderly patients and children may respond with CNS excitation rather than depression

521

Generic Name and Selected Trade Names	Normal Adult Dosage	Major Adverse Effects/Cautions	Key Counselling Points	Miscellaneous Issues
Phenobarbital (continued)			may be habit forming; if you develop sores on the lips or mouth, chest pain, fever, muscle or joint pain, changes in your skin (including rash), sore throat, fever, swelling of eyelids, face, or lips, or difficulty breathing contact the prescriber; it is important that the prescriber checks your progress regularly; take the medication as directed; do not discontinue without first checking with the physician; if you miss a dose take it as soon as possible, if it is almost time for your next dose, skip the missed one and return to regular schedule — do not double doses	

Generic Name and Selected Trade Names	Normal Adult Dosage	Major Adverse Effects/Cautions	Key Counseling Points	Miscellaneous Issues
Phenytoin Dilantin Dilantin Kapseals Dilantin Infatabs Dilantin-125 Diphenylan	Individualize dosage <u>Capsules</u>: For epilepsy, usually start with 100 mg TID; titrate dose based upon patient response and blood levels at 7–10 day intervals; usual maintenance dose is 100 to 400 mg/day <u>Suspension</u>: For epilepsy, usually start with 125 mg (5 mL) TID; may adjust at 7–10 day intervals up to 625 mg/day <u>Chewable tablets</u>: For epilepsy, 100 to 125 mg TID; may adjust at 7–10 day intervals Injectable form available — SEE PI	<u>Considerations</u>: Abrupt withdrawal can aggravate seizures; lymphadenopathy has occurred; discontinue if skin rash occurs; may produce birth defects if taken during pregnancy Most common AEs include nystagmus, ataxia, slurred speech, decreased coordination and confusion, nausea/vomiting, constipation, gingival hyperplasia, bleeding or tender gums <u>Pregnancy category</u>: C	Tell the prescriber if you have any other medical conditions; check with the physician or pharmacist before taking any other medication; if you are pregnant or plan on becoming pregnant, discuss this with the physician; may alter the effectiveness of oral contraceptives, so an additional or different method of birth control is recommended; this agent may cause drowsiness, vision problems, or dizziness early in therapy so do not drive or use machinery until you know how you react; maintaining good dental hygiene while taking this medication is important, inform your dentist you are taking this medication;	Serum levels should be monitored; many drug interactions are possible — SEE Prescribing Information (PI)

Generic Name and Selected Trade Names	Normal Adult Dosage	Key Counseling Points
Phenytoin (continued) Dilantin Dilantin Kapseals Dilantin Infatabs Dilantin-125 Diphenylan		if you develop bleeding, tender or enlarged gums, clumsiness or unsteadiness, confusion, uncontrolled rolling of the eyes, enlarged glands, fever or sore throat, increase in seizures, mood or mental changes, muscle weakness or pain, or skin rash or itching contact the prescriber; it is important that the prescriber checks your progress regularly; take as directed; if it upsets your stomach it may be taken with food, it should always be taken at the same time in relationship to meals; do not stop taking the medication on your own; if you miss a dose take it as soon as possible, but if you are on a once a day regimen and you remember the next day, skip the dose and go back to regular dosing schedule; if you are taking more than one dose a day and you miss a dose take it as soon as possible, but if it is within 4 hrs of the next dose, skip the missed one and go back to regular dosing schedule; if you miss doses for more than 2 days in a row, contact the prescriber — do not double doses For capsule form, must be swallowed whole, do not crush, chew, or break; for chewable tablets, may be chewed or crushed before swallowed or may be swallowed whole

Generic Name and Selected Trade Names	Normal Adult Dosage	Major Adverse Effects/Cautions	Key Counseling Points	Miscellaneous Issues
Primidone Mysoline	Individualize dosage For epilepsy, 100 to 125 mg HS days 1–3; 100 to 125 mg BID days 4–6; 100 to 125 mg TID days 7–9; then 250 mg TID; dosage different if used in combination — SEE Prescribing Information (PI)	<u>Contraindication</u>: Porphyria <u>Considerations</u>: Abrupt withdrawal may precipitate seizures; may cause birth defects Most common AEs include ataxia and vertigo, nausea/vomiting, fatigue, emotional disturbances, impotence, diplopia <u>Pregnancy category</u>: Not specified	Tell the prescriber if you have any respiratory disorders, hyperactivity (children), kidney or liver disease, or porphyria; check with the physician or pharmacist before taking any other medication; if you are pregnant or plan on becoming pregnant, discuss this with the physician; may alter the effectiveness of oral contraceptives, so an additional or different method of birth control is recommended; this agent may cause drowsiness, so do not drive a car or use machinery until you know how you react;	

Generic Name and Selected Trade Names	Normal Adult Dosage	Major Adverse Effects/Cautions	Key Counseling Points	Miscellaneous Issues
Primidone (continued) Mysoline			if you develop unusual excitement or restlessness contact the prescriber; it is important that the prescriber checks your progress regularly; take the medication as directed; do not discontinue without first discussing it with the physician; if you miss a dose take it as soon as possible but if it is within an hour of your next dose, skip the missed one and go back to regular dosing schedule — do not double doses	

Generic Name and Selected Trade Names	Normal Adult Dosage	Major Adverse Effects/Cautions	Key Counseling Points	Miscellaneous Issues
Topiramate Topamax	Individualize dosage For add-on therapy in epilepsy, usually start with 400 mg/day in divided doses (usually BID); may titrate slowly begin with 50 mg and increase by 50 mg each week	<u>Considerations:</u> Elimination decreased in patients with kidney or liver dysfunction; kidney stones have formed in some patients; should not be abruptly discontinued <u>Most common AEs</u> include somnolence, speech disturbances, psychomotor slowing, dizziness, ataxia, nausea <u>Pregnancy category:</u> C	Tell the prescriber if you have liver or kidney disease; check with the physician or pharmacist before taking any other medication; take as directed and do not stop taking without discussing it with the prescriber; some people may become drowsy or unsteady, so do not drive a car or use machinery until you know how you react	

Generic Name and Selected Trade Names	Normal Adult Dosage	Major Adverse Effects/Cautions	Key Counseling Points	Miscellaneous Issues
Valproic Acid Depakene	Individualize dosage For epilepsy, start with 5 to 15 mg/kg/day; increased at 1 week intervals by 5 to 10 mg/kg/day; maximum dosage 60 mg/kg/day	SEE divalproex sodium	SEE divalproex sodium and for capsules, swallow whole, do not break, crush, or chew to prevent irritation of the mouth or throat; for syrup may be mixed with any liquid	

*As a general rule, a medication should not be administered to a patient with a known hypersensitivity to it or a similar agent.
[1] Patients should be warned to avoid alcohol or other CNS depressants such as antihistamines while receiving antiepileptic agents.
[2] SEE anti-panic agents.

Migraine Preparations

Table: Migraine Preparations*

Generic Name and Selected Trade Names	Normal Adult Dosage	Major Adverse Effects/Cautions	Key Counseling Points	Miscellaneous Issues
Divalproex Sodium[1] Depakote				

Generic Name and Selected Trade Names	Normal Adult Dosage	Major Adverse Effects/Cautions	Key Counselling Points	Miscellaneous Issues
Ergotamine Tartrate Ergomar Ergostat Medihaler Ergotamine	Individualize dosage *Sublingual tablets* To abort or prevent vascular headaches such as migraine, at the first sign of an attack administer 2 mg (1 tab) SL; then 1 tab at half-hour intervals if necessary but do not exceed 3 tabs/24 hr period *Inhaler* Usually, start with 1 inhalation at first sign of an attack; then repeat every 5 minutes if necessary but do not exceed 6 inhalations/24 hr period or 15 inhalations/week	Contraindications: Hypersensitivity to any ergot alkaloid, women who are or may become pregnant, and patients with sepsis, hypertension, peripheral vascular disease (eg, thromboangitis obliterans, thrombophlebitis, Raynaud's disease), coronary heart disease, impaired hepatic or renal function Considerations: Do not exceed recommended dosage due to risk of ergotism; signs and symptoms of overdose occur with as little as 5 mg ingested — if occurs, seek immediate assistance; found in breast milk (may cause adverse effects to infant) and may inhibit lactation	*Sublingual tablets* Tell the prescriber if you have any of the listed contraindications, and whether you previously had an allergic reaction to any ergot product; take only as directed — do not exceed the recommended dosage under any condition; take the medication at first sign of a headache or at warning signs of migraine; place the tablet under the tongue and allow it to dissolve — do not chew or swallow it; contact the prescriber if your headaches appear to be getting worse or occur more frequently than before you started this agent, or if you notice an irregular heart beat, nausea/vomiting, numbness of the fingers or toes, or pain/weakness of an extremity;	

Generic Name and Selected Trade Names	Normal Adult Dosage	Major Adverse Effects/Cautions	Key Counselling Points
Ergotamine Tartrate (continued) Ergomar Ergostat Medihaler Ergotamine		Most common AEs include nausea/vomiting, weakness of the legs, pain in limb muscles, numbness and tingling of fingers and toes, precordial pain, transient changes in heart rate, localized edema and itching <u>Pregnancy category</u>: X	do not take any other medication without first discussing it with your physician or pharmacist; keep the medication away from children because accidental overdose is very dangerous; drinking alcoholic beverages and/or smoking may make headaches worse; if you are prescribed another agent to prevent headaches, remember to take it routinely; you may be more sensitive to cold temperatures so dress warmly *Inhaler* Same as for ergotamine tartrate tablets, except: agent administered via an inhaler not SL; should not be used more often than 2 times/week, at least 5 days apart; ensure patient knows how to use inhaler; give patient the product instructions provided by the manufacturer

Generic Name and Selected Trade Names	Normal Adult Dosage	Major Adverse Effects/Cautions	Key Counselling Points	Miscellaneous Issues
Ergotamine Tartrate & Caffeine Cafergot Wigraine	Individualize dosage To abort or prevent vascular headaches such as migraine, the average adult dose is 2 tablets at the first sign of an attack; then 1 tab every one-half hour if necessary but do not exceed 6 tabs/attack or 10 tabs/week	<u>Contraindications</u>: SEE ergotamine tartrate <u>Considerations</u>: Do not exceed recommended dosage due to risk of ergotism — if occurs, seek immediate assistance; some ergot preparations pass into breast milk (may cause adverse effects to infant) and caffeine will pass into breast milk, so may need to avoid breast feeding Most common AEs include diarrhea; also SEE ergotamine tartrate <u>Pregnancy category</u>: X	SEE ergotamine tartrate, except this product is taken orally	

Generic Name and Selected Trade Names	Normal Adult Dosage	Major Adverse Effects/Cautions	Key Counseling Points	Miscellaneous Issues
Dihydroergotamine Mesylate Injection D.H.E. 45	Individualize dosage To abort or prevent vascular headaches such as migraine, give 1 mL (1 mg) IM at the first sign of an attack; then additional doses at 1 hr intervals but do not exceed 3 mL; may be administered IV to a maximum dosage of 2 mL; for either IM or IV, do not exceed 6 mL/week	Contraindications: Use with vasoconstrictors, patients with shock or vascular surgery, women who are breast feeding; also SEE ergotamine tartrate Considerations: May cause vasospastic reactions (eg, angina and signs/symptoms of vascular ischemia) that may be dose-related; do not exceed recommended dosage due to risk of ergotism — if occurs, seek immediate assistance; pleural and retroperitoneal fibrosis reported Most common AEs include injection site reactions, headache, leg cramps and soreness, vasospasm, paresthesia, hypertension, dizziness, anxiety, dyspnea, flushing, diarrhea, rash, increased sweating; also, SEE ergotamine tartrate Pregnancy category: X	This medication is only for vascular headaches of the migraine type, it is not effective against other types of headaches, and is not a pain reliever; if patient or caregiver is administering the medication, ensure he/she is familiar with proper aseptic injection technique; also SEE ergotamine tartrate except that this medication is given via injection	For IM route, titrate dose over the course of several headaches to determine optimal dosage; numerous drug interactions are possible — SEE Prescribing Information (PI)

Generic Name and Selected Trade Names	Normal Adult Dosage	Major Adverse Effects/Cautions	Key Counseling Points	Miscellaneous Issues
Naritriptan HCl Amerge	Individualize dosage For the acute treatment of migraine attacks, controlled trials showed that single doses of 1 and 2.5 mg taken with fluid were effective but the 2.5 mg dose was associated with greater response; may repeat dose once after 4 hrs if needed but do not exceed 5 mg/24 hr period Contraindicated in severe renal and hepatic impairment but may be used in mild-to-moderate impairment — SEE Prescribing Information (PI)	Contraindications: Patients with history, symptoms, or signs of ischemic cardiac/ cerebrovascular/peripheral vascular syndromes, and uncontrolled hypertension; other significant underlying cardiovascular disease such as angina, MI, and strokes; patients with severe renal and/or hepatic impairment, hemiplegic or basilar migraine; within 24 hrs of treatment with another 5-HT$_1$ agonist Considerations: There is a risk of causing myocardial ischemia or MI; do not use or use very cautiously in persons with unrecognized coronary artery disease such as those with risk factors including hypercholesterolemia, smoker, obesity, diabetes mellitus, positive family history;	Tell the prescriber if you have any of the listed contraindications and all the other medications you are taking; evaluate whether patient has any risk factors for coronary artery disease such as high cholesterol, diabetes mellitus, history of smoking, is post-menopausal, or male more than 40 years of age, and family history of cardiac disease; medication is used to treat an attack not to prevent one; do not take any other prescription or non-prescription medication without discussing it first with your physician or pharmacist; take only as directed — do not exceed the recommended dosage under any condition;	

Generic Name and Selected Trade Names	Normal Adult Dosage	Major Adverse Effects/Cautions	Key Counselling Points	Miscellaneous Issues
Naritriptan HCl (continued) Amerge		administer first dose in physician's or other equipped office; may cause coronary vasospasm, chest discomfort, cerebrovascular events such as strokes and TIAs, increases in blood pressure, and hypersensitivity reactions; not recommended in elderly Most common AEs include paresthesias, dizziness, drowsiness, malaise/fatigue, throat/neck symptoms, nausea Pregnancy category: C	contact the prescriber if you develop pain or discomfort in your chest or throat, abdominal pain, shortness of breath, wheezes, palpitations	

Generic Name and Selected Trade Names	Normal Adult Dosage	Major Adverse Effects/Cautions	Key Counseling Points	Miscellaneous Issues
Propranolol HCl[2] Inderal Inderal LA				

Generic Name and Selected Trade Names	Normal Adult Dosage	Major Adverse Effects/Cautions	Key Counseling Points	Miscellaneous Issues
Rizatriptan Benzoate Maxalt Maxalt-MLT	Individualize dosage Maxalt: For the acute treatment of migraine attacks, controlled trials showed that single doses of 5 and 10 mg were effective but the 10 mg dose may provide greater effect; repeat doses should be separated by at least 2 hrs if needed but do not exceed 30 mg/24 hr period Maxalt MLT: These orally disintegrating tablets do not need to be administered with liquid; dosing is the same as Maxalt	<u>Contraindications</u>: Patients with history, symptoms, or signs of ischemic cardiac/cerebrovascular/peripheral vascular syndromes, and uncontrolled hypertension; other significant underlying cardiovascular disease such as angina, MI, and strokes; patients with hemiplegic or basilar migraine; within 24 hrs of treatment with another 5-HT₁ agonist or an ergot-type/ergotamine-containing medication; concurrent use or within 2 weeks of stopping an MAO inhibitor	This medication may make you dizzy, tired, or drowsy so do not drive or use machinery until you know how you react; give patient the product instructions provided by the manufacturer; also SEE naritriptan HCl For Maxalt-MLT: In addition to above, instruct patient not to remove the blister from the outer pouch until just prior to dosing, then peel open the blister with dry hands, allow the tablet to dissolve on the tongue — do not crush or chew	Patients taking propranolol should receive the 5 mg dose of rizatriptan benzoate and should take a maximum of 3 doses/24 hr period — SEE Prescribing Information (PI); Maxalt-MLT contains phenylalanine, which may be an important concern in persons with phenylketonuria

Generic Name and Selected Trade Names	Normal Adult Dosage	Major Adverse Effects/Cautions	Key Counseling Points	Miscellaneous Issues
Rizatriptan Benzoate (continued) Maxalt Maxalt-MLT	Reduced dosage may be required in patients with renal or hepatic impairment — SEE Prescribing Information (PI)	<u>Considerations</u>: Only use in persons confirmed to have migraine headaches; safety of treating, on average, more than 4 headaches/30 day period is not established; use cautiously in persons undergoing hemodialysis or with moderate hepatic insufficiency; also, SEE naritriptan HCl except for geriatric concern Most common AEs include asthenia/fatigue, somnolence, pain/pressure sensation, dizziness, nausea <u>Pregnancy category</u>: C		

Generic Name and Selected Trade Names	Normal Adult Dosage	Major Adverse Effects/Cautions	Key Counseling Points	Miscellaneous Issues
Sumatriptan Succinate Imitrex	Individualize dosage *Injection* For the acute treatment of migraine headache and the acute treatment of cluster headache episodes, the maximum single recommended dose is 6 mg administered subcutaneously (SC); repeat doses must be separated by at least 1 hr but should not exceed two 6-mg injections/24 hr period; patients receiving MAO inhibitors may require lower dosages — SEE Prescribing Information (PI)	<u>Contraindications for injection</u>: Intravenous (IV) administration, also SEE rizatriptan benzoate except for statement concerning use with MAO inhibitor <u>Contraindications for tablets</u>: SEE rizatriptan benzoate except for statement concerning use with another 5-HT$_1$ agonist <u>Considerations</u>: Use only when diagnosis of migraine or cluster headaches clearly established; there is a risk of causing myocardial ischemia, increased BP, MI, coronary artery vasospasm, ventricular tachycardia/fibrillation, cardiac arrest and death; strongly recommended not to use in persons with unrecognized coronary artery disease such as those with risk factors including hypercholesterolemia,	SEE naritriptan HCl; also <u>Injection</u>: Ensure patient and/or caregiver is familiar with proper injection technique and, if appropriate, the auto-injector; give patient the product instructions provided by the manufacturer <u>Tablets</u>: Swallow tablets whole with a full glass of water — do not break, crush, or chew <u>Nasal spray</u>: Ensure patient knows how to administer dose; give patient the product instructions provided by the manufacturer	Injection: An auto-injection device (autoinjector) is available for 6 mg doses; in patients receiving lower doses only the single-dose vial dosage form should be used

Generic Name and Selected Trade Names	Normal Adult Dosage	Major Adverse Effects/Cautions
Sumatriptan Succinate (continued) Imitrex	*Tablets* For the acute treatment of migraine headache, give a single 25-mg tablet with fluids; maximum single recommended dose is 100 mg; if needed, a second dose of up to 100 mg may be administered after 2 hrs; if headache returns, additional doses may be given at least 2 hrs apart but should not exceed 300 mg/24 hr period; if headache returns following use of sumatriptan injection, additional doses of the tablet form (up to 200 mg/day) may be given with dosage interval of at least 2 hrs between tablet doses *Nasal spray* Administer a single dose of 5, 10, or 20 mg in one nostril (or, for example, a 10 mg dose may be administered as 5 mg in each nostril); if headache returns, the dose may be repeated once after 2 hrs but should not exceed 40 mg/24 hr period	smoker, obesity, diabetes mellitus, positive family history; if patient has cardiovascular risk factors but has a satisfactory cardiovascular evaluation, administer first dose in physician's or other equipped office; regular users of this medication should have cardiac status evaluated periodically; may cause coronary vasospasm, chest discomfort, cerebrovascular events such as strokes and TIAs, increases in blood pressure, and hypersensitivity reactions Most common AEs include atypical sensations such as tingling, flushing, chest or throat discomfort/tightness, drowsiness, vertigo; and injection site reactions for injectable form; and bad taste for tablets <u>Pregnancy category</u>: C

Generic Name and Selected Trade Names	Normal Adult Dosage	Major Adverse Effects/Cautions	Key Counseling Points	Miscellaneous Issues
Timolol Maleate[2] Blocadren				
Zolmitriptan Zomig	Individualize dosage For the acute treatment of migraine headache, controlled trials showed that single doses of 1, 2.5, and 5 mg were effective but a greater proportion of patients responded to the 2.5 and 5 mg doses than the 1 mg dose; usually start patients on 2.5 mg; repeat doses should be separated by at least 2 hrs if needed but do not exceed 10 mg/24 hr period	<u>Contraindications</u>: SEE rizatriptan benzoate <u>Considerations</u>: Only use in persons confirmed to have migraine headaches; safety of treating, on average, more than 3 headaches/30 day period is not established; use cautiously in persons with hepatic disease; also, SEE naritriptan HCl except for geriatric concern Most common AEs include atypical sensations such as paresthesia, asthenia, nausea, dizziness, pain, chest/neck/throat tightness or heaviness, somnolence, warm sensation <u>Pregnancy category</u>: C	SEE rizatriptan benzoate	Doses <2.5 mg may be obtained by breaking the 2.5 mg tablet in half

Generic Name and Selected Trade Names	Normal Adult Dosage	Major Adverse Effects/Cautions	Key Counseling Points	Miscellaneous Issues
Zolmitriptan (continued) Zomig	Lower dosages may be required in patients with moderate to severe hepatic impairment — SEE Prescribing Information (PI)			

*As a general rule, a medication should not be administered to a patient with a known hypersensitivity to it or a similar agent.
[1]SEE antiepileptic medications.
[2]SEE beta adrenergic blocking agents.

Hormones

Table 1: Androgens*

Generic Name and Selected Trade Names	Normal Adult Dosage	Major Adverse Effects/Cautions	Key Counseling Points	Miscellaneous Issues
Fluoxy-mesterone[1] Halotestin	Individualize dosage For male hypogonadism, usual dosage is 5 to 20 mg daily For use in women — SEE Prescribing Information (PI)	Contraindications: Males with breast carcinoma or known or suspected cancer of the prostate, and in patients with serious cardiac, renal, or liver disease Considerations: Use caution in persons with cardiac, renal, or hepatic disease; may cause allergic reactions, edema, oligospermia, priapism, excessive sexual stimulation, cholestatic hepatitis and jaundice; geriatric males are more likely to develop prostatic hypertrophy and carcinoma Most common AEs include acne, gynecomastia, edema, nausea, GI upset, excessive frequency and duration of penile erections Pregnancy category: X	Tell the prescriber if you have any type of cancer, or a heart, kidney, or liver problem; for women, do not take if you are pregnant and notify the prescriber immediately if you become pregnant while taking this agent; for males, tell the prescriber if you develop frequent or persistent erections of the penis; take with food unless otherwise directed; while taking this agent, notify the prescriber if you develop nausea, vomiting, changes in skin color, or ankle edema (swelling); do not exceed the prescribed dosage; if you miss a dose take it as soon as you remember, but if it is almost time for the next dose skip the missed one — do not double doses	Should not be used to enhance athletic performance; if priapism develops, temporarily discontinue therapy and then re-institute at a lower dosage; contains the dye tartrazine (FD&C yellow No. 5), which may cause allergic reactions; due to risk of liver toxicity, routine laboratory testing should be performed periodically

Generic Name and Selected Trade Names	Normal Adult Dosage	Major Adverse Effects/Cautions	Key Counseling Points	Miscellaneous Issues
Methyltestosterone Android Oreton Methyl Testred	Individualize dosage For replacement therapy in androgen-deficient males, administer 10 to 50 mg daily; lower dosages used in delayed puberty and to treat metastatic breast cancer in women — SEE Prescribing Information (PI)	Contraindications: Men with carcinoma of the breast or prostate, women who are or may become pregnant Considerations: May cause hypercalcemia in patients with breast cancer; prolonged high doses may cause edema (with or without CHF), gynecomastia, and liver disease; cholestatic hepatitis and jaundice may occur with relatively low dosages; geriatric males are more likely to develop prostatic hypertrophy and carcinoma; monitor women for signs of virilization Most common AEs in men include gynecomastia, excessive frequency and duration of penile erections, oligospermia with high dosages, nausea	SEE fluoxymesterone	Should not be used to enhance athletic performance; due to risk of liver toxicity, routine laboratory testing should be performed periodically; if used in adolescent males, check bone development every six months

Generic Name and Selected Trade Names	Normal Adult Dosage	Major Adverse Effects/Cautions	Key Counseling Points	Miscellaneous Issues
Methyltestosterone (continued) Android Oreton Methyl Testred		Most common AEs in women include amenorrhea and other menstrual irregularities, virilization, nausea Pregnancy category: X		

Generic Name and Selected Trade Names	Normal Adult Dosage	Major Adverse Effects/Cautions	Key Counseling Points	Miscellaneous Issues
Testosterone (injectable)	Individualize dosage *Short-acting, aqueous* Administered IM only (not IV); for androgen replacement therapy, 25 to 50 mg IM 2-3 times per week; for other uses, dosage is dependent on condition being treated — SEE Prescribing Information (PI) *Long-acting, oil* (enanthate, cypionate, and propionate salts available) Administered IM only (not IV); usually <400 mg/month — SEE PI	SEE methyltestosterone testosterone	If patient or caregiver is administering the medication, ensure he/she is familiar with proper injection technique; also SEE fluoxymesterone	SEE methyltestosterone testosterone

Generic Name and Selected Trade Names	Normal Adult Dosage	Major Adverse Effects/Cautions	Key Counseling Points	Miscellaneous Issues
Testosterone (scrotal system) Testoderm Testoderm with Adhesive	Individualize dosage For testosterone replacement, usually start with a 6 mg/day system (patch) applied to the scrotal area daily; patch to be worn 22–24 hrs/day	<u>Contraindications</u>: Men with carcinoma of the breast or known or suspected carcinoma of the prostate, women <u>Considerations</u>: Prolonged high doses may cause edema (with or without CHF), gynecomastia, and liver disease; geriatric males are more likely to develop prostatic hypertrophy and carcinoma; may cause fetal harm if administered to pregnant women; may cause frequent or persistent penile erections, virilization of female partners	Tell the prescriber if you have any type of cancer, or a heart, kidney, or liver disease; apply patch to the scrotal area because the medicine gets into the body better this way; ensure patient knows how to apply patch properly (SEE PI); before applying, wash your hands well, then dry shave the area — do not use soap, water, or chemical agents to get rid of hair; when you are finished wearing the patch, fold it in half with the sticky sides together, place it in the protective pouch or aluminum foil, and throw it away out of the reach of children or animals;	Should not be used to enhance athletic performance; due to risk of liver toxicity, routine laboratory testing should be performed periodically; scrotal hair should be removed before applying system, do not use chemical depilatories

Generic Name and Selected Trade Names	Normal Adult Dosage	Major Adverse Effects/Cautions	Key Counseling Points	Miscellaneous Issues
Testosterone (scrotal system) (continued) Testoderm Testoderm with Adhesive		Most common AEs include local effects such as scrotal itching, discomfort, irritation; gynecomastia, acne, prostatitis/urinary tract infections, breast tenderness <u>Pregnancy category</u>: X	while taking this agent, notify the prescriber if you develop nausea, vomiting, changes in skin color, or ankle edema (swelling); tell the prescriber if you develop frequent or persistent erections of the penis; do not exceed the prescribed dosage; if you miss a dose take it as soon as you remember, but if it is almost time for the next dose skip the missed one — do not double doses	

Generic Name and Selected Trade Names	Normal Adult Dosage	Major Adverse Effects/Cautions	Key Counselling Points	Miscellaneous Issues
Testosterone (topical system) Androderm	Individualize dosage. For testosterone replacement, start with one 5 mg system or two 2.5 mg systems applied nightly for 24 hrs — apply to a dry, clean area of the back, abdomen, upper arms or thighs, but NOT to a bony area of the body or to scrotal area	<u>Contraindications, considerations and pregnancy category:</u> SEE Testosterone Scrotal System <u>Most common AEs</u> include pruritus, erythema, or burning at application site, burn-like blister under the system, rash, prostate abnormalities, headache, allergic reactions, depression	Ensure patient knows how to apply patch properly — see Prescribing Information (PI); for other issues, SEE Testosterone Scrotal System	Should not be used to enhance athletic performance; due to risk of liver toxicity, routine laboratory testing should be performed periodically

*As a general rule, a medication should not be administered to a patient with a known hypersensitivity to it or a similar agent.

†Used for other conditions as well; refer to Prescribing Information and other sources.

Table 2: Estrogens and Select Estrogen Combinations*

Generic Name and Selected Trade Names	Normal Adult Dosage	Major Adverse Effects/Cautions	Key Counseling Points	Miscellaneous Issues
Conjugated Estrogens Premarin	Individualize dosage For vasomotor symptoms due to menopause: Usually 1.25 mg QD For atrophic vaginitis due to menopause: Usually 0.3 to 1.25 mg or more QD For hypoestrogenism: Dosing is complex and a wide range is possible — SEE Prescribing Information (PI) For osteoporosis: Usually, 0.625 mg QD perhaps on a cyclic basis — 3 weeks on and 1 off	Contraindications: Known or suspected pregnancy, known or suspected cancer of the breast except when used for metastatic disease, known or suspected estrogen-dependent neoplasia, undiagnosed abnormal genital bleeding, active thrombophlebitis or thromboembolic disease Considerations: Estrogens (without progestin) reported to increase risk of endometrial carcinoma in postmenopausal women; should not be used during pregnancy; possible increased risk of breast cancer, gall-bladder disease, thrombophlebitis and other thromboembolic disorders, hypercalcemia in patients with breast cancer and bone metastases;	Product is marketed with a leaflet designed for patients — dispense with medication; tell the prescriber if you have any type of cancer, fibroid tumors of the uterus, a liver or kidney disorder, abnormal genital bleeding, history of forming blood clots; do not use if you are pregnant and if you get pregnant while taking this agent contact the prescriber immediately; ensure patient understands the risks of cancer, gallbladder disease, thromboembolism, etc associated with therapy; try to take the medicine at the same time each day;	In many situations, it may be advisable to add a progestin — SEE Prescribing Information (PI)

554

Generic Name and Selected Trade Names	Normal Adult Dosage	Major Adverse Effects/Cautions	Key Counselling Points	Miscellaneous Issues
Conjugated Estrogens (continued) Premarin	For cancer: SEE PI Vaginal cream and parenteral formulations available — SEE PI	addition of progestin decreases risk of endometrial hyperplasia; may elevate blood pressure and plasma triglycerides; may cause fluid retention, uterine bleeding, increase the size of uterine fibroids; use with caution in persons with liver or kidney impairment Most common AEs include changes in vaginal bleeding, vaginal candidiasis, breast tenderness/enlargement, nausea, vomiting, abdominal cramps, bloating, jaundice, pancreatitis, venous thromboembolism, pulmonary embolism, intolerance to contact lenses, headache, dizziness, depression Pregnancy category: X	if you miss a dose take it as soon as you remember, but if it is almost time for the next dose skip the missed one — do not double doses	

Generic Name and Selected Trade Names	Normal Adult Dosage	Major Adverse Effects/Cautions	Key Counseling Points	Miscellaneous Issues
Conjugated Estrogens plus Medroxyprogesterone Premphase Prempro	Indivdualize dosage For moderate to severe vasomotor symptoms and vulvar/vaginal atrophy associated with menopause, and osteoporosis prevention *Premphase* Consists of 2 separate tabs — 1 tab is conjugated estrogens 0.625 mg and other tab is conjugated estrogens 0.625 mg plus 5 mg medroxyprogesterone; tab 1 is taken on days 1–14 and tab 2 on days 15–28	<u>Contraindications</u>: Liver dysfunction or disease, also SEE conjugated estrogens <u>Considerations, most common AEs, and pregnancy category</u>: SEE conjugated estrogens	SEE conjugated estrogens	

Generic Name and Selected Trade Names	Normal Adult Dosage	Major Adverse Effects/Cautions	Key Counselling Points	Miscellaneous Issues
Conjugated Estrogens plus Medroxyprogesterone (continued) Premphase Prempro	*Prempro* Consists of 1 tab with conjugated estrogens 0.625 mg plus 2.5 mg medroxyprogesterone			

Generic Name and Selected Trade Names	Normal Adult Dosage	Major Adverse Effects/Cautions	Key Counseling Points	Miscellaneous Issues
Esterified Estrogens Estratab Menest	Individualize dosage For vasomotor symptoms due to menopause: Usually 1.25 mg QD perhaps cyclically — eg, 3 weeks on and 1 off For atrophic vaginitis and kraurosis vulvae due to menopause: Usually 0.3 to 1.25 mg or more QD perhaps cyclically For female hypogonadism: Dosing is complex and a wide range is possible — SEE Prescribing Information (PI) For cancer: SEE PI	SEE conjugated estrogens	SEE conjugated estrogens	SEE conjugated estrogens

558

Generic Name and Selected Trade Names	Normal Adult Dosage	Major Adverse Effects/Cautions	Key Counseling Points	Miscellaneous Issues
Estradiol Transdermal System Alora Climara Estraderm FemPatch Vivelle	Individualize dosage All transdermal systems ("patches") provide continuous estradiol administration; some patches are applied once per week, others twice; doses and indications vary somewhat — SEE Prescribing Information	Adverse effects at site of application (eg, irritation) are possible; also SEE conjugated estrogens	Product is marketed with a leaflet designed for patients — dispense with medication; tell the prescriber if you have any type of cancer, fibroid tumors of the uterus, a liver or kidney disorder, abnormal genital bleeding, history of forming blood clots; do not use if you are pregnant and if you get pregnant while taking this agent contact the prescriber immediately; ensure patient understands the risks of cancer, gallbladder disease, thromboembolism, etc associated with therapy; ensure patient understands the proper way to apply and ultimately dispose of patch;	SEE conjugated estrogens; agents are not interchangeable

Generic Name and Selected Trade Names	Normal Adult Dosage	Major Adverse Effects/Cautions	Key Counseling Points	Miscellaneous Issues
Estradiol Transdermal System (continued) Alora Climara Estraderm FemPatch Vivelle			if you forget to apply a new patch at the prescribed time do so as soon as possible but if it is time for the next patch skip the missed one and return to usual dosing regimen, always remove the old patch before applying a new one, do not apply more than one patch at a time unless directed to do so	

Generic Name and Selected Trade Names	Normal Adult Dosage	Major Adverse Effects/Cautions	Key Counseling Points	Miscellaneous Issues
Estropipate Ogen Ortho-est	Individualize dosage <u>For vasomotor symptoms and/or vulval and vaginal atrophy due to menopause:</u> Usually 0.75 to 6 mg QD perhaps cyclically; use lowest effective dose <u>For prevention of osteoporosis:</u> 0.75 mg QD for 25 days out of a 31 day cycle per month <u>For female hypogonadism:</u> Dosing is complex and a wide range is possible — SEE Prescribing Information (PI) <u>For cancer:</u> SEE PI	SEE conjugated estrogens	SEE conjugated estrogens	Supplied as 0.625 tablet (0.75 mg estropipate; calculated as sodium estrone sulfate 0.625); similarly, 1.25 mg tablet equivalent to 1.5 mg of estropipate; also SEE conjugated estrogens

*As a general rule, a medication should not be administered to a patient with a known hypersensitivity to it or a similar agent.

Table 3: Selected Oral Contraceptives*

Generic Name and Selected Trade Names	Normal Adult Dosage	Major Adverse Effects/Cautions	Key Counseling Points	Miscellaneous Issues
Monophasic Products (contains an estrogen [eg, mestranol or ethinyl estradiol] & a progestin [eg, ethynodiol norethindrone, or norgestrel]) Brevicon Demulen 1/50, 1/35 Desogen Genora 1/50, 1/35 Levlen Loestrin 21 Loestrin Fe	Individualize dosage	Contraindications: Thrombophlebitis or thromboembolic disorders, past history of deep vein thrombophlebitis (DVT) or thromboembolic disorders, cerebrovascular or coronary artery disease, known or suspected carcinoma of the breast, carcinoma of the endometrium or other known or suspected estrogen-dependent neoplasia, undiagnosed abnormal genital bleeding. cholestatic jaundice or pregnancy or jaundice with prior oral contraceptive (OC) use, hepatic adenoma/carcinoma or benign liver tumors, known or suspected pregnancy Considerations: Cigarette smoking increases the risk of serious cardiovascular side effects from OCs and the risk	Product is marketed with a leaflet designed for patients — dispense with medication and ensure patient knows when to start, what to do if she missed a dose, potential side effects, and difference between 21- and 28-day packs; ensure patient understands the risk of OC use — SEE Contraindications and Consideration sections of this monograph, as well as Prescribing Information (PI); tell the prescriber if patient has any of the contraindications/ considerations noted; strongly advise woman not to smoke	Drug interactions are possible, some of which may decrease efficacy of the OC — SEE Prescribing Information (PI)

Generic Name and Selected Trade Names	Normal Adult Dosage	Major Adverse Effects/Cautions	Key Counseling Points	Miscellaneous Issues
Monophasic Products (continued) Lo/Ovral Modicon Nelova 1/50M, 1/35 Nordette Norethin 1/35E Norethin 1/50M Norinyl 1 + 35 Norinyl 1 + 50 Ortho-Cyclen Ortho-Novum 1/50, 1/35 Ovcon-50 Ovral		increases with age and heavy smoking (ie, 15 or more cigarettes per day); OC use associated with increased risk of several serious conditions such as MI, thromboembolism, stroke, vascular disorders, hepatic neoplasia, and gallbladder disease — risk is enhanced when other risk factors are present; may increase blood pressure, cause headache, cause jaundice, cause ocular lesions, increase fluid retention, and cause breakthrough and other bleeding abnormalities; may elevate low density lipoproteins; may affect tolerance to contact lenses Most common AEs include a wide number of potential problems — SEE Prescribing Information (PI) Pregnancy category: X		

Generic Name and Selected Trade Names	Normal Adult Dosage	Major Adverse Effects/Cautions	Key Counseling Points	Miscellaneous Issues
Biphasic Products Jenest-28 Nelova 10/11 Ortho-Novum 10/11	Individualize dosage	SEE Monophasic Products	SEE Monophasic Products	SEE Monophasic Products
Triphasic Products Ortho-Novum 7/7/7 Ortho Tri-Cyclen Tri-Levlen Tri-Norinyl Triphasil	Individualize dosage	SEE Monophasic Products	SEE Monophasic Products	SEE Monophasic Products

*As a general rule, a medication should not be administered to a patient with a known hypersensitivity to it or a similar agent.

Table 4: Thyroid Hormones*

Generic Name and Selected Trade Names	Normal Adult Dosage	Major Adverse Effects/Cautions	Key Counseling Points	Miscellaneous Issues
Levothyroxine Sodium (T$_4$) Eltroxin Levo-T Levothroid Levoxyl Synthroid	Individualize dosage For hypothyroidism: Usually, start with 50 mcg daily, and titrate based upon clinical response and appropriate laboratory tests — SEE Prescribing Information (PI); alternatively, in young/healthy persons, full replacement dose is about 1.6 mcg/kg/day; usual maintenance dose is <200 mcg/day but some patients require more; elderly and others may need lower dosages —SEE (PI)	Contraindications: Untreated thyrotoxicosis, uncorrected adrenal insufficiency Considerations: Use caution in the elderly, persons with diabetes mellitus or insipidus, and patients with cardiovascular disorders such as angina, coronary artery disease, and hypertension; has caused seizures; may enhance anticoagulant therapy; patients receiving lithium may require altered dosages of thyroid hormones	Tell the prescriber if you have a heart disorder such as angina or hypertension, a seizure disorder, diabetes mellitus, or an adrenal disorder; notify the prescriber if while taking this agent you develop chest pain, shortness of breath, a skin rash or reaction, irregular heartbeat, irritability, nervousness, sleeplessness, diarrhea, heat intolerance, changes in appetite; if patient is hypertensive monitor BP more frequently, if patient has diabetes monitor blood glucose more frequently; do not increase or decrease the prescribed dose without discussing it first with the prescriber;	Should not be used in the treatment of obesity unless patient is hypothyroid; numerous drug interactions are possible — SEE Prescribing Information (PI); tablets may contain dyes that may cause allergic reactions, other tablets may contain lactose — SEE PI

Generic Name and Selected Trade Names	Normal Adult Dosage	Major Adverse Effects/Cautions	Key Counseling Points	Miscellaneous Issues
Levothyroxine Sodium (T₄) (continued) Eltroxin Levo-T Levothroid Levoxyl Synthroid	For myxedema coma: Preferably treat IV, but may treat via nasogastric tube; usual initial dose is 300 to 500 mcg, and 75 to 100 mcg/day thereafter; titrate according to response and laboratory tests; certain patients require less — SEE PI For thyroid cancer and pediatric use: SEE PI	Most common AEs include those associated with the disease (eg, hypothyroidism), therapeutic overdose (ie, hyperthyroidism); hypersensitivity reactions such as rash and urticaria Pregnancy category: A	it may take a few weeks for this medicine to work; if you miss a dose take it as soon as you remember, but if it is almost time for the next dose skip the missed one — do not double doses	

Generic Name and Selected Trade Names	Normal Adult Dosage	Major Adverse Effects/Cautions	Key Counseling Points	Miscellaneous Issues
Liothyronine Sodium (T_3) Cytomel Triostat	Individualize dosage For mild hypothyroidism: Usually start with 25 mcg daily and titrate in increments of 5 to 25 mcg every 1–2 weeks; usual maintenance dose is 25 to 75 mcg/day For myxedema: Usually start with 5 mcg daily and titrate in increments of 5 to 10 mcg every 1–2 weeks until 25 mcg/day is reached at which point may titrate in increments of 5 to 25 mcg every 1–2 weeks; usual maintenance is 50 to 100 mcg/day	SEE levothyroxine sodium	SEE levothyroxine sodium	Should not be used in the treatment of obesity unless patient is hypothyroid; numerous drug interactions are possible — SEE Prescribing Information (PI)

Generic Name and Selected Trade Names	Normal Adult Dosage	Major Adverse Effects/Cautions	Key Counseling Points	Miscellaneous Issues
Liothyronine Sodium (T₃) (continued) Cytomel Triostat	<u>For myxedema coma</u>: SEE Prescribing Information (PI) <u>Dosage adjustments</u>: Elderly and pediatric patients require lower dosages — SEE PI			

*As a general rule, a medication should not be administered to a patient with a known hypersensitivity to it or a similar agent.

Table 5: Glucocorticoids (systemic)*

Generic Name and Selected Trade Names	Normal Adult Dosage	Major Adverse Effects/Cautions	Key Counseling Points	Miscellaneous Issues
Betamethasone, Betamethasone Acetate & Betamethasone Sodium Phosphate Celestone	Individualize dosage Initial oral dosage may be 0.6 to 7.2 mg/day and initial IM dosage may vary from 0.5 to 9 mg per day depending on use — SEE Prescribing Information (PI); maintenance dose depends on patient response and use — SEE PI	<u>Contraindication</u>: Systemic fungal infections <u>Considerations</u>: Certain products to be given orally, intranasally, IM not IV, etc — SEE Prescribing Information (PI); while receiving therapy, do not vaccinate against smallpox and other vaccinations should be done cautiously as should use in persons with TB or ocular herpes simplex — SEE (PI); patients in stressful situations may require increased dosage; may mask signs of infection; long-term use may lead to cataracts, glaucoma, and ocular infections due to fungi or viruses; may increase fluid retention, blood pressure, and potassium excretion;	Patients receiving immunosuppressant doses should avoid exposure to chickenpox or measles; ensure patients understand the Considerations section of this table; dose must be tapered (stopped) slowly, so do not stop therapy without discussing it first with the prescriber; if the prescriber asks you to follow a low-sodium and/or high-potassium diet, please do so; for oral dosage forms, take with food or antacids unless otherwise directed; procedure for missed doses depends on route, dosage form, and use — consider individually; ensure	Glucocorticoids are marketed in a variety of strengths and dosage forms

Generic Name and Selected Trade Names	Normal Adult Dosage	Major Adverse Effects/Cautions	Key Counseling Points	Miscellaneous Issues
Betamethasone, Betamethasone Acetate & Betamethasone Sodium Phosphate (continued) Celestone		consider other conditions patient might have that would be affected by low potassium (eg, CHF and arrhythmias); infections more likely in immunosuppressed patients; parenteral use has caused allergic reactions; psychiatric derangements are possible; if patient has hypoprothrombinemia use aspirin cautiously; intraarticular injection may cause systemic effects; may cause or worsen GI ulcers; may worsen diabetes mellitus; do not inject into previously infected joints or into unstable joints; always use lowest possible dose Most common AEs are numerous and affect virtually all body systems — SEE PI <u>Pregnancy category</u>: Not specified	patient knows the manner in which alternative dosage forms (eg, intranasal, inhalation) are used if applicable	

Generic Name and Selected Trade Names	Normal Adult Dosage	Major Adverse Effects/Cautions	Key Counseling Points	Miscellaneous Issues
Cortisone Acetate Cortone	Individualize dosage Initial and maintenance dosage depends on dosage form, route of administration, therapeutic need, and a variety of individual patient concerns — SEE Prescribing Information (PI)	SEE Betamethasone	SEE Betamethasone	SEE Betamethasone
Dexamethasone & Dexamethasone Phosphate Decadron	SEE Cortisone Acetate	SEE Betamethasone	SEE Betamethasone	SEE Betamethasone

Generic Name and Selected Trade Names	Normal Adult Dosage	Major Adverse Effects/Cautions	Key Counseling Points	Miscellaneous Issues
Hydrocortisone, Hydrocortisone Acetate, Hydrocortisone Cypionate, Hydrocortisone Sodium Phosphate, & Hydrocortisone Sodium Succinate Cortef Hydrocortone Solu-Cortef	SEE Cortisone Acetate	SEE Betamethasone	SEE Betamethasone	SEE Betamethasone

Generic Name and Selected Trade Names	Normal Adult Dosage	Major Adverse Effects/Cautions	Key Counselling Points	Miscellaneous Issues
Methylpred-nisolone & Methylpred-nisolone Sodium Succinate Medrol Solu-Medrol	SEE Cortisone Acetate	SEE Betamethasone	SEE Betamethasone	SEE Betamethasone

Generic Name and Selected Trade Names	Normal Adult Dosage	Major Adverse Effects/Cautions	Key Counseling Points	Miscellaneous Issues
Prednisolone, Prednisolone Sodium Phosphate, & Prednisolone Tebutate Delta-Cortef Hydeltrasol Hydeltra-T.B.A. Pediapred Prelone	SEE Cortisone Acetate	SEE Betamethasone	SEE Betamethasone	SEE Betamethasone
Prednisone Deltasone Meticorten Orasone	SEE Cortisone Acetate	SEE Betamethasone	SEE Betamethasone	SEE Betamethasone

Generic Name and Selected Trade Names	Normal Adult Dosage	Major Adverse Effects/Cautions	Key Counseling Points	Miscellaneous Issues
Triamcino-lone, Triamcinolone Acetonide, & Triamcinolone Diacetate Aristocort Kenacort Kenalog-40 Triamolone 40 Triamonide 40 Trilone	SEE Cortisone Acetate	SEE Betamethasone	SEE Betamethasone	SEE Betamethasone

*As a general rule, a medication should not be administered to a patient with a known hypersensitivity to it or a similar agent.

Table 6: Miscellaneous Hormones*

Generic Name and Selected Trade Names	Normal Adult Dosage	Major Adverse Effects/Cautions	Key Counseling Points	Miscellaneous Issues
Danazol Danocrine	Individualize dosage For endometriosis: In moderate to severe disease or in infertility due to endometriosis start with 800 mg/day in two divided doses and then titrate down; in mild disease, start with 200 to 400 mg/day in two doses; continue therapy uninterrupted for 3–6 months and may extend to 9 months For fibrocystic breast disease: Dose ranges from 100 to 400 mg/day in two divided doses	Contraindications: Undiagnosed abnormal genital bleeding, markedly impaired hepatic/renal/cardiac function, pregnancy, breast feeding, porphyria Considerations: Use a sensitive test to ensure patient is not pregnant before beginning therapy; may cause decreased high density lipoproteins and increased low density lipoproteins; elevated liver function tests reported; if used for fibrocystic breast disease ensure patient does not have breast carcinoma; monitor patient for androgenic effects; may cause photosensitivity reactions; may cause fluid retention so use cautiously in persons with cardiac or renal dysfunction, seizure disorder, migraine	Tell the prescriber if you are pregnant, have any abnormal genital bleeding, have a seizure disorder or migraine headaches, or have any liver, kidney or heart disease; while taking this medication, do not breast feed and use a non-hormonal method of birth control to ensure that you do not become pregnant; while taking this medication, if you think you have become pregnant contact the prescriber immediately; stay out of direct sunlight, and if you go into sunlight wear sunblock;	

Generic Name and Selected Trade Names	Normal Adult Dosage	Major Adverse Effects/Cautions	Key Counseling Points	Miscellaneous Issues
Danazol (continued) Danocrine	For hereditary angioedema: Start with 200 mg BID or TID and titrate — SEE Prescribing Information (PI)	Most common AEs include androgenic effects such as weight gain, acne, mild hirsutism and changes in voice, menstrual abnormalities such as spotting, flushing, sweating, vaginal dryness, hepatic dysfunction Pregnancy category: X	If you miss a dose of this medication take it as soon as you remember, but if it is almost time for the next dose skip the missed one and return to your normal schedule — do not double doses	

Generic Name and Selected Trade Names	Normal Adult Dosage	Major Adverse Effects/Cautions	Key Counseling Points	Miscellaneous Issues
Desmopressin (vasopressin) DDAVP Injection, Nasal Spray, & Tablets	Individualize dosage *Injectable* For diabetes insipidus: Usual range in adults is 2 mcg (0.5 mL) to 4 mcg (1 mL) daily IV or SC in two divided doses For hemophilia A and von Willebrand's Disease: Given as IV infusion — SEE Prescribing Information (PI) *Nasal Spray* For central cranial diabetes insipidus: Usual adult dose is 0.1 to 0.4 mL daily as a single dose or divided into 2 or 3 doses, most adults need 0.2 mL daily in 2 doses	Considerations: Usually need to adjust fluid intake downward to decrease potential for water intoxication and hyponatremia; use caution in patients with cardiovascular disorders and conditions associated with fluid and electrolyte imbalance such as cystic fibrosis; Injectable: can increase or decrease blood pressure and thrombotic events rarely reported; Nasal Spray: can increase blood pressure Most common AEs in adults include rhinitis, abdominal pain, headaches, nausea, nostril pain (nasal form) local reactions (injectable) Pregnancy category: B	Tell the prescriber if you have a heart disease of any kind, suffer from migraine headaches, or have cystic fibrosis; if patient or caregiver is giving the injectable or nasal formulation, ensure he/she is familiar with proper administration technique	For injectable and nasal spray, morning and evening doses should be adjusted separately; for nasal spray, pump delivers 10 mcg/spray

Generic Name and Selected Trade Names	Normal Adult Dosage	Major Adverse Effects/Cautions	Key Counseling Points	Miscellaneous Issues
Desmopressin (vasopressin) DDAVP Injection, Nasal Spray, & Tablets	For pediatric use in primary nocturnal enuresis: SEE PI *Tablets* For central cranial diabetes insipidus: Start with 0.05 mg (one-half of the 0.1 mg tab) two times a day and adjust doses individually; usual dosage range is 0.1 to 0.8 mg daily in divided doses; if previously received nasal spray, begin therapy 12 hrs after last intranasal dose For pediatric use: SEE PI			

Generic Name and Selected Trade Names	Normal Adult Dosage	Major Adverse Effects/Cautions	Key Counselling Points	Miscellaneous Issues
Fludrocortisone Acetate Florinef	Individualize dosage For Addison's disease: The usual dose is 0.1 mg QD although range is 0.1 mg three times a week to 0.2 mg QD For salt-losing adrenogenital syndrome: Usually 0.1 to 0.2 mg QD	Contraindication: Systemic fungal infections Considerations: May cause *marked* sodium retention; also except for route of administration data, SEE Betamethasone Most common AEs include those related to potent mineralocorticoid effects — eg, retention of sodium and water; may cause hypertension, CHF, potassium loss, and many others — SEE Prescribing Information (PI) Pregnancy category: C	Tell the prescriber if you have any type of cardiac disorder including hypertension; do not stop therapy without discussing it first with the prescriber; if the prescriber asks you to follow a low-sodium and/or high-potassium diet, please do so; if you miss a dose of this medication take it as soon as you remember, but if it is almost time for the next dose skip the missed one and return to your normal schedule — do not double doses	Numerous drug interactions are possible — SEE Prescribing Information (PI)

Generic Name and Selected Trade Names	Normal Adult Dosage	Major Adverse Effects/Cautions	Key Counselling Points	Miscellaneous Issues
Leuprolide Acetate Lupron Lupron Depot	Individualize dosage Dosage depends on the specific dosage form selected and the therapeutic use (eg, prostate cancer vs endometriosis) — SEE Prescribing Information (PI)	Contraindications: Certain formulations are not to be used in women — SEE Prescribing Information (PI), undiagnosed abnormal vaginal bleeding, women who are or may become pregnant, women who are breast feeding Considerations: Signs/symptoms of disease have worsened when therapy first initiated; in women, menstrual periods may not be regular or may stop; certain formulations provide continuous therapy for several months — select dosage form carefully Most common AEs include hot flashes/sweats, edema, headache, nausea/vomiting, depression, and many others that are indication and dosage form specific — SEE PI Pregnancy category: X	For women, ensure patient is not pregnant and if she becomes pregnant while taking this agent must notify the prescriber immediately; if patient or caregiver is administering the injections, ensure he/she is familiar with proper injection technique; do not stop taking this medication without discussing it first with the prescriber; if you are using this medication daily and miss a dose give it as soon as possible, but if you remember the next day skip the missed one and return to normal schedule — do not double doses	Several different depot formulations are available

Generic Name and Selected Trade Names	Normal Adult Dosage	Major Adverse Effects/Cautions	Key Counseling Points	Miscellaneous Issues
Somatropin (Growth Hormone) Humatrope Norditropin Nutropin Protropin	Individualize dosage For growth hormone deficits in adults: Dosages are based on patient weight, but differ by specific product — SEE Prescribing Information (PI) for individual products For pediatric and other uses: SEE the PI for individual products	Contraindications: Differ by product and formulation (eg, due to different diluents for the injection and whether product indicated in adults only) — SEE Prescribing Information (PI) Most common AEs in adults include edema, arthralgia, paresthesia, myalgia, pain, rhinitis, peripheral edema, back pain, headache, hypertension Pregnancy category: C	If patient or caregiver is administering the injections, ensure he/she is familiar with proper injection technique; adverse effects, etc differ by product — SEE Prescribing Information (PI)	Certain products indicated for children only, and other products have additional indications — SEE Prescribing Information (PI) for individual agents as they are different

*As a general rule, a medication should not be administered to a patient with a known hypersensitivity to it or a similar agent.

Fertility Agents

Table: Fertility Agents*

Generic Name and Selected Trade Names	Normal Adult Dosage	Major Adverse Effects/Cautions	Key Counseling Points	Miscellaneous Issues
Bromocriptine Mesylate[1] Parlodel Parlodel Snap Tabs	Individualize dosage For hyperprolactinemic conditions, start with 1.25 to 2.5 mg daily; may titrate in 2.5 mg increments every 3-7 days; usual maintenance range is 2.5 to 15 mg/day	Contraindications: Uncontrolled hypertension, sensitivity to any ergot alkaloid; stop therapy if patient becomes pregnant Considerations: May cause hypotension, hypertension, seizures, stroke; rarely caused acute MI; do not use with other ergot alkaloids; long-term therapy (6-36 months) with doses of 20-100 mg/day occasionally associated with pulmonary infiltrates, pleural effusion, and pleural thickening; safety in renal or liver disease not established; use caution in patients with history of psychosis or cardiovascular disease	Tell the prescriber if you have or had a cardiovascular disease, high blood pressure, a seizure disorder, kidney disease, liver disease, or a psychiatric problem, or if you are allergic to ergot medications such as ergotamine; contact the prescriber if you develop a severe headache, blurred vision, severe nausea or vomiting; may be taken with food; when starting therapy this medication may make you tired, dizzy, or lightheaded so do not drive a car or use machinery until you know how you are affected;	Ensure patient does not have a pituitary tumor before therapy is initiated — SEE Prescribing Information (PI); monitor blood pressure (especially during first few weeks of therapy) and be alert for unremitting headache

Generic Name and Selected Trade Names	Normal Adult Dosage	Major Adverse Effects/Cautions	Key Counselling Points	Miscellaneous Issues
Bromocriptine Mesylate[1] **(continued)** Parlodel Parlodel Snap Tabs		Most common AEs include nausea, headache, dizziness, fatigue, lightheadedness, vomiting, abdominal cramps, nasal congestion, diarrhea, constipation, drowsiness Pregnancy category: B	if you miss a dose and remember it within 4 hrs take the missed dose, but if a longer time has passed, skip the dose and return to regular schedule — do not double doses	

Generic Name and Selected Trade Names	Normal Adult Dosage	Major Adverse Effects/Cautions	Key Counseling Points	Miscellaneous Issues
Clomiphene Citrate[1] Clomid Serophene	Individualize dosage To treat ovulatory dysfunction, start with 50 mg QD for 5 days; the dose should be increased only in patients who do not ovulate in response to this therapy; dosages above 100 mg per day for 5 days are not recommended — For more information, SEE Prescribing Information (PI)	<u>Contraindications</u>: Pregnancy (as fetal harm may occur), liver disease or history of same, abnormal uterine bleeding, patients with ovarian cysts, uncontrolled thyroid or adrenal dysfunction, presence of an organic intracranial lesion such as a pituitary tumor <u>Considerations</u>: May cause blurred vision or other visual disturbances such as flashes, and ovarian hyperstimulation syndrome <u>Most common AEs</u> include ovarian enlargement, vasomotor flushes, abdominal/pelvic discomfort, nausea/vomiting, breast discomfort, visual disturbances, headache, abnormal uterine bleeding <u>Pregnancy category</u>: X	Tell the prescriber if you have a liver, thyroid, or adrenal disorder; contact the prescriber if blurred vision or any other type of visual disturbance occurs, or if abdominal/pelvic discomfort or distention develops; if you become pregnant while on this medication, stop the therapy and call prescriber immediately; begin on the day of your menstrual cycle told to you by the prescriber; this medication may give you blurred/altered vision or make you dizzy or lightheaded so do not drive a car or use machinery until you know how you are affected:	Patient needs to be evaluated carefully to exclude pregnancy, ovarian enlargement, ovarian cyst between treatment cycles; therapy is associated with an increased chance of multiple birth pregnancy — SEE Prescribing Information (PI)

Generic Name and Selected Trade Names	Normal Adult Dosage	Major Adverse Effects/Cautions	Key Counselling Points	Miscellaneous Issues
Clomiphene Citrate[1] **(continued)** Clomid Serophene			if you miss a dose take it as soon as possible, if you remember when it is time for the next dose take both doses together then return to regular schedule — if you miss more than one dose, contact prescriber	

Generic Name and Selected Trade Names	Normal Adult Dosage	Major Adverse Effects/Cautions	Key Counseling Points	Miscellaneous Issues
Gonadorelin Acetate[1] (synthetic gonadotropin-releasing hormone [GnRH]) Lutrepulse	Individualize dosage In primary hypothalamic amenorrhea, start with 5 mcg every 90 minutes (via pump — SEE pump manual with product); dosages between 1 and 20 mcg have been successful	Contraindications: Any condition that would be worsened by pregnancy or worsened by increased amounts of reproductive hormones, ovarian cysts, causes of anovulation other than those of hypothalamic origin Considerations: May cause multiple birth pregnancy, serious hypersensitivity reactions, ovarian hyperstimulation Most common AEs include those at the injection site — rash, itching, hives, inflammation, infection, mild phlebitis, hematoma at catheter site Pregnancy category: B	This medication is administered by injection; stop the medication and seek medical attention at first sign of skin rash, hives, rapid heart rate, difficulty in swallowing or breathing	Lutrepulse pump is required; reconstitute the medication according to instructions provided immediately prior to use; only physicians experienced with pulsatile GnRH delivery should use this product; do not administer ovulation stimulators concurrently

Generic Name and Selected Trade Names	Normal Adult Dosage	Major Adverse Effects/Cautions	Key Counseling Points	Miscellaneous Issues
(Human) Chorionic Gonadotropin[1] **(HCG)** A.P.L. Pregnyl Profasi	Individualize dosage To induce ovulation, 5,000 to 10,000 USP units IM one day following the last dose of menotropins has been successful	Contraindications: Precocious puberty, pregnancy Considerations: May cause ovarian hyper-stimulation, enlargement of preexisting ovarian cysts or rupture of ovarian cysts, multiple birth pregnancy, arterial thromboembolism, hypersensitivity reactions; as fluid retention may occur, administer cautiously to persons with cardiac or renal disease, epilepsy, migraine, or asthma Most common AEs include headache, irritability, restlessness, depression, fatigue, edema, precocious puberty, gynecomastia, pain at injection site Pregnancy category: X	Tell the prescriber if you have a heart or kidney disorder, epilepsy, asthma, or suffer from migraine headache; this medication is administered by injection; stop the medication and seek medical attention at first sign of skin rash, hives, rapid heart rate, difficulty in swallowing or breathing; do not take this medication if you become pregnant	Should be prescribed by experienced clinicians only

Generic Name and Selected Trade Names	Normal Adult Dosage	Major Adverse Effects/Cautions	Key Counseling Points	Miscellaneous Issues
Menotropins[1] **(FSH/LH)** Humegon Pergonal Repronex	Individualize dosage Women Administered in a sequential manner with human chorionic gonadotropin (HCG) to induce ovulation; initial dose of menotropins is 75 IU IM per day — As dosing is complex, SEE Prescribing Information (PI)	Contraindications, Women: High FSH level, uncontrolled thyroid and adrenal dysfunction, an organic intracranial lesion such as a pituitary tumor, any cause of infertility other than anovulation unless the patient is a candidate for in vitro fertilization, abnormal bleeding of undetermined origin, pregnancy Contraindications, Men: Normal or elevated gonadotropin levels, infertility disorders other than hypogonadotropic hypogonadism Considerations: May cause ovarian enlargement, serious pulmonary conditions such as atelectasis and acute respiratory distress syndrome, thromboembolic events, multiple birth pregnancy	This medication is administered by injection; stop the medication and seek medical attention at first sign of skin rash, hives, rapid heart rate, difficulty in swallowing or breathing; ensure patient understands potential adverse effects; if you become pregnant while on this medication, stop the therapy and call prescriber immediately	Should be prescribed by experienced clinicians only

Generic Name and Selected Trade Names	Normal Adult Dosage	Major Adverse Effects/Cautions	Key Counseling Points	Miscellaneous Issues
Menotropins[1] **(FSH/LH) (continued)** Humegon Pergonal Repronex	Men Administered following pretreatment with HCG and then with HCG to induce spermatogenesis in men with primary hypogonadotropic hypogonadism — SEE PI; initial dose of menotropins is 75 IU IM three times a week — As dosing is complex, SEE PI	Most common AEs in women include pulmonary and vascular complications, ovarian hyperstimulation syndrome, hemoperitoneum, mild-to-moderate ovarian enlargement, ovarian cysts, abdominal pain, sensitivity reactions, dizziness/lightheadedness Most common AEs in men include gynecomastia, breast pain, elevated liver enzymes Pregnancy category: X		

Generic Name and Selected Trade Names	Normal Adult Dosage	Major Adverse Effects/Cautions	Key Counseling Points	Miscellaneous Issues
Progesterone Gel[1] Crinone 4% gel Crinone 8% gel	Individualize dosage For assisted reproductive technology in women, use the 8% product to administer 90 mg QD or BID depending on condition — SEE Prescribing Information (PI)	Contraindications: Undiagnosed vaginal bleeding, liver dysfunction or disease, known or suspected malignancy of breast or genital organs, missed abortion, active or history of hormone-associated thrombophlebitis or thromboembolic disorder Considerations: May cause fluid retention, so use caution in conditions that might be affected by this such as cardiac or renal dysfunction, asthma, migraine; use caution in persons with history of depression	Tell the prescriber if you are allergic to testosterone or testosterone-like products, if you suffer from vaginal bleeding, have a liver disorder, cancer of the breast or someplace else, if you have or have had blood clots, if you ever suffered from clinical depression; ensure patient knows how to administer the product — instructions provided with product; notify the prescriber if you develop pain in the calves or sudden shortness of breath, dizziness, severe nausea/vomiting/or constipation	Patient information leaflet provided in Product Information (PI) and with product

Generic Name and Selected Trade Names	Normal Adult Dosage	Major Adverse Effects/Cautions	Key Counseling Points	Miscellaneous Issues
Progesterone Gel[1] **(continued)** Crinone 4% gel Crinone 8% gel		Most common AEs include cramps, headache, breast pain, genital monilia, bloating, pain, nausea, dizziness, vaginal discharge, constipation, arthralgia, depression, nervousness, somnolence Pregnancy category: Not specified		

*As a general rule, a medication should not be administered to a patient with a known hypersensitivity to it or a similar agent.
[1]Used for other conditions as well; refer to Prescribing Information.

Osteoporosis Treatments

Table: Medications for Osteoporosis*

Generic Name and Selected Trade Names	Normal Adult Dosage	Major Adverse Effects/Cautions	Key Counseling Points	Miscellaneous Issues
Alendronate Sodium Fosamax	Individualize dosage Osteoporosis in postmenopausal women: Dosage to treat osteoporosis is 10 mg QD; for prevention of osteoporosis dosage is 5 mg QD For Paget's disease of bone: Recommended dosage is 40 mg QD for 6 months — SEE Prescribing Information (PI)	Contraindications: Abnormalities of the esophagus such as stricture that may delay esophageal emptying, inability to stand or sit upright for at least 30 minutes, hypocalcemia Considerations: May cause local irritation of the upper GI mucosa — esophageal erosions/ulcers could be serious; has caused gastric and duodenal ulcers; should not be used in persons with creatinine clearance <35 mL/ minute; hypocalcemia must be corrected before therapy with alendronate is started Most common AEs include abdominal pain, nausea, constipation, diarrhea, flatulence, musculoskeletal pain, headache Pregnancy category: C	Tell the prescriber if you have any trouble swallowing solids or liquids, or if you have a renal disorder; while taking this agent, tell the prescriber if you develop difficulty swallowing or pain/ burning in your esophagus; medication must be taken at least one-half hour before the first food, beverage, or medication of the day; take the medication with a full glass (6–8 oz) of plain water on an empty stomach — don't use any other beverage; do not take before going to bed; do not lie down for at least 30 minutes after taking a dose;	Risk of severe esophageal erosions is greater in patients who lie down after taking a dose and/or fail to take the dose with a full 6–8 ounce glass of water, and/or continue to take this agent after developing symptoms

597

Generic Name and Selected Trade Names	Normal Adult Dosage	Major Adverse Effects/Cautions	Key Counselling Points	Miscellaneous Issues
Alendronate Sodium (continued) Fosamax			do not chew or suck on the tablet; if calcium supplements and/or vitamin D were prescribed, it is very important to take them; if you miss a dose, do not take it later but do resume normal dosing schedule the next day — do not double doses	

Generic Name and Selected Trade Names	Normal Adult Dosage	Major Adverse Effects/Cautions	Key Counseling Points	Miscellaneous Issues
Calcitonin Salmon Calcimar Miacalcin	Individualize dosage *Injectable* For postmenopausal osteoporosis: Minimum dosage not established; consider giving 100 International Units (I.U.) SC or IM every other day; may need calcium and vitamin D simultaneously — SEE Prescribing Information (PI) For hypercalcemia: Usually start with 4 I.U./kG of body weight SC or IM Q12H; may titrate after 1–2 days to 8 I.U./kG Q12H, and then to a maximum of 8 I.U./kG Q6H	Considerations: Possibility of allergic systemic reaction exists — may need to consider skin testing as described in Prescribing Information (PI); hypocalcemic tetany is theoretically possible; for nasal spray, also need to conduct routine nasal examinations Most common AEs with injection include nausea with or without vomiting, local inflammatory reactions at the site of injection Most common AEs with nasal spray include rhinitis, various nasal symptoms (eg, nasal crusts, dryness, redness, sores), back pain, skin rash, myalgia, bronchospasm, angina, dyspepsia, constipation, abdominal pain, nausea, diarrhea, dizziness, abnormal eye tearing, depression Pregnancy category: C	Tell the prescriber if you had an allergic reaction to this medication before; if patient is self-injecting, ensure she is instructed in proper injection technique; *missed doses*: if you are taking two doses a day, and remember within 2 hrs of the missed dose take it right away and return to normal schedule but if you remember more than 2 hrs later skip the dose; if you are taking one dose a day, take the missed dose as soon as possible but if is already the next day skip the dose and return to normal schedule; if you are taking one dose every other day, take the missed dose as soon as you remember,	For nasal spray: Before using, maintain at room temperature and prime the pump by holding the bottle upright with the two white side arms of the pump depressed toward the bottle until a full spray is produced — SEE Prescribing Information (PI)

Generic Name and Selected Trade Names	Normal Adult Dosage	Major Adverse Effects/Cautions	Key Counseling Points
Calcitonin Salmon (continued) Calcimar Miacalcin	<u>For Paget's disease of bone</u>: Start with 100 I.U. SC or IM daily; other doses may be useful — SEE PI *Nasal spray* In postmenopausal osteoporosis, usually one spray (200 I.U.) per day intranasally, alternating nostrils daily		but if you remember the next day take a dose, then skip a day and start the dosing regimen again — do not double doses <u>For nasal spray</u>: Tell the prescriber if you had an allergic reaction to this medication before; ensure patient knows how to use pump properly — SEE Prescribing Information (PI); store unassembled bottles in the refrigerator but do not freeze; before priming and using, allow the bottle to reach room temperature and store the bottle in use at room temperature in an upright position for up to 30 days; before using, blow your nose gently then keeping your head in an upright position carefully place the nozzle into one nostril and spray only one time; if you miss a dose take it as soon as you remember, but if it is almost time for the next dose, skip the missed one and return to regular schedule — do not double doses

Generic Name and Selected Trade Names	Normal Adult Dosage	Major Adverse Effects/Cautions	Key Counseling Points	Miscellaneous Issues
Conjugated Estrogens[1] Premarin				
Conjugated Estrogens plus Medroxyprogesterone[1] Premphase Prempro				
Estropipate[1] Ortho-est				

*As a general rule, a medication should not be administered to a patient with a known hypersensitivity to it or a similar agent.
[1] SEE hormones.

Antidiabetic Agents

Table 1: Oral Hypoglycemics and Related Agents*

Generic Name and Selected Trade Names	Normal Adult Dosage	Major Adverse Effects/Cautions	Key Counseling Points	Miscellaneous Issues
Acarbose Precose	Individualize dosage As an adjunct in NIDDM initially, 25 mg at the start of each meal, may be increased at 4–8 week intervals up to 100 mg TID, based upon postprandial glucose levels	Contraindications: Cirrhosis, ketoacidosis, intestinal obstructions or inflammatory bowel disorders Consideration: May elevate liver enzyme levels Most common AEs include abdominal pain, diarrhea, flatulence Pregnancy category: B	This medication should be taken with the first bite of each meal, if it occurs, GI upset should lessen over time; continue with your diet and exercise regimen and monitoring of blood glucose; the agent itself will not cause hypoglycemia but may potentiate that caused by your oral hypoglycemic, therefore you should carry glucose or fruit juice with you; it is important not to miss any doses; if you finish a meal and forget to take the medicine, skip the missed dose and return to regular schedule — do not double doses	

Generic Name and Selected Trade Names	Normal Adult Dosage	Major Adverse Effects/Cautions	Key Counseling Points	Miscellaneous Issues
Chlorpropamide Diabinese	Dosage individualized based upon urinary and blood glucose, and glycosylated hemoglobin Usually, start with 250 mg/day; maintenance 100 to 500 mg/day usually as a single daily dose Dosage adjustments may be required in patients with renal or liver disease, the elderly, debilitated or malnourished patients	<u>Contraindication</u>: Diabetic ketoacidosis <u>Considerations</u>: Use of oral hypoglycemics has been reported to increase cardiovascular mortality as compared to treatment with diet alone or diet plus insulin; hypoglycemia is more likely in patients with renal or liver disease, elderly, debilitated or malnourished patients; patients exposed to stresses (eg, fever, trauma, infection) may lose glucose control and may require insulin therapy; response to the medication may diminish over time	Many medical conditions can affect this agent, inform the prescriber if you have any serious medical conditions or have had an unusual or allergic reaction to any sulfa-type agent; generally not recommended for use during pregnancy, contact the prescriber if you are or plan to become pregnant; if you develop seizures, fainting, or unconsciousness contact the prescriber; it is important to follow your diet and exercise plans and to monitor blood/urine glucose as directed; ensure patient is aware of the signs, symptoms, and treatment of hypoglycemia and hyperglycemia; it is important to wear a medical ID bracelet at all times;	

Generic Name and Selected Trade Names	Normal Adult Dosage	Major Adverse Effects/Cautions	Key Counseling Points	Miscellaneous Issues
Chlorpropamide (continued) Diabinese		Most common AEs include hypoglycemia, weight gain, dermatologic complaints, photosensitivity, changes in sensation of taste, dizziness, drowsiness, GI distress, cholestatic jaundice Pregnancy category: C	It is important to take this agent as directed even if you feel well; it is best to take your entire daily dose each morning with breakfast; if you miss a dose take it as soon as possible, but if it is almost time for the next dose skip the missed dose — do not double doses	

Generic Name and Selected Trade Names	Normal Adult Dosage	Major Adverse Effects/Cautions	Key Counseling Points	Miscellaneous Issues
Glimepiride Amaryl	Dosage individualized based upon urinary and blood glucose, and glycosylated hemoglobin <u>Initial</u>: Administer 1 to 2 mg with breakfast or first main meal <u>Maintenance</u>: Usually, 1 to 4 mg QD with a maximum of 8 mg; after reaching 2 mg/day, titrate in increments of no more than 2 mg at 1–2 week intervals Use with insulin: SEE Prescribing Information (PI)	<u>Contraindications and considerations</u>: SEE chlorpropamide Most common AEs include hypoglycemia, dizziness, asthenia, headache, nausea <u>Pregnancy category</u>: C	SEE chlorpropamide	

Generic Name and Selected Trade Names	Normal Adult Dosage	Major Adverse Effects/Cautions	Key Counseling Points	Miscellaneous Issues
Glipizide Glucotrol Glucotrol XL	Dosage individualized based upon urinary and blood glucose, and glycosylated hemoglobin <u>Initial</u>: Usually, 5 mg before breakfast; for Glucotrol only, geriatric patients or those with liver disease may start on 2.5 mg QD <u>Maintenance with Glucotrol</u>: Titrate in increments of 2.5 to 5 mg as determined by blood glucose; maximum QD dose is 15 mg, higher doses should be divided	<u>Contraindications and considerations</u>: SEE chlorpropamide <u>Most common AEs</u> include hypoglycemia, dizziness, headache, nausea, diarrhea, constipation, gastralgia, skin reactions <u>Pregnancy category</u>: C	SEE chlorpropamide For Glucotrol XL, swallow whole, do not break, crush, or chew; patient may notice what looks like a tablet in their stool, it is the sustained release mechanism	

Generic Name and Selected Trade Names	Normal Adult Dosage	Major Adverse Effects/Cautions	Key Counseling Points	Miscellaneous Issues
Glipizide (continued) Glucotrol Glucotrol XL	Maintenance with Glucotrol XL: Administer 5 to 10 mg with breakfast and titrate based on blood glucose; maximum recommended dose is 20 mg Use with insulin: SEE Prescribing Information (PI) All Products: Dosage adjustments may be required in patients with renal or liver disease, the elderly, debilitated or malnourished patients — SEE PI			

Generic Name and Selected Trade Names	Normal Adult Dosage	Major Adverse Effects/Cautions	Key Counseling Points	Miscellaneous Issues
Glyburide Diabeta Micronase Glynase PresTab (Micronized)	Dosage individualized based upon urinary and blood glucose, and glycosylated hemoglobin *Diabeta and Micronase* <u>Initial</u>: Usually, 2.5 to 5 mg with breakfast or first main meal <u>Usual maintenance</u>: Range is 1.25 to 20 mg/day; titrate in increments of no more than 2.5 mg weekly based on blood glucose *Glynase PresTab* <u>Initial</u>: Usually, 1.5 to 3 mg daily with breakfast or first main meal	<u>Contraindications and considerations</u>: SEE chlorpropamide Most common AEs include hypoglycemia, dizziness, headache, nausea, heartburn, skin reactions, cholestatic jaundice and hepatitis, elevation of liver enzymes <u>Pregnancy category</u>: C for Diabeta, and category B for Micronase and Glynase PresTab	SEE chlorpropamide	Products should not be used interchangeably, as the dosage recommendations are different

Generic Name and Selected Trade Names	Normal Adult Dosage	Major Adverse Effects/Cautions	Key Counseling Points	Miscellaneous Issues
Glyburide (continued) Diabeta Micronase Glynase PresTab (Micronized)	<u>Usual maintenance</u>: 0.75 to 12 mg daily; titrate in increments of no more than 1.5 mg weekly based upon blood glucose <u>All Products</u>: Dosage adjustments may be required in patients with renal or liver disease, the elderly, debilitated or malnourished patients — SEE Prescribing Information (PI)			

Generic Name and Selected Trade Names	Normal Adult Dosage	Major Adverse Effects/Cautions	Key Counseling Points	Miscellaneous Issues
Metformin HCl Glucophage	Individualize dosage based upon blood glucose and glycosylated hemoglobin levels Usually, start with 500 mg BID with morning meal and evening meal, or 850 mg with morning meal; in general, clinical response not seen with dosages <1500 mg/day; may titrate by 500 mg per week or 850 mg every other week up to a maximum of 2550 mg/day divided with meals	<u>Contraindications</u>: Renal disease, patients undergoing radiologic studies with iodine, acute or chronic metabolic acidosis including diabetic ketoacidosis <u>Considerations</u>: Rarely lactic acidosis has occurred, more common in patients with renal and/or liver disease; use of oral hypoglycemics has been reported to increase cardiovascular mortality as compared to treatment with diet alone or diet plus insulin, renal function must be monitored; not recommended for use in patients with impaired liver function, in pregnancy, or in pediatric patients	Many medical conditions can affect this agent, inform the prescriber if you have any serious medical conditions; generally not recommended for use during pregnancy, contact the prescriber if you are or plan to become pregnant; if you develop breathing problems, diarrhea, muscle pain or cramping, unusual tiredness or weakness consult the prescriber; it is important to follow your diet and exercise plans and to monitor blood/urine glucose as directed; patients should be aware of the signs, symptoms, and treatment of hypoglycemia and hyperglycemia; it is important to wear a medical ID bracelet at all times;	

Generic Name and Selected Trade Names	Normal Adult Dosage	Major Adverse Effects/Cautions	Key Counseling Points	Miscellaneous Issues
Metformin HCl (continued) Glucophage	Dosage adjustments may be required in patients with renal disease, the elderly, debilitated or malnourished patients — SEE Prescribing Information (PI)	Most common AEs include diarrhea, nausea, vomiting, bloating, flatulence, anorexia, metallic taste, rash, lactic acidosis (rare, but severe) Pregnancy category: B	It is important to take this agent as directed even if you feel well; you will start on a low dose which will be gradually increased to decrease the likelihood that you will experience side effects; it is best to take with meals; if you miss a dose take it as soon as possible, but if it is almost time for the next dose skip the missed dose — do not double doses	

Generic Name and Selected Trade Names	Normal Adult Dosage	Major Adverse Effects/Cautions	Key Counseling Points	Miscellaneous Issues
Tolazamide Tolinase	Individualize dosage based upon blood glucose and glycosylated hemoglobin levels Initial: 100 to 250 mg with breakfast, increase by 100 to 250 mg at weekly intervals as needed Maintenance: Administer 250 to 500 mg daily with breakfast	<u>Contraindications and considerations</u>: SEE chlorpropamide Most common AEs include hypoglycemia, dizziness, headache, nausea, diarrhea, constipation, gastralgia, skin reactions <u>Pregnancy category</u>: C	SEE chlorpropamide	

Generic Name and Selected Trade Names	Normal Adult Dosage	Major Adverse Effects/Cautions	Key Counseling Points	Miscellaneous Issues
Tolbutamide Orinase	Individualized dosage based upon blood glucose and glycosylated hemoglobin levels Initial: 1000 to 2000 mg as a single morning dose or in divided doses Maintenance: 250 to 2000 mg as a single morning dose or in divided doses	Contraindications and considerations: SEE chlorpropamide Most common AEs include hypoglycemia, dizziness, headache, nausea, diarrhea, constipation, gastralgia, skin reactions Pregnancy category: C	SEE chlorpropamide	

Generic Name and Selected Trade Names	Normal Adult Dosage	Major Adverse Effects/Cautions	Key Counseling Points	Miscellaneous Issues
Troglitazone Rezulin	Individualize dosage Patients on insulin <u>initial</u>: 200 mg daily, may be increased after 2–4 weeks if response is inadequate <u>Range of maintenance dose</u>: 200 to 600 mg QD	<u>Considerations</u>: Effective only in the presence of insulin, do not use in Type I diabetes or diabetic ketoacidosis; use with caution in patients with hepatic disease; may counteract the effects of oral contraceptives <u>Most common AEs include</u> headache, asthenia dizziness, jaundice (rare) <u>Pregnancy category</u>: B	Tell the prescriber if you have a liver disorder or are taking an oral contraceptive; risk of hypoglycemia from insulin may be greater when combined with troglitazone; it is important to adhere to your diet and exercise regimen and to monitor your blood/urine glucose as directed by the prescriber; take with meals, take missed doses with the next meal — do not double doses	

*As a general rule, a medication should not be administered to a patient with a known hypersensitivity to it or a similar agent.

Table 2: Insulin*,1,2

Generic Name and Selected Trade Names	Normal Adult Dosage	Major Adverse Effects/Cautions	Key Counseling Points	Miscellaneous Issues
Regular Human Insulin — Rapid Acting (Recombinant DNA Origin) Humulin R Novolin R	Individualize dosage	Considerations: Insulin doses may be affected by changes in food intake, activity, work schedule, illnesses, pregnancy, medications, exercise, and travel across multiple time zones Most common AEs include hypoglycemia, lipoatrophy or lipohypertrophy at injection site; local or systemic allergic reactions may occur, but are rare Pregnancy category: Not specified	If you develop signs of hypoglycemia such as sweating, dizziness, palpitations, tremors, hunger, restlessness, tingling of hands, feet, lips, or tongue, lightheadedness, or inability to concentrate, eat or drink sugar containing foods; if you develop disorientation, unconsciousness, or seizures seek medical attention immediately, family members should be aware of these signs and symptoms; changes in your diet, activity, work schedule, medication regimen or general health can affect your insulin requirements, consult with the prescriber if any of these changes occur;	Store in refrigerator or if not possible keep as cool as possible (below 86° F) but do not freeze Pharmacokinetic Properties <u>Onset</u>: 0.5–1 hrs <u>Peak</u>: 5–10 hrs <u>Duration</u>: 8–12 hrs May be mixed with all other insulins; if mixed with longer-acting insulins, draw Regular insulin into the syringe first to prevent clouding, inject immediately, do not administer IV

Generic Name and Selected Trade Names	Normal Adult Dosage	Major Adverse Effects/Cautions	Key Counseling Points	Miscellaneous Issues
Regular Human Insulin — Rapid Acting (Recombinant DNA Origin) (continued) Humulin R Novolin R			you will need to monitor your blood glucose levels frequently; it is very important that you follow the dosage and monitoring schedule determined by the prescriber; you may want you to wear a medical alert bracelet/necklace or carry an ID card to indicate you have diabetes mellitus; ensure patient or caregiver has read the patient information leaflet provided with the medication; ensure patient or caregiver is aware of proper aseptic injection technique	

619

Generic Name and Selected Trade Names	Normal Adult Dosage	Major Adverse Effects/Cautions	Key Counselling Points	Miscellaneous Issues
Semilente Human Insulin — Rapid Acting (Recombinant DNA Origin)	Individualize dosage	SEE regular human insulin	SEE regular human insulin	SEE Regular human insulin except the following: Pharmacokinetic Properties <u>Onset</u>: 1–1.5 hrs <u>Peak</u>: 5–10 hrs <u>Duration</u>: 12–16 hrs May be mixed with Lente insulin

Generic Name and Selected Trade Names	Normal Adult Dosage	Major Adverse Effects/Cautions	Key Counselling Points	Miscellaneous Issues
NPH Human Insulin — Intermediate Acting (Recombinant DNA Origin) Humulin N Novolin N	Individualize dosage	SEE regular human insulin	SEE regular human insulin	SEE Regular human insulin except the following: Pharmacokinetic Properties <u>Onset</u>: 1–1.5 hrs <u>Peak</u>: 4–12 hrs <u>Duration</u>: 24 hrs May be mixed with Regular insulin; draw Regular insulin into the syringe first to prevent clouding, inject immediately, do not administer IV

621

Generic Name and Selected Trade Names	Normal Adult Dosage	Major Adverse Effects/Cautions	Key Counseling Points	Miscellaneous Issues
Lente Human Insulin — Intermediate Acting (Recombinant DNA Origin) Humulin L Novolin L	Individualize dosage	SEE regular human insulin	SEE regular human insulin	SEE Regular human insulin except the following: Pharmacokinetic properties <u>Onset</u>: 1–2.5 hrs <u>Peak</u>: 7–15 hrs <u>Duration</u>: 24 hrs May be mixed with Regular or Semilente insulin; draw Regular insulin into the syringe first to prevent clouding, inject immediately, do not administer IV

Generic Name and Selected Trade Names	Normal Adult Dosage	Major Adverse Effects/Cautions	Key Counseling Points	Miscellaneous Issues
Ultralente Human Insulin — Slow Acting (Recombinant DNA Origin) Humulin U	Individualize dosage	SEE regular human insulin	SEE regular human insulin	SEE Regular human insulin except the following: Pharmacokinetic Properties <u>Onset</u>: 4–8 hrs <u>Peak</u>: 14–24 hrs <u>Duration</u>: 36 hrs May be mixed with Regular insulin; draw Regular insulin into the syringe first to prevent clouding, inject immediately, do not administer IV

Generic Name and Selected Trade Names	Normal Adult Dosage	Major Adverse Effects/Cautions	Key Counseling Points	Miscellaneous Issues
Insulin Lispro Humalog	Individualize dosage	<u>Contraindication</u>: During episodes of hypoglycemia <u>Consideration</u>: Rapid onset of action and short duration of action as compared with other insulin; also SEE human insulin Most common AEs SEE human insulin <u>Pregnancy category</u>: B	This insulin differs from other insulins, it has a rapid onset of action and a shorter duration of action, it should be administered 15 minutes before a meal; type I diabetics will also require a longer lasting insulin, and SEE human insulin — rapid acting	Store in refrigerator or if not possible keep as cool as possible (below 86° F) but do not freeze Pharmacokinetic Properties <u>Onset</u>: 0.25 hrs <u>Peak</u>: 0.5–1.5 hrs <u>Duration</u>: 6–8 hrs May be mixed with Ultralente or NPH (only studied with Humulin brand);

Generic Name and Selected Trade Names	Normal Adult Dosage	Major Adverse Effects/Cautions	Key Counseling Points	Miscellaneous Issues
Insulin Lispro (continued) Humalog				if mixed with longer-acting insulins, draw Humalog into the syringe first to prevent clouding, inject immediately, do not administer IV

*As a general rule, a medication should not be administered to a patient with a known hypersensitivity to it or a similar agent.

[1] All patients receiving insulin should preferably conduct blood glucose monitoring or, if not feasible, urine monitoring.

[2] Combination products are available — SEE Prescribing Information (PI).

625

Gastrointestinal Agents

Table 1: Antidiarrheals*

Generic Name and Selected Trade Names	Normal Adult Dosage	Major Adverse Effects/Cautions	Key Counseling Points	Miscellaneous Issues
Difenoxin HCl and Atropine Sulfate Motofen	Individualize dosage. To treat diarrhea, start with two tabs (2 mg of difenoxin HCl), then take 1 tab after each loose stool or 1 tab Q3–4H as needed up to 8 tabs per day	Contraindications: Children under 2 years of age, diarrhea associated with organisms that penetrate the intestinal mucosa such as *E. coli*, *Salmonella*, and *Shigella* species, jaundiced patients Considerations: Overdose may lead to severe respiratory depression, coma, and perhaps permanent brain damage or death; if patient is severely dehydrated or has electrolyte abnormalities, hold therapy until these are corrected; use with caution in patients with renal or liver impairment; may cause toxic megacolon in patients with acute ulcerative colitis	Tell the prescriber if you have a kidney or liver disorder, ulcerative colitis, glaucoma, myasthenia gravis, or difficulty with urination; keep the tablets out of the reach of children; may cause drowsiness/sedation, which may be enhanced by other sedatives such as alcohol or antihistamines; due to risk of sedation, use caution if driving or using machinery; do not exceed prescribed dosage	In the treatment of diarrhea, if clinical improvement is not seen in 48 hrs do not continue this medication; for acute diarrhea, therapy beyond 48 hrs is rarely needed; use caution in individuals who should not receive anticholinergic agents such as atropine

Generic Name and Selected Trade Names	Normal Adult Dosage	Major Adverse Effects/Cautions	Key Counseling Points	Miscellaneous Issues
Difenoxin HCl and Atropine Sulfate (continued) Motofen		Most common AEs include nausea, vomiting, dry mouth, dizziness, lightheadedness, drowsiness, headache Pregnancy category: C		

Generic Name and Selected Trade Names	Normal Adult Dosage	Major Adverse Effects/Cautions	Key Counseling Points	Miscellaneous Issues
Diphenoxylate HCl and Atropine Sulfate Lomotil	Individualize dosage To treat diarrhea, 2 tabs or 10 mL (2 teaspoonfuls) QID until control achieved, then reduce dose as needed Reduced dosage required in children — SEE Prescribing Information (PI)	<u>Contraindications</u>: Patients with obstructive jaundice, diarrhea associated with pseudomembranous enterocolitis or enterotoxin-producing bacteria <u>Considerations</u>: Should not be used in children under 2 years of age and should be used very cautiously in children of other ages; overdose may lead to severe respiratory depression, coma, and perhaps permanent brain damage or death; if patient is severely dehydrated or has electrolyte abnormalities, hold therapy until these are corrected; do not use in diarrhea associated with organisms that penetrate the intestinal wall such as toxigenic *E. coli*, *Salmonella*, and *Shigella*, or in pseudo-membranous colitis due to antibiotics;	SEE difenoxin HCl	Clinical improvement of acute diarrhea is usually observed within 48 hrs; if clinical improvement of chronic diarrhea is not seen within 10 days, the medication is not likely to be successful; use caution in individuals who should not receive anticholinergic agents

Generic Name and Selected Trade Names	Normal Adult Dosage	Major Adverse Effects/Cautions	Key Counseling Points	Miscellaneous Issues
Diphenoxylate HCl and Atropine Sulfate (continued) Lomotil		use with caution in patients with renal or liver impairment; may cause toxic megacolon in patients with acute ulcerative colitis; should not be used with monoamine oxidase inhibitors Most common AEs include numbness of extremities, depression, malaise, lethargy, confusion, sedation, drowsiness, nausea, vomiting, toxic megacolon, anorexia, abdominal discomfort, hyperthermia, tachycardia, urinary retention, flushing, drying of skin and mucous membranes Pregnancy category: C		

Generic Name and Selected Trade Names	Normal Adult Dosage	Major Adverse Effects/Cautions	Key Counseling Points	Miscellaneous Issues
Furazolidone Furoxone	Individualize dosage To treat diarrhea due to susceptible bacteria and protozoa, 100 mg QID (tablets or liquid) Reduced dosage required in children — SEE Prescribing Information (PI)	Contraindications: Ingestion of alcohol during or within 4 days after therapy (due to possible disulfiram-like reaction), use of monoamine oxidase (MAO) inhibitors, infants under 1 month of age Considerations: May produce orthostatic hypotension, hypoglycemia, and mild reversible intravascular hemolysis in certain ethnic groups — SEE Prescribing Information (PI) Most common AEs include hypersensitivity reactions (eg, a fall in blood pressure, urticaria, fever), nausea, vomiting, headache, malaise Pregnancy category: C	Tell the prescriber if you are taking a monoamine oxidase (MAO) inhibitor; do not drink alcoholic beverages or take medications that contain alcohol while taking this agent or within at least four days after finishing therapy; if you are of Mediterranean or Near-eastern descent or are black, speak with the prescriber before taking this medication; may take with food; if you miss a dose take it as soon as you remember, but if it is almost time for the next dose, skip the missed one and return to regular schedule — do not double doses	If satisfactory clinical response is not seen within 7 days, the pathogen may be resistant to this medication and alternative therapy should be considered; avoid foods and medications that interact with monoamine oxidase (MAO) inhibitors

Generic Name and Selected Trade Names	Normal Adult Dosage	Major Adverse Effects/Cautions	Key Counseling Points	Miscellaneous Issues
Loperamide HCl Imodium capsules	Individualize dosage For treatment of acute diarrhea: Start with 4 mg (2 caps), then 2 mg (1 cap) after each loose bowel movement; dosage should not exceed 16 mg/day For treatment of chronic diarrhea: Start with 4 mg, then 2 mg after each unformed stool until diarrhea controlled, after which reduce dosage as needed Dosage adjustment: Reduced dosage required in children — SEE Prescribing Information (PI)	Contraindication: Patients in whom constipation must be avoided Considerations: Not recommended in children less than 2 years of age; if patient is severely dehydrated or has electrolyte abnormalities, these need to be corrected; should not be used in acute dysentery; toxic megacolon reported in patients with acute ulcerative colitis and drug-induced pseudomembranous colitis; use caution in liver dysfunction Most common AEs include hypersensitivity reactions, abdominal pain/discomfort/distention, nausea and vomiting, constipation, tiredness, drowsiness, dizziness, dry mouth Pregnancy category: B	Contact the prescriber if diarrhea does not improve after a couple of days, if blood is seen in the stool, or if you develop a fever; if you are taking this medication on a regular schedule and miss a dose take it as soon as you remember, but if it is almost time for the next dose, skip the missed one and return to regular schedule — do not double doses	Clinical improvement of acute diarrhea is usually observed within 48 hrs; if clinical improvement of chronic diarrhea is not seen within 10 days, the medication is not likely to be successful

Generic Name and Selected Trade Names	Normal Adult Dosage	Major Adverse Effects/Cautions	Key Counselling Points	Miscellaneous Issues
Octreotide Acetate[1] Sandostatin	Individualize dosage <u>For treatment of diarrhea due to carcinoid tumor</u>: Start with 100 to 600 mcg/day subcutaneously in 2–4 divided doses for 2 weeks; median daily maintenance dose in studies was 450 mcg/day but patients may require more or less	<u>Considerations</u>: Shown to inhibit gallbladder contractility and decrease bile secretion; may cause biliary abnormalities such as sludge or gallstones; may cause hypothyroidism, hypoglycemia, hyperglycemia, cardiac conduction abnormalities (especially in acromegaly), pancreatitis, depressed vitamin B_{12} levels <u>Most common AEs</u> include gallbladder abnormalities, hypo- and hyperglycemia, hypothyroidism, pain at injection site, headache, dizziness <u>Pregnancy category</u>: B	Tell the prescriber if you have any heart, kidney, gallbladder, or thyroid disorder or if you have diabetes mellitus; instruct patient and/or caregiver in proper injection technique; if you miss a dose take it as soon as you remember, but if it is almost time for the next dose, skip the missed one and return to normal schedule — do not double doses; space the doses evenly during the day unless advised differently by prescriber	

Generic Name and Selected Trade Names	Normal Adult Dosage	Major Adverse Effects/Cautions	Key Counseling Points	Miscellaneous Issues
Octreotide Acetate[1] **(continued)** Sandostatin	For diarrhea due to vasoactive intestinal peptide tumors (VIPomas): Start with 200 to 300 mcg/day subcutaneously in 2–4 divided doses for 2 weeks; for maintenance, doses above 450 mcg/day rarely needed Dosage adjustments: May be required in patients with severe renal failure requiring hemodialysis — SEE Prescribing Information (PI)			

Generic Name and Selected Trade Names	Normal Adult Dosage	Major Adverse Effects/Cautions	Key Counselling Points	Miscellaneous Issues
Opium Tincture (Deodorized opium tincture)	Individualize dosage For diarrhea, usual dosage is 0.6 mL QID, but may range from 0.3–1 mL QID; single doses should not exceed 1 mL and daily dosage should not exceed 6 mL	<u>Considerations</u>: Use with caution in patients with asthma, severe prostatic hyperplasia, hepatic disease, or persons with history of opiate dependence; may cause nausea and other GI disturbances as well as drowsiness, dizziness, lightheadedness, fainting <u>Pregnancy category</u>: Not specified	Take this medication as directed — do not take more than the prescribed dosage; keep the container tightly closed so that the alcohol does not evaporate; may cause drowsiness/sedation, which may be enhanced by other sedatives such as alcohol or antihistamines; due to risk of sedation, use caution if driving or using machinery; if you are taking this medication on a regular schedule and miss a dose take it as soon as you remember, but if it is almost time for the next dose, skip the missed one and return to regular schedule — do not double doses	Use extreme caution NOT to confuse this with paregoric

Generic Name and Selected Trade Names	Normal Adult Dosage	Major Adverse Effects/Cautions	Key Counseling Points	Miscellaneous Issues
Paregoric (**Camphorated opium tincture**)	Individualize dosage To treat diarrhea, usual dosage is 5 to 10 mL 1–4 times per day Dosage reductions required in pediatric patients — SEE Prescribing Information (PI)	SEE Opium Tincture	SEE Opium Tincture	Use extreme caution NOT to confuse this with opium tincture

*As a general rule, a medication should not be administered to a patient with a known hypersensitivity to it or a similar agent.
†Is used for other conditions as well; refer to Prescribing Information (PI).

Table 2: Antiemetics*

Generic Name and Selected Trade Names	Normal Adult Dosage	Major Adverse Effects/Cautions	Key Counseling Points	Miscellaneous Issues
Chlorpromazine[1] Thorazine				
Diphenhydramine HCl[2] Benadryl				

Generic Name and Selected Trade Names	Normal Adult Dosage	Major Adverse Effects/Cautions	Key Counseling Points	Miscellaneous Issues
Dronabinol[3] Marinol	Individualize dosage To treat nausea and vomiting, administer 5 mg/m² 1–3 hrs prior to chemotherapy then every 2–4 hrs after chemotherapy for a total of 4–6 doses per day; may titrate dose upward by 2.5 mg/m² increments up to 15 mg/m² per dose (although this maximum dose may lead to psychiatric symptoms)	<u>Contraindications:</u> Hypersensitivity to any cannabinoid or sesame oil <u>Considerations:</u> Has potential to be abused and use caution in persons with a history of drug abuse; use with caution in patients with cardiovascular disorder due to possible hypotension, hypertension, syncope, or tachycardia; may exacerbate mania, depression, and schizophrenia; may increase sedation caused by other CNS depressants Most common AEs include abdominal pain, nausea, vomiting, dizziness, euphoria, paranoid reaction, diarrhea, somnolence, hypotension, flushing <u>Pregnancy category:</u> C	Contact the prescriber if you develop nervousness, anxiety, paranoia, changes in mood, or other type of altered behavior; do not exceed the prescribed dose as side effects are more likely to occur; may cause drowsiness/sedation, which may be enhanced by other sedatives such as alcohol or antihistamines; dizziness, lightheadedness, or fainting may occur, especially when you get up from a lying or seated position — getting up slowly may prevent this from happening; due to risk of sedation, use caution if driving or using machinery; if you miss a dose take it as soon as you remember, but if it is almost time for the next dose, skip the missed one and return to normal schedule — do not double doses	Patients should be supervised when beginning therapy

Generic Name and Selected Trade Names	Normal Adult Dosage	Major Adverse Effects/Cautions	Key Counseling Points	Miscellaneous Issues
Granisetron HCl Kytril	*Injection* To prevent nausea and vomiting associated with oncology therapy, 10 mcg/kG IV within 30 minutes before cancer chemotherapy; administer undiluted over 30 seconds or diluted over 5 minutes For use in children — SEE Prescribing Information (PI) *Tablet* To prevent nausea and vomiting associated with oncology therapy, administer 1 mg up to 1 hr before chemotherapy and 1 mg 12 hrs after the first dose (administer only on days chemotherapy is given)	Consideration: Has been shown to produce tumors in rats Most common AEs include headache, asthenia (weakness), somnolence, diarrhea, constipation, abdominal pain (tabs), numerous CNS effects such as agitation and anxiety, fever, leukopenia, decreased appetite, anemia, alopecia Pregnancy category: B	Tell the prescriber if you previously had an adverse effect from a medication used to treat nausea and vomiting; medication is to be used only on the days that you are receiving chemotherapy	Medications that inhibit or induce the cytochrome P-450 enzyme system may interact with this agent

Generic Name and Selected Trade Names	Normal Adult Dosage	Major Adverse Effects/Cautions	Key Counselling Points	Miscellaneous Issues
Hydroxyzine HCl[2] Atarax				
Hydroxyzine Pamoate[2] Vistaril				
Meclizine HCl[2] Antivert				

Generic Name and Selected Trade Names	Normal Adult Dosage	Major Adverse Effects/Cautions	Key Counselling Points	Miscellaneous Issues
Metoclo-pramide[3] Reglan	Individualize dosage. For the prevention of nausea and vomiting due to cancer chemotherapy: Administer slowly IV 30 minutes before chemotherapy and repeat Q2H for 2 doses, then Q3H for 3 doses — for highly emetogenic agents, the initial 2 doses should be 2 mg/kG; for less emetogenic agents, give 1mg/kG/dose	Contraindications: Whenever stimulation of GI motility may be dangerous (eg, presence of GI bleeding), persons with seizure disorder or pheochromocytoma, along with other agents known to cause extrapyramidal effects Considerations: May cause mental depression; usually should not be administered to persons with history of depression, extrapyramidal symptoms, Parkinsonian-like syndrome, and tardive dyskinesia; use caution in hypertension	Tell the prescriber if you have hypertension, Parkinson's disease or a seizure disorder such as epilepsy; contact the prescriber if you develop nervousness, anxiety, paranoia, changes in mood, or other type of altered behavior; do not exceed the prescribed dose as side effects are more likely to occur; may cause drowsiness/ sedation, which may be enhanced by other sedatives such as alcohol or antihistamines; due to risk of sedation, use caution if driving or using machinery; if you miss a dose take it as soon as you remember, but if it is almost time for the next dose, skip the missed one and return to normal schedule — do not double doses	

643

Generic Name and Selected Trade Names	Normal Adult Dosage	Major Adverse Effects/Cautions	Key Counselling Points	Miscellaneous Issues
Metoclopramide[3] **(continued)** Reglan	For prevention of <u>postoperative nausea and vomiting</u>: Usually, 10 mg IM although 20 mg IM may be used Reduced dosage may be required in renal or liver impairment — SEE Prescribing Information (PI)	Most common AEs include CNS effects such as insomnia/restlessness/fatigue/ drowsiness; suicidal tendencies, extrapyramidal reactions, amenorrhea, gynecomastia, impotence, hypo- and hypertension, arrhythmias, nausea, diarrhea <u>Pregnancy category</u>: B		

Generic Name and Selected Trade Names	Normal Adult Dosage	Major Adverse Effects/Cautions	Key Counselling Points	Miscellaneous Issues
Ondansetron Zofran	*Injection* To prevent cancer chemotherapy-induced nausea and vomiting, administer 32 mg IV as a single dose infused over 15 minutes beginning 30 minutes before the start of emetogenic chemotherapy OR three 0.15 mg/kg doses, with the first dose before chemotherapy and then 4 and 8 hrs later Dosage may need to be reduced in liver dysfunction and in pediatric patients — SEE Prescribing Information (PI)	<u>Considerations</u>: Hypersensitivity reactions have occurred in patients hypersensitive to other 5-HT$_3$ receptor antagonists; may mask progressive ileus and/or gastric distention Most common AEs include headache, malaise/fatigue, constipation, diarrhea, dizziness, abdominal pain, rash, elevation of liver enzymes; specifically with injectable — musculoskeletal pain, shivers, drowsiness/sedation, injection site reaction, urinary retention <u>Pregnancy category</u>: B	Tell the prescriber if you previously had an adverse effect from a medication used to treat nausea and vomiting; depending on circumstances, may be used only on the days that you are receiving chemotherapy or undergoing radiation; if you miss a dose of this medication and do not feel nauseous, skip the dose and return to regular dosing schedule but if you miss a dose and feel nauseous take the missed dose as soon as possible	Medications that inhibit or induce the cytochrome P-450 enzyme system may interact with this agent; refer to Prescribing Information (PI) for preparation and other considerations for the IV formulation

Generic Name and Selected Trade Names	Normal Adult Dosage	Key Counseling Points	Miscellaneous Issues
Ondansetron (continued) Zofran	*Tablets and oral solution* To prevent nausea and vomiting associated with moderately emetogenic cancer chemotherapy, administer 8 mg twice daily — administer the first dose 30 minutes before chemotherapy and the second dose 8 hrs later, then administer Q12H for 1–2 days following chemotherapy To prevent nausea and vomiting due to radiotherapy, administer 8 mg TID; SEE PI for more complete data To prevent postoperative nausea and vomiting, administer 16 mg 1 hour before induction of anesthesia Dosage may need to be reduced in liver dysfunction and in pediatric patients — SEE (PI)		

Generic Name and Selected Trade Names	Normal Adult Dosage	Major Adverse Effects/Cautions	Key Counseling Points	Miscellaneous Issues
Perfenazine[1] Trilafon				
Prochlor-perazine[1] Compazine				
Promethazine HCl[1] Phenergan				

Generic Name and Selected Trade Names	Normal Adult Dosage	Major Adverse Effects/Cautions	Key Counseling Points	Miscellaneous Issues
Scopolamine Transderm Scop	To prevent nausea and vomiting due to motion sickness, apply 1 patch to the hairless area behind the ear at least 4 hrs before the antiemetic effect is required; if therapy needed for more than 3 days, discard the patch and apply a fresh one behind the other ear	Contraindications: Hypersensitivity to belladonna alkaloids, angle-closure (narrow-angle) glaucoma Considerations: Do not use in children; idiosyncratic reactions may occur; use with caution in patients with pyloric obstruction, urinary bladder neck obstruction, the elderly, impaired metabolic/liver/or kidney function, history of seizures or psychosis Most common AEs include dryness of the mouth, drowsiness, transient impairment of eye accommodation, blurred vision, dilation of the pupils Pregnancy category: C	Tell the prescriber if you are allergic to scopolamine and similar agents, have glaucoma, a kidney or liver disorder, a seizure disorder, myasthenia gravis, obstruction in the stomach or intestine, difficulty in urination, enlarged prostate, history of a psychiatric ailment; contact the prescriber if you develop blurred vision, pain in the eye, widening of the pupil, difficulty urinating, dizziness, confusion, skin rash; ensure patient knows how to apply the patch and wash hands properly, and dispose of used patches — SEE Prescribing Information (PI) for instructions;	After the patch is applied, wash hands thoroughly with soap and water; upon patch removal, wash/dry hands and the application site thoroughly

Generic Name and Selected Trade Names	Normal Adult Dosage	Major Adverse Effects/Cautions	Key Counselling Points	Miscellaneous Issues
Scopolamine (continued) Transderm Scop			may cause drowsiness/sedation, which may be enhanced by other sedatives such as alcohol or antihistamines; due to risk of sedation, use caution if driving or using machinery; do NOT apply more than 1 patch at a time	

Generic Name and Selected Trade Names	Normal Adult Dosage	Major Adverse Effects/Cautions	Key Counseling Points	Miscellaneous Issues
Thiethyl-perazine Maleate Torecan	Individualize dosage To treat nausea and vomiting, usual oral dosage range is 10 mg to 30 mg QD to TID, usual IM dosage is 10 mg (2 mL) QD to TID	<u>Contraindications</u>: Severe CNS depression and comatose states, hypersensitivity to phenothiazines, IV use, pregnancy <u>Considerations</u>: May potentiate other CNS depressants and atropine; restlessness and postoperative CNS depression during anesthesia recovery may occur; if hypotension occurs, avoid epinephrine; may cause abnormal movements such as extrapyramidal symptoms Most common AEs include movement disorders, drowsiness, dryness of the mouth and nose, blurred vision, tinnitus, peripheral edema; consider all other AEs that phenothiazines cause <u>Pregnancy category</u>: Not specified, but product is contraindicated in pregnancy	Tell the prescriber if you are pregnant; this medication is used only to treat nausea and vomiting — do not use more than the prescribed amount; tablets may be taken with food or an 8-ounce glass of water; may cause drowsiness/ sedation, which may be enhanced by other sedatives such as alcohol or antihistamines; due to risk of sedation use caution if driving or using machinery; if using this agent regularly and you miss a dose, take it as soon as you remember, but if it is almost time for the next dose, skip the missed one and return to normal schedule — do not double doses	Injectable contains sodium metabisulfite and tablets contain FD & C Yellow #5, which may cause allergic-type reactions

Generic Name and Selected Trade Names	Normal Adult Dosage	Major Adverse Effects/Cautions	Key Counseling Points	Miscellaneous Issues
Trimetho-benzamide HCl Tebamide T-Gen Tigan Trimazide	Individualize dosage For the control of nausea and vomiting, usual adult dosage is 250 mg capsule TID or QID; 200 mg suppository TID or QID; 200 mg IM TID or QID Reduced dosage required for pediatric patients — SEE Prescribing Information (PI)	<u>Contraindications</u>: Injectable form in children, suppository form in newborn infants (contains benzocaine so avoid in sensitive patients) <u>Considerations</u>: Use caution if using in children — SEE Prescribing Information (PI); may produce drowsiness; has been associated with Reye's syndrome; may interact with alcohol; for other AEs, SEE PI <u>Pregnancy category</u>: Not specified	Depending on prescription, ensure patient knows how to use suppositories or inject IM; do not use in children unless specified by physician; may cause drowsiness/sedation, which may be enhanced by other sedatives such as alcohol or antihistamines; due to risk of sedation, use caution if driving or using machinery; if using this agent regularly and you miss a dose, take it as soon as you remember, but if it is almost time for the next dose, skip the missed one and return to normal schedule — do not double doses	

*As a general rule, a medication should not be administered to a patient with a known hypersensitivity to it or a similar agent.
[1] SEE Psychotherapeutic agents.
[2] SEE Antihistamines.
[3] Used for other conditions as well; SEE Prescribing Information (PI).

Table 3: Antispasmodics

Generic Name and Selected Trade Names	Normal Adult Dosage	Major Adverse Effects/Cautions	Key Counselling Points	Miscellaneous Issues
Belladonna Alkaloids plus Other Ingredients (eg, phenobarbital) in Combination Donnatal	Individualize dosage As adjunctive therapy, usually, 1 or 2 tabs or caps, or 1 or 2 teaspoonfuls of elixir TID or QID; 1 extended release tablet Q8H or Q12H Reduced dosage required in children — SEE Prescribing Information (PI)	<u>Contraindications</u>: Glaucoma, obstructive uropathy, GI obstruction, paralytic ileus, intestinal atony of elderly or debilitated, unstable cardiac status in acute hemorrhage, severe ulcerative colitis, myasthenia gravis, hiatal hernia associated with reflux esophagitis, acute intermittent porphyria, and patients in whom phenobarbital produces restlessness and/or excitement <u>Considerations</u>: In high temperature environment may cause heat prostration; diarrhea may be early sign of intestinal obstruction; may produce drowsiness and blurred vision;	Tell the prescriber if you have glaucoma, any type of GI problem such as an obstruction, urinary retention, benign prostatic hyperplasia, myasthenia gravis, whether you are taking an anticoagulant ("blood thinner"); this medication may make you less likely to perspire so be careful not to become over-heated; may cause drowsiness/sedation, which may be enhanced by other sedatives such as alcohol or antihistamines; due to risk of sedation, use caution if driving or using machinery;	Phenobarbital may be habit forming; phenobarbital may decrease effect of anticoagulants

Generic Name and Selected Trade Names	Normal Adult Dosage	Major Adverse Effects/Cautions	Key Counselling Points	Miscellaneous Issues
Belladonna Alkaloids plus Other Ingredients (eg, phenobarbital) in Combination (continued) Donnatal		use caution in persons with liver or renal dysfunction, coronary artery disease, CHF, cardiac arrhythmias, hypertension, autonomic neuropathy, hyperthyroidism; may delay gastric emptying Most common AEs include dry mouth, urinary hesitancy/retention, blurred vision, tachycardia, palpitations, mydriasis, cyclopegia, increased ocular tension, loss of taste, headache, insomnia, nervousness, drowsiness, impotence, allergic reactions <u>Pregnancy category</u>: C	If you miss a dose take it as soon as you remember, but if it is almost time for the next dose, skip the missed one and return to normal schedule — do not double doses	

Generic Name and Selected Trade Names	Normal Adult Dosage	Major Adverse Effects/Cautions	Key Counseling Points	Miscellaneous Issues
Clidinium Bromide and Chlordiazepoxide HCl Clindex Librax	Individualize dosage As adjunctive therapy, the usual maintenance dose is 1 or 2 caps TID or QID administered before meals and at bedtime Reduce dosage in elderly or debilitated — SEE Prescribing Information (PI)	<u>Contraindications</u>: Glaucoma, prostatic hypertrophy, bladder neck obstruction <u>Considerations</u>: Usually avoid in pregnancy due to increased risk of congenital abnormalities; limit dose to smallest possible one in elderly and debilitated to preclude ataxia, over-sedation, or confusion; paradoxical reactions to chlordiazepoxide (eg, excitement) are possible Most common AEs include dryness of mouth, blurred vision, urinary hesitancy, drowsiness, ataxia, confusion, skin eruptions, edema, nausea, constipation <u>Pregnancy category</u>: Not specified, but product should be avoided due to increased risk of congenital anomalies	Tell the prescriber if you have glaucoma, myasthenia gravis, history of a drug abuse problem, or any type of urinary disorder; this medication may make you less likely to perspire so be careful not to become over-heated; may cause drowsiness/sedation, which may be enhanced by other sedatives such as alcohol or antihistamines; due to risk of sedation, use caution if driving or using machinery; if you miss a dose take it as soon as you remember, but if it is almost time for the next dose, skip the missed one and return to normal schedule — do not double doses	

Generic Name and Selected Trade Names	Normal Adult Dosage	Major Adverse Effects/Cautions	Key Counseling Points	Miscellaneous Issues
Dicyclomine HCl Bentyl	Individualize dosage For the treatment of functional bowel/ irritable bowel syndrome: for oral therapy start with 80 mg per day in 4 equally divided doses, then may titrate to 160 mg per day (the only dose shown to be effective) in 4 equally divided doses; the IM formulation is about twice as bioavailable as the oral form, recommended dosage is 80 mg per day in 4 equally divided doses	Contraindications: Obstructive uropathy, obstructive disease of the GI tract, severe ulcerative colitis, reflux esophagitis, unstable cardiovascular status in acute hemorrhage, glaucoma, myasthenia gravis, infants less than 6 months of age, nursing mothers Considerations: In high environmental temperature, heat prostration may occur; diarrhea may be early sign of intestinal obstruction; may produce drowsiness, blurred vision, psychosis (eg, confusion, disorientation, short-term memory loss); use with caution in autonomic neuropathy, hepatic or renal disease, ulcerative colitis, hyperthyroidism, coronary artery disease, CHF, tachyarrhythmias, hiatal hernia, prostatic hypertrophy	Tell the prescriber if patient has any of the conditions listed under "contraindications"; do not use in infants less than 6 months of age; this medication may make you less likely to perspire and in general may make you more prone to heat prostration so be careful to stay out of very hot areas and not to become over-heated; may cause blurred vision, constipation, and dryness of the mouth, nose, and throat; may cause drowsiness/ sedation, which may be enhanced by other sedatives such as alcohol or antihistamines; due to risk of sedation, use caution if driving or using machinery;	Do not use the parenteral formulation IV

Generic Name and Selected Trade Names	Normal Adult Dosage	Major Adverse Effects/Cautions	Key Counselling Points	Miscellaneous Issues
Dicyclomine HCl (continued) Bentyl		Most common AEs include dry mouth, dizziness, blurred vision, nausea, lightheadedness, drowsiness, weakness, nervousness Pregnancy category: B	If you miss a dose take it as soon as you remember, but if it is almost time for the next dose, skip the missed one and return to normal schedule — do not double doses	

Generic Name and Selected Trade Names	Normal Adult Dosage	Major Adverse Effects/Cautions	Key Counselling Points	Miscellaneous Issues
Glycopyrrolate Robinul Robinul Forte	Individualize dosage As adjunctive therapy: Regular tablets: Start with 1 mg TID — morning, afternoon, and at bedtime; some patients need 2 mg hs Longer-acting tablets (eg, Robinul Forte): Start with 2 mg two or three times a day in equally divided doses Injectable: Depends on use — SEE Prescribing Information (PI)	Contraindications: Glaucoma, obstructive uropathy (eg, bladder neck obstruction due to prostatic hypertrophy), obstruction of GI tract, paralytic ileus, atony of the elderly or debilitated, severe ulcerative colitis, reflux esophagitis, unstable cardiovascular status in acute hemorrhage, toxic megacolon complicating ulcerative colitis, myasthenia gravis; for injectable form, do not use in infants <1 month of age Considerations: In high environmental temperature, heat prostration may occur; diarrhea may be early sign of intestinal obstruction; may produce drowsiness, blurred vision;	Tell the prescriber if patient has any of the conditions listed under "contraindications"; this medication may make you less likely to perspire and in general may make you more prone to heat prostration so be careful to stay out of very hot areas and not to become over-heated; may cause blurred vision, constipation, and dryness of the mouth, nose and throat; may cause drowsiness/ sedation, which may be enhanced by other sedatives such as alcohol or antihistamines;	

Generic Name and Selected Trade Names	Normal Adult Dosage	Major Adverse Effects/Cautions	Key Counseling Points	Miscellaneous Issues
Glycopyrrolate (continued) Robinul Robinul Forte		use with caution in autonomic neuropathy, hepatic or renal disease, asthma, ulcerative colitis, hyperthyroidism, coronary artery disease, CHF, tachyarrhythmias, hypertension, hiatal hernia, prostatic hypertrophy Most common AEs include dry mouth, decreased sweating, urinary hesitancy and retention, blurred vision, tachycardia, palpitations, dilation of pupil, increased ocular tension, loss of taste, headaches, nervousness, mental confusion, dizziness, insomnia, nausea, vomiting, allergic reactions <u>Pregnancy category</u>: Oral form, not specified; injectable is Category B	due to risk of sedation, use caution if driving or using machinery; if you miss a dose take it as soon as you remember, but if it is almost time for the next dose, skip the missed one and return to normal schedule — do not double doses	

Generic Name and Selected Trade Names	Normal Adult Dosage	Major Adverse Effects/Cautions	Key Counseling Points	Miscellaneous Issues
Hyoscyamine Sulfate Cytospaz Levbid Levsin Levsinex	Individualize dosage Each dosage form (tablets, extended release tablets, sublingual tablets, elixir, drops, injectable, etc) provides different quantities of the active ingredient, hyoscyamine sulfate — SEE Prescribing Information (PI) for specific schedules	Contraindications: Glaucoma, obstructive uropathy (eg, bladder neck obstruction due to prostatic hypertrophy), obstruction of GI tract, paralytic ileus, atony of the elderly or debilitated, severe ulcerative colitis, reflux esophagitis, unstable cardiovascular status in acute hemorrhage, toxic megacolon complicating ulcerative colitis and myasthenia gravis Considerations: SEE glycopyrrolate Pregnancy category: C	SEE glycopyrrolate	

Generic Name and Selected Trade Names	Normal Adult Dosage	Major Adverse Effects/Cautions	Key Counselling Points	Miscellaneous Issues
Propantheline Bromide Pro-Banthine	Individualize dosage As adjunctive therapy, usually start with 15 mg 30 minutes before each meal (TID) and 30 mg at bedtime, then titrate as needed; for smaller persons and geriatric patients, usually 7.5 mg 30 minutes before each meal and HS is sufficient	<u>Considerations, adverse effects, and pregnancy category</u>: SEE hyoscyamine sulfate	SEE glycopyrrolate	

*As a general rule, a medication should not be administered to a patient with a known hypersensitivity to it or a similar agent.

Table 4: Agents for Peptic Ulcer Disease, Gastroesophageal Reflux Disease (GERD), and Related Conditions

Generic Name and Selected Trade Names	Normal Adult Dosage	Major Adverse Effects/Cautions	Key Counseling Points	Miscellaneous Issues
Cimetidine and Cimetidine HCl[1] Tagamet	Individualize dosage *Oral formulations* For active duodenal ulcer: Most patients respond to 800 mg hs, although some patients respond to less (eg, 400 mg hs) and some more (1600 mg hs); other regimens include 300 mg with meals and hs, and 400 mg BID For maintenance therapy of duodenal ulcer: Usually, 400 mg hs	Considerations: Rapid IV injection has caused cardiac arrhythmias and hypotension; reversible confusion state has occurred, especially in older persons and those with liver and/or kidney impairment Most common AEs include headache, confusion, gynecomastia, increased liver enzymes, small increases in plasma creatinine, hypersensitivity reactions Pregnancy category: B	Tell the prescriber if you have a liver or kidney disorder; tell the physician and/or pharmacist all other medications that you are taking; contact the prescriber if you develop breast tenderness or enlargement, become confused or disoriented; take the medicine for the entire prescribed regimen even if you feel better sooner; smoking cigarettes or taking aspirin and similar products may worsen your condition — speak with the physician and/or pharmacist;	Ensure patient does not have gastric malignancy; numerous important drug interactions reported (eg, interference with cytochrome P-450 system), SEE Prescribing Information (PI)

Generic Name and Selected Trade Names	Normal Adult Dosage	Key Counseling Points	Miscellaneous Issues
Cimetidine and **Cimetidine HCl**[1] **(continued)** Tagamet	For active benign gastric ulcer: Usually, 800 mg hs or 300 mg with meals and hs For erosive GERD: Usually, 800 mg BID or 400 mg QID for 12 weeks For pathological hypersecretory conditions such as Zollinger-Ellison Syndrome: Usually, 300 mg with meals and hs; some patients require up to 2400 mg/day *Parenteral formulations* IM: Usually, 300 mg Q6–8H IV injection, intermittent IV infusion, continuous IV infusion: SEE Prescribing Information (PI)	speak with the physician and/or pharmacist; if you miss a dose take it as soon as you remember, but if it is almost time for the next dose, skip the missed one and return to normal schedule — do not double doses	

Generic Name and Selected Trade Names	Normal Adult Dosage	Major Adverse Effects/Cautions	Key Counseling Points	Miscellaneous Issues
Cisapride Propulsid	Individualize dosage For nocturnal heartburn due to GERD, start with 10 mg QID, at least 15 minutes ac and hs; some patients require 20 mg QID	Contraindications: Concomitant administration of ketoconazole, itraconazole, miconazole, fluconazole, erythromycin, clarithromycin, or troleandomycin; patients in whom increase in GI motility could be harmful; GI hemorrhage, mechanical obstruction, or perforation Considerations: Potential drug interactions are severe, and may lead to severe cardiac problems including torsades de pointes — SEE Prescribing Information (PI); use caution in persons with QT prolongation on ECG Most common AEs include headache, diarrhea, abdominal pain, constipation, dyspepsia Pregnancy category: C	Tell the prescriber if you have any type of a heart or GI problem, or are taking any other medications; while receiving this agent, do not take any other medications without notifying the prescriber and the pharmacist that you are taking this agent; unless otherwise instructed, take at least 10 minutes before meals and at bedtime; if you miss a dose take it as soon as you remember, but if it is almost time for the next dose, skip the missed one and return to normal schedule — do not double doses	Numerous important drug interactions reported (eg, interference with cytochrome P-450 system), SEE Prescribing Information (PI)

Generic Name and Selected Trade Names	Normal Adult Dosage	Major Adverse Effects/Cautions	Key Counseling Points	Miscellaneous Issues
Famotidine[1] Pepcid	Individualize dosage *Oral formulations* For acute duodenal ulcer: Usually, 40 mg hs; 20 mg BID is also used For maintenance therapy of duodenal ulcer: Usually, 20 mg hs For acute benign gastric ulcer: Usually, 40 mg hs For GERD: Usually, 20 mg BID for up to 6 weeks	Most common AEs include headache, dizziness, constipation, diarrhea Pregnancy category: B	Tell the prescriber if you have any type of kidney disease; if using the suspension, shake the bottle well for at least 10 to 15 seconds before removing a dose, and discard any unused suspension after 30 days; take the medicine for the entire prescribed regimen even if you feel better sooner; smoking cigarettes or taking aspirin and similar products may worsen your condition — speak with your physician and/or pharmacist; if you miss a dose take it as soon as you remember, but if it is almost time for the next dose, skip the missed one and return to normal schedule — do not double doses	Ensure patient does not have gastric malignancy; unused constituted oral suspension should be discarded after 30 days

Generic Name and Selected Trade Names	Normal Adult Dosage	Major Adverse Effects/Cautions	Key Counseling Points	Miscellaneous Issues
Famotidine[1] **(continued)** Pepcid	For Pathological hypersecretory conditions such as Zollinger-Ellison Syndrome: Usually, 20 mg Q6H but some patients require up to 160 mg Q6H *Parenteral formulations* Are available — SEE Prescribing Information (PI) Patients with renal impairment may require lower dosages — SEE PI			

Generic Name and Selected Trade Names	Normal Adult Dosage	Major Adverse Effects/Cautions	Key Counseling Points	Miscellaneous Issues
Lansoprazole Prevacid	Individualize dosage For duodenal ulcer: Usually, 15 mg QD for 4 weeks For maintenance of duodenal ulcer: Usually, 15 mg QD To treat gastric ulcer: Usually, 30 mg QD for up to 8 weeks To treat erosive esophagitis: Usually, 30 mg QD for up to 8 weeks; if not effective, use additional 8 weeks For maintenance of erosive esophagitis: Usually, 15 mg QD	Most common AEs include abdominal pain, diarrhea, nausea, headache Pregnancy category: B	Unless otherwise directed, take before eating; do not break, chew, or crush capsule but if you have difficulty swallowing the delayed-release capsule, open it and sprinkle on a tablespoonful of applesauce and swallow; take the medicine for the entire prescribed regimen even if you feel better sooner; smoking cigarettes or taking aspirin and similar products may worsen your condition — speak with your physician and/or pharmacist; if you miss a dose take it as soon as you remember, but if it is almost time for the next dose, skip the missed one and return to normal schedule — do not double doses	Ensure patient does not have gastric malignancy; if patient has difficulty swallowing delayed-release capsules, open the capsules and sprinkle on a tablespoonful of applesauce and swallow; if used in patient on an nasogastric (NG) tube, open capsule and mix with 40 mL of apple juice and inject into NG tube; metabolized by cytochrome P-450 system, so drug interactions are possible;

Generic Name and Selected Trade Names	Normal Adult Dosage	Major Adverse Effects/Cautions	Key Counseling Points	Miscellaneous Issues
Lansoprazole (continued) Prevacid	Pathological hypersecretory conditions such as Zollinger-Ellison Syndrome: Start with 60 mg QD and titrate; dosages >120 mg should be given in divided doses Use in double or triple therapy to eradicate H. pylori: Refer to Prescribing Information (PI) Dosage adjustments: May need reduced dosage in liver impairment			commonly used in conjunction with antibiotics such as amoxicillin and clarithromycin — refer to appropriate sections in this text and to respective Prescribing Information (PI)

Generic Name and Selected Trade Names	Normal Adult Dosage	Major Adverse Effects/Cautions	Key Counseling Points	Miscellaneous Issues
Misoprostol Cytotec	Individualize dosage For the prevention of NSAID-induced gastric ulcer, usually use 200 mcg QID with food; if dose cannot be tolerated, use 100 mcg instead	<u>Contraindications</u>: Women who are pregnant, women of child-bearing potential unless NSAID must be given and patient is at high risk for NSAID-induced adverse events, but ensure patient is not pregnant and is not likely to become pregnant; nursing women <u>Most common AEs</u> include diarrhea, abdominal pain, nausea, flatulence, headache, dyspepsia, vomiting, constipation <u>Pregnancy category</u>: X	Tell the prescriber if you are pregnant; do not become pregnant while taking this medication, but if you do, contact the prescriber immediately (also, this drug may cause incomplete miscarriage); if diarrhea or abdominal pain is severe contact prescriber, but mild diarrhea may be self-limiting; unless otherwise instructed take with food; do not give this drug to anyone else; if you miss a dose take it as soon as you remember, but if it is almost time for the next dose, skip the missed one and return to normal schedule — do not double doses	Diarrhea is usually dose-related and may be self-limiting

Generic Name and Selected Trade Names	Normal Adult Dosage	Major Adverse Effects/Cautions	Key Counseling Points	Miscellaneous Issues
Nizatidine Axid	Individualize dosage To treat duodenal ulcer: Usually, 300 mg hs; alternatively, 150 mg BID For maintenance of duodenal ulcer: Usually, 150 mg hs To treat GERD: Usually, 150 mg BID For acute benign gastric ulcer: Either 150 mg BID or 300 mg hs Dosage adjustments: Patients with moderate to severe renal insufficiency may require lower dosages — SEE Prescribing Information (PI)	Contraindication: Hypersensitivity to any H_2 antagonist Considerations: Reduce dosage in persons with moderate to severe renal impairment; probably should avoid in nursing women Most common AEs include anemia, urticaria, and a variety of effects no more common than placebo — SEE Prescribing Information (PI) Pregnancy category: B	Tell the prescriber if you have a kidney disorder; take the medicine for the entire prescribed regimen even if you feel better sooner; smoking cigarettes or taking aspirin and similar products may worsen your condition — speak with your physician and/or pharmacist; if you miss a dose take it as soon as you remember, but if it is almost time for the next dose, skip the missed one and return to normal schedule — do not double doses	Ensure patient does not have gastric malignancy

Generic Name and Selected Trade Names	Normal Adult Dosage	Major Adverse Effects/Cautions	Key Counselling Points	Miscellaneous Issues
Omeprazole Prilosec	Individualize dosage For treatment of duodenal ulcer: Usually, 20 mg QD To treat gastric ulcer: Usually, 40 mg QD for 4–8 weeks To treat GERD: If no esophageal lesions, 20 mg QD for up to 4 weeks; with erosive esophagitis, 20 mg QD for 4–8 weeks For maintenance of erosive esophagitis: Usually, 20 mg QD	Consideration: Atrophic gastritis has been reported in patients using medication long-term Most common AEs include headache, diarrhea, dizziness, rash, constipation, back pain, and a variety of effects no more common than placebo — SEE Prescribing Information (PI) Pregnancy category: C	SEE lansoprazole	Ensure patient does not have gastric malignancy; capsules should not be opened, crushed, or chewed, and should be swallowed whole; drug interactions are possible — SEE Prescribing Information (PI); commonly used in conjunction with antibiotics — refer to appropriate sections in this text and to respective PIs

Generic Name and Selected Trade Names	Normal Adult Dosage	Major Adverse Effects/Cautions	Key Counseling Points	Miscellaneous Issues
Omeprazole (continued) Prilosec	For pathological hypersecretory conditions such as Zollinger-Ellison Syndrome: Start with 60 mg QD and titrate; dosages as high as 120 mg TID have been used; daily dosages >80 mg should be given in divided doses Use with antibiotics to eradicate H. pylori; Refer to Prescribing Information (PI)			

Generic Name and Selected Trade Names	Normal Adult Dosage	Major Adverse Effects/Cautions	Key Counseling Points	Miscellaneous Issues
Ranitidine HCl[1] Zantac	Individualize dosage *Oral formulations* To treat duodenal ulcer: Usually, 150 mg BID; alternatively, 300 mg QD after evening meal or hs; other doses have been used — SEE Prescribing Information (PI) For maintenance therapy of duodenal or gastric ulcer: Usually, 150 mg hs To treat acute benign gastric ulcer or GERD: Usually, 150 mg BID	<u>Considerations</u>: Avoid in patients with history of acute porphyria Most common AEs include headache and a wide variety of effects not clearly shown to be due to ranitidine — SEE Prescribing Information (PI); for parenteral form, pain has been reported at injection site; local burning or itching reported with IV administration <u>Pregnancy category</u>: B	Tell the prescriber if you have a history of the blood disorder acute porphyria; also, SEE nizatidine	Ensure patient does not have gastric malignancy; regular tablets and EFFERdose Granules contain phenylalanine

Generic Name and Selected Trade Names	Normal Adult Dosage	Key Counseling Points	Miscellaneous Issues
Ranitidine HCl[1] (continued) Zantac	To treat erosive esophagitis: Usually, 150 mg QID Maintenance therapy of erosive esophagitis: Usually, 150 mg BID Pathological hypersecretory conditions such as Zollinger-Ellison Syndrome: Start with 150 mg BID and titrate; up to 6 g/day have been used Dosage adjustments: Patients with impaired renal function may need reduced dosages — SEE PI *Parenteral formulations* IM: Usually, 50 mg Q6–8H IV injection, intermittent IV infusion, continuous IV infusion: SEE PI Dosage adjustments: Patients with impaired renal function may need reduced dosages — SEE PI		

Generic Name and Selected Trade Names	Normal Adult Dosage	Major Adverse Effects/Cautions	Key Counselling Points	Miscellaneous Issues
Sucralfate Carafate	Treat active duodenal ulcer: administer 1 G QID on an empty stomach for 4-8 weeks unless healing noted by x-ray or endoscopy Maintenance duodenal ulcer (tablets only): Usually, 1 G BID	Considerations: In patients with chronic renal failure, aluminum build-up is possible, especially if patient is taking aluminum-containing antacids; may interfere with the absorption of other medications used simultaneously — separate doses Most common AEs include constipation and a wide variety of rare effects — SEE Prescribing Information (PI) Pregnancy category: B	If you are taking antacids to treat pain, do not take them within one-half hour before or after sucralfate; unless otherwise directed, take this medication with water on an empty stomach; do not take any other medication at the same time as this agent — separate doses; if using the suspension, shake well before using; also, SEE nizatidine	

*As a general rule, a medication should not be administered to a patient with a known hypersensitivity to it or a similar agent.
†Nonprescription dosage forms/strengths are available as well.

Topical Corticosteroids

Table: Topical Corticosteroids*

Generic Name and Selected Trade Names	Normal Adult Dosage	Major Adverse Effects/Cautions	Key Counseling Points	Miscellaneous Issues
Very High Potency **Augmented Betamethasone Dipropionate** Diprolene **Clobetasol Propionate** Cormax Temovate **Diflorasone Diacetate** Florone Maxiflor **Halobetasol Propionate** Ultravate	Topical corticosteroids are classified based upon potency; agent and strength selected needs to be based on specific clinical situation; dosage forms available include cream, gel, lotion, ointment, topical aerosol foam, topical solution	The following are general issues, for specific data SEE Product Information (PI) <u>Considerations</u>: Usually should not be used as monotherapy to treat infections, rosacea, perioral dermatitis or acne; not recommended for ophthalmic use; for very-high potency agents, avoid application to face, groin, or axilla; systemic effects are possible, use special caution in children; do not use as sole therapy for psoriasis; avoid contact with eyes; occlusive dressings are usually avoided with very high potency agents and many others as well; may cause local irritation	Tell the prescriber if you have diabetes mellitus, an infection, tuberculosis, any type of a skin disorder, a cataract, or glaucoma; contact the prescriber if you develop a rash or blisters while taking this agent; children and teenagers should not use long-term without being evaluated by prescriber frequently; do not bandage the skin being treated or use an occlusive dressing (eg, plastic wrap) unless directed to do so by the prescriber; if applicable, ensure patient knows how to apply bandage or an occlusive dressing; for pediatric patients, don't use tight diapers;	

677

Generic Name and Selected Trade Names	Normal Adult Dosage	Major Adverse Effects/Cautions	Key Counseling Points	Miscellaneous Issues
Very High Potency (continued) **Augmented Betamethasone Dipropionate** (continued) Diprolene **Clobetasol Propionate** Cormax Temovate **Diflorasone Diacetate** Florone Maxiflor **Halobetasol Propionate** Ultravate		Most common AEs include local reactions (eg, itching, burning, stinging, redness, dry skin, and pruritus) Pregnancy category: C	don't get this medicine in your eyes; use only as directed, do not use more or less frequently, or for a longer time than prescribed; apply creams, ointments, and gels sparingly to affected areas — rub in gently; wash your hands after applying the medication; if you are applying the medicine on a regular basis and miss a dose, apply it as soon as possible but if it is almost time for the next dose, skip the missed one and apply it at the next regularly scheduled time	

Generic Name and Selected Trade Names	Normal Adult Dosage	Major Adverse Effects/Cautions	Key Counseling Points	Miscellaneous Issues
High Potency **Amcinonide** Cyclocort **Augmented Betamethasone Dipropionate** Diprolene AF **Betamethasone Valerate** Betatrex Beta-Val Valisone **Desoximetasone** Topicort **Diflorasone Diacetate** Florone Maxiflor	SEE Very High Potency topical corticosteroids	SEE Very High Potency topical corticosteroids	SEE Very High Potency topical corticosteroids	

Generic Name and Selected Trade Names	Normal Adult Dosage	Major Adverse Effects/Cautions	Key Counselling Points	Miscellaneous Issues
High Potency (continued) **Flucinolone Acetonide** Synalar Synemol **Fluocinonide** Fluonex Lidex **Halcinonide** Halog **Triamcinolone Acetonide** Aristocort Flutex Kenalog				

Generic Name and Selected Trade Names	Normal Adult Dosage	Major Adverse Effects/Cautions	Key Counseling Points	Miscellaneous Issues
Medium Potency **Betamethasone Benzoate** Unicort **Betamethasone Dipropionate** Alphatrex Diprosone Maxivate Telador **Betamethasone Valerate** Betatrex Beta-Val Valisone **Clocortolone Pivalate** Cloderm	SEE Very High Potency topical corticosteroids	SEE Very High Potency topical corticosteroids	SEE Very High Potency topical corticosteroids	

Generic Name and Selected Trade Names	Major Adverse Effects/Cautions	Key Counseling Points	Miscellaneous Issues
Medium Potency (continued) **Desoximetasone** Topicort-LP **Fluocinolone Acetonide** Synalar Synemol **Flurandrenolide** Cordran **Fluticasone Propionate** Cutivate **Hydrocortisone Butyrate** Locoid **Hydrocortisone Valerate** Westcort **Mometasone Furoate** Elocon **Triamcinolone Acetonide** Aristocort Flutex Kenalog			

Generic Name and Selected Trade Names	Normal Adult Dosage	Major Adverse Effects/Cautions	Key Counseling Points	Miscellaneous Issues
Low Potency **Aclometasone Dipropionate**	SEE Very High Potency topical corticosteroids	SEE Very High Potency topical corticosteroids	SEE Very High Potency topical corticosteroids	
Aclovate				
Desonide				
DesOwen				
Tridesilon				
Dexamethasone				
Dexamethasone Sodium Phosphate				
Hydrocortisone				
Hydrocortisone Acetate				

*As a general rule, a medication should not be administered to a patient with a known hypersensitivity to it or a similar agent.

Alzheimer's Disease Agents

Table: Alzheimer's Disease Agents*

Generic Name and Selected Trade Names	Normal Adult Dosage	Major Adverse Effects/Cautions	Key Counseling Points	Miscellaneous Issues
Donepezil HCl Aricept	Individualize dosage For treatment of mild to moderate dementia of Alzheimer's type; start with 5 mg HS; may titrate to 10 mg HS after 4–6 weeks	<u>Considerations</u>: Use with caution in patients with sick sinus syndrome or other cardiac conduction problems, asthma or obstructive pulmonary disease; may aggravate peptic ulcers, urinary hesitancy, and epilepsy Most common AEs include diarrhea, nausea/vomiting, anorexia, insomnia, muscle cramps, fatigue <u>Pregnancy category</u>: C	Tell the prescriber if the patient has any of the conditions listed under "contraindications" or "considerations"; may cause some people to become dizzy or unsteady, so know how you react before driving a car or using machinery; it is important that the prescriber checks your progress regularly; if you develop clumsiness, diarrhea, loss of appetite, nausea or vomiting check with the prescriber; take as directed, do not take more or less of it; it is best if the medication is taken right before bedtime; may be taken with or without food; if you miss a dose skip the missed one and return to regular schedule — do not double doses	

687

Generic Name and Selected Trade Names	Normal Adult Dosage	Major Adverse Effects/Cautions	Key Counseling Points	Miscellaneous Issues
Tacrine HCl Cognex	Individualize dosage For treatment of mild to moderate dementia of Alzheimer's type, start with 10 mg QID for at least 6 weeks; may titrate to 20 mg QID if there are no significant liver enzyme (transaminase) elevations and patient is tolerating the agent; then, may increase to 30 mg QID in 6 weeks and then to 40 mg QID 6 weeks later based upon tolerability	<u>Contraindication</u>: Patients previously treated with tacrine who developed treatment-associated jaundice, confirmed by elevated total bilirubin greater than 3.0 mg/dL <u>Considerations</u>: SEE donepezil HCl and use with caution in patients with a history of or current liver abnormalities Most common AEs include nausea/vomiting, anorexia, agitation, confusion, rash, elevation of liver enzymes Pregnancy category: C	SEE donepezil; also, it is important that the prescriber checks your progress regularly, including regular blood tests; it is important for the medication to be taken 4 times a day at evenly spaced intervals; it is best if the medication is taken between meals, but if stomach upset occurs may be taken with meals; if you miss a dose take it as soon as possible, but if it is within 2 hrs of the next dose skip the missed one and return to regular schedule — do not double doses	Transaminase levels must be measured every other week during the first 16 weeks of therapy then monthly

Generic Name and Selected Trade Names	Normal Adult Dosage	Major Adverse Effects/Cautions	Key Counseling Points	Miscellaneous Issues
Tacrine HCl (continued) Cognex	If elevations of liver enzymes occur, adjustments in the dosage and monitoring schedule are necessary — SEE Prescribing Information (PI)			

*As a rule, a medication should not be administered to a patient with a known hypersensitivity to it or a similar agent.

Agents for Glaucoma

Table: Selected Glaucoma Agents*

Generic Name and Selected Trade Names	Normal Adult Dosage	Major Adverse Effects/Cautions	Key Counseling Points	Miscellaneous Issues
Acetazolamide Dazamide Diamox Diamox Sequels	Individualize dosage <u>For chronic open-angle glaucoma</u>: Administer 250 mg to 1 G daily usually in divided doses <u>For secondary glaucoma and preoperative use</u>: Short-term, 250 mg Q4H or BID <u>For epilepsy</u>: 8 to 30 mg/kg/day in divided doses; optimum range reported to be 375 mg to 1 G daily but use smaller doses when used in combination For other uses and parenteral dosage form — SEE Prescribing Information (PI)	<u>Contraindications</u>: Hepatic insufficiency, renal failure, adrenocortical insufficiency, hyperchloremic acidosis, hyponatremia, and hypokalemia <u>Considerations</u>: Hypokalemia with brisk diuresis may occur if cirrhosis is present, if there is inadequate electrolyte intake, or if steroids or ACTH are being used; increasing the dosage above 1 G/day usually does not increase efficacy and may increase drowsiness or paresthesia; there is cross sensitivity (allergy) with sulfonamides Most common AEs include nausea/vomiting, anorexia, drowsiness, paresthesia <u>Pregnancy category</u>: C	Tell the prescriber if you have diabetes mellitus, respiratory disease, gout, low blood levels of potassium or sodium, a kidney or liver disease, or Addison's disease; may produce drowsiness, or dizziness in some patients, so make sure you know how you react before driving a car or using machinery; if you develop shortness of breath or trouble breathing or unusual tiredness contact the prescriber; may produce a loss of potassium, so the prescriber may want you to eat or drink foods that have a high potassium content (eg, orange or citrus juices) or take a potassium supplement.	

Generic Name and Selected Trade Names	Normal Adult Dosage	Major Adverse Effects/Cautions	Key Counseling Points	Miscellaneous Issues
Acetazolamide (continued) Dazamide Diamox Diamox Sequels			so follow the diet recommended by the prescriber; the prescriber may want you to increase your fluid intake while taking this agent; it is important to take only as directed; take with meals; for single daily doses take in the morning to decrease night-time urination, for twice a day dosing take the evening dose before 6 PM; if you miss a dose take it as soon as possible, but if it is almost time for the next dose, skip the missed one and return to regular schedule — do not double doses	

Generic Name and Selected Trade Names	Normal Adult Dosage	Major Adverse Effects/Cautions	Key Counseling Points	Miscellaneous Issues
Betaxolol HCl Betoptic Betoptic S	Individualize dosage For ocular hypertension and open-angle glaucoma, usually instill 1 to 2 drops in affected eye(s) BID	<u>Contraindications</u>: Patients with sinus bradycardia, greater than a first degree A-V block, cardiogenic shock, or over cardiac failure <u>Considerations</u>: Systemic effects (eg, bronchospasm in asthmatic patients, cardiac failure) are rare, but can occur; use with caution in patients with cardiac disease, diabetes mellitus, hyperthyroidism, muscle weakness, asthma Most common AEs include eye discomfort (short lasting), tearing, local irritation <u>Pregnancy category</u>: C	Tell the prescriber if you have asthma or other respiratory diseases, diabetes mellitus, hypoglycemia, heart or blood vessel disease, or an overactive thyroid; if you develop redness of eyes, blurred vision, different size pupils, discoloration of the eyeball, droopy upper eyelid or eye pain, contact the prescriber; ensure that the patient understands proper technique for use of eye drops; use as directed and do not use more of it or use it more often; if you miss a dose take it as soon as possible but if it is almost time for the next dose, skip the missed one and return to regular schedule — do not double doses	If used in narrow-angle glaucoma must be used with a miotic agent

Generic Name and Selected Trade Names	Normal Adult Dosage	Major Adverse Effects/Cautions	Key Counseling Points	Miscellaneous Issues
Carbachol Isopto Carbachol	Individualize dosage For open-angle glaucoma, usually 1 drop QD to TID Intraocular solution available for miosis — SEE Prescribing Information (PI)	<u>Contraindication</u>: Conditions such as iritis where pupillary constriction is undesirable <u>Considerations</u>: Use with caution in patients with asthma, acute cardiac failure, corneal abrasion or injury, GI spasm, peptic ulcer, urinary tract obstruction, or Parkinson's disease Most common AEs include blurred vision or change in vision, eye pain, stinging or burning of the eye <u>Pregnancy category</u>: C	Tell the prescriber if you have asthma, other eye problems, heart disease, overactive thyroid, Parkinson's disease or urinary tract blockage; may cause your pupils to become unusually small which can decrease your ability to see at night or in dim light, so make sure you know how you react before driving a car or using machinery; if you develop a veil or curtain appearing across part of your vision contact the prescriber immediately; ensure that patient knows how to administer eye drops; use as directed; if you miss a dose instill as soon as possible, if it is almost time for the next dose, skip the missed one and go back to regular schedule — do not double doses	

Generic Name and Selected Trade Names	Normal Adult Dosage	Major Adverse Effects/Cautions	Key Counseling Points	Miscellaneous Issues
Demecarium Bromide Humorsol	Individualize dosage For open-angle glaucoma, maintenance therapy ranges from 1 or 2 drops twice a week to 1 or 2 drops BID; initial therapy should be conducted under the supervision of an experienced practitioner Additional indications exist — SEE Prescribing Information (PI)	<u>Contraindications</u>: Pregnancy, active uveal inflammation and/or glaucoma associated with iridocyclitis <u>Considerations</u>: Gonioscopy recommended prior to use; use with caution in patients with narrow angle glaucoma, bradycardia with or without hypotension, recent MI, bronchial asthma, spastic GI disturbances, epilepsy, or Parkinson's disease <u>Most common AEs</u> include stinging, burning, lacrimation, lid muscle twitching, conjunctival and ciliary redness, brow ache, headache, induced myopia, visual blurring <u>Pregnancy category</u>: X	Tell the prescriber if you have any serious medical conditions; patients should be warned to avoid contact with insecticides or pesticides, may produce blurred vision in some patients, so make sure your vision is clear before driving a car or using machinery; if you develop salivation, urinary incontinence, diarrhea, profuse sweating, muscle weakness, respiratory difficulties, or cardiac irregularities discontinue the medication and contact the prescriber; following instillation of the drops apply gentle pressure on the lacrimal duct with the index finger for several seconds; use only as directed; if you miss a dose check with the prescriber — do not double doses	Agent should be discontinued prior to eye surgery; preservative may be absorbed by soft contact lens, so patient should wait at least 15 min following instillation before inserting contact lens; many drug interactions are possible — SEE Prescribing Information (PI)

Generic Name and Selected Trade Names	Normal Adult Dosage	Major Adverse Effects/Cautions	Key Counseling Points	Miscellaneous Issues
Dichlorphenamide Daranide	Individualize dosage For adjunctive treatment of glaucoma, priming dose of 100 to 200 mg; then 100 mg Q12H until desired response is obtained; maintenance dosage 25 to 50 mg QD to TID Generally given in combination with other agents — SEE Prescribing Information (PI)	<u>Contraindications</u>: SEE acetazolamide <u>Considerations</u>: Hypokalemia with brisk diuresis may occur if cirrhosis is present, inadequate electrolyte intake, or steroids or ACTH are being used; use caution in patients with severe respiratory acidosis; there is cross sensitivity (allergy) with sulfonamides <u>Most common AEs</u>: SEE acetazolamide Pregnancy category: C	SEE acetazolamide	

Generic Name and Selected Trade Names	Normal Adult Dosage	Major Adverse Effects/Cautions	Key Counseling Points	Miscellaneous Issues
Dorzolamide HCl Trusopt	For ocular hypertension and open-angle glaucoma 1 drop in affected eye(s) TID	Considerations: Sulfonamide-like systemic reactions are possible; not recommended for use in patients with narrow angle glaucoma or with severe renal impairment or concurrently with systemic carbonic anhydrase inhibitors Most common AEs include ocular burning, stinging, or discomfort, bitter taste, superficial punctate keratitis, ocular allergic reactions, blurred vision, tearing, dryness, photophobia Pregnancy category: C	Tell the prescriber if you have kidney or liver disease; if you develop conjunctivitis, itching or red eyes, rash, or fever discontinue the medication and contact the prescriber; may produce blurred vision in some patients, so make sure your vision is clear before driving a car or using machinery; may cause your eyes to become more sensitive to light than normal, so wear sunglasses to decrease the discomfort; it is important to use the medication only as directed; ensure patient understands proper technique for administration of eye drops; if you miss a dose take it as soon as possible but if it is almost time for the next dose, skip the missed one and return to regular schedule — do not double doses	If more than one ophthalmic agent is being used administer at least 10 minutes apart; preservative may be absorbed by soft contact lens, so not for use in patients wearing soft contact lens

Generic Name and Selected Trade Names	Normal Adult Dosage	Major Adverse Effects/Cautions	Key Counselling Points	Miscellaneous Issues
Epinephrine Epifrin Glaucon	Individualize dosage For open-angle glaucoma, usually 1 drop in affected eye(s) QD or BID	<u>Contraindications</u>: Narrow angle glaucoma, cardiovascular diseases <u>Considerations</u>: Use with caution in patients with aphakia, asthma, diabetes mellitus, or hyperthyroidism Most common AEs include headache or brow-ache, stinging, redness, or other eye irritations, tearing, blurred vision <u>Pregnancy category</u>: C	Tell the prescriber if you have bronchial asthma, diabetes mellitus, heart or blood vessel disease, high blood pressure, overactive thyroid, or any other eye disease; if you develop blurred or decreased vision, fast irregular or pounding heartbeat, dizziness, increased sweating, paleness or trembling, contact the prescriber; use as directed; do not use more of it or use it more often; ensure patient understand proper technique for administering eye drops; following instillation apply gentle pressure to the lacrimal sac for 1 to 2 minutes; if you miss a dose apply it as soon as possible, but if it is almost time for the next dose, skip the missed one, return to regular schedule — do not double doses	

Generic Name and Selected Trade Names	Normal Adult Dosage	Major Adverse Effects/Cautions	Key Counseling Points	Miscellaneous Issues
Pilocarpine Isopto Carpine Pilocar Ocusert Pilo-20 Ocusert Pilo-40	Individualize dosage Ocular system for open-angle glaucoma: Usually one 20 or 40 mcg/hr ocular system once every 7 days Ophthalmic gel for open-angle glaucoma: Usually 1.5 cm HS Ophthalmic solution for open-angle glaucoma: Usually 1 drop BID to QID Other indications are possible — SEE Prescribing Information (PI)	SEE carbachol	SEE carbachol and for ocular system dosage form, ensure patient has read the patient instruction leaflet	

Generic Name and Selected Trade Names	Normal Adult Dosage	Major Adverse Effects/Cautions	Key Counselling Points	Miscellaneous Issues
Timolol Maleate Timoptic Timoptic Ocudose Timoptic-XE	Individualize dosage For ocular hypertension and open-angle glaucoma, start with 1 drop of 0.25% in affected eye(s) BID; may increase to 1 drop of 0.5% BID if needed	<u>Contraindications</u>: Bronchial asthma or a history of or severe chronic obstructive pulmonary disease plus SEE betaxolol HCl <u>Considerations, most common AEs, and pregnancy category</u>: SEE betaxolol HCl	SEE betaxolol HCl, also, ensure patient understands proper technique for use of ophthalmic gels	SEE betaxolol HCl and Ocudose is preservative free and contains a single dose per unit

*As a rule, a medication should not be administered to a patient with a known hypersensitivity to it or a similar agent.

Agent for Erectile Dysfunction

Table: Agent for Erectile Dysfunction*

Generic Name and Selected Trade Names	Normal Adult Dosage	Major Adverse Effects/Cautions	Key Counseling Points	Miscellaneous Issues
Sildenafil Citrate Viagra	Individualize dosage For erectile dysfunction, usual recommended dose is 50 mg pm about 1 hr before sexual intercourse; may be taken 4 hrs to 0.5 hrs before intercourse; may titrate down to 25 mg QD or up to 100 mg QD but maximum dosing frequency is QD; in men ≥65 years of age, consider a starting dose of 25 mg QD	Contraindications: Concomitant use of nitrates (regular or PRN usage) Considerations: The following patients may have significantly higher plasma levels of sildenafil than normal — >65 years of age, hepatic and severe renal impairment, concomitant use of potent cytochrome P-450 3A4 inhibitors (eg, cimetidine and erythromycin); do not generally use in men with preexisting cardiovascular disease; due to vasodilatory effects, may decrease BP; priapism reported; safety in patients with bleeding disorders and active peptic ulceration unknown; use with other therapies for erectile dysfunction not studied	Tell the prescriber if you have or had a cardiovascular disease, high or low blood pressure, kidney disease, or liver disease; tell your prescriber and pharmacist all other medications you are taking; contact prescriber if cardiovascular symptoms such as angina or dizziness occur; ensure patient understands the contraindication with nitrates; priapism (painful and sustained erection) has been reported, and if this occurs seek medical attention immediately as penile damage may occur;	Not to be used in women; ensure patient has been evaluated properly for erectile dysfunction — SEE Prescribing Information (PI); many drug interactions are possible — SEE PI; provide patient package insert

Generic Name and Selected Trade Names	Normal Adult Dosage	Major Adverse Effects/Cautions	Key Counseling Points	Miscellaneous Issues
Sildenafil Citrate (continued) Viagra		Most common AEs include headache, flushing, dyspepsia, nasal congestion, urinary tract infection, abnormal vision (eg, blurred vision, sensitivity to light, changes in color change perception), diarrhea, dizziness, rash; post-marketing, severe cardiovascular events including MI, arrhythmias, and sudden death reported <u>Pregnancy category:</u> B	medication usually begins to work within 30 minutes and may last for up to 4 hrs but response usually is less after 2 hrs; it is very important not to exceed prescribed dosage; medication does not provide protection against sexually transmitted diseases	

*As a general rule, a medication should not be administered to a patient with a known hypersensitivity to it or a similar agent

Appendices

Appendix A: Common Medical Abbreviations

AAO	alert, awake, and oriented
AAO X 3	alert, and oriented to time, place, and person
A_1	aortic first heart sound
A_2	aortic second heart sound
abd	abdomen
ABGs	arterial blood gases
ABR	absolute bed rest
ABS	absent
ABW	actual body weight
ACE	angiotensin converting enzyme
ACLS	advanced cardiac life support
ADA	American Diabetes Association
ADR	adverse drug reaction
AE	adverse effect
AF	atrial fibrillation
A fib	atrial fibrillation
A/G	albumin to globulin ratio
AGVHD	acute graft-versus-host disease
AKA	also known as; above the knee amputation; all known allergies
ALL	acute lymphocytic leukemia; acute lymphoblastic leukemia
ALT	alanine aminotransferase; alanine transferase
AMA	against medical advice; American Medical Association
AMI	acute myocardial infarction
AML	acute myelogenous leukemia
ANA	antinuclear antibody/ies
A & O	alert and oriented
A & O X 3	alert and oriented to person, place, and time
AOM	acute otitis media
AP	anteroposterior
APACHE	Acute Physiology and Chronic Health Evaluation
APTT	activated partial thromboplastin time
ARC	AIDS related complex
ASAP	as soon as possible
AST	aspartate aminotransferase; aspartate transferase
ASCVD	arteriosclerotic cardiovascular disease
ASHD	arteriosclerotic heart disease
AV	atrioventricular
A & W	alive and well
BBB	bundle branch block; blood brain barrier
B↑E	both upper extremities
B↓E	both lower extremities
BKA	below the knee amputation
BM	bowel movement
BMI	body mass index
BMR	basal metabolic rate
BP; B/P	blood pressure
BPH	benign prostatic hyperplasia

Appendix A (continued): Common Medical Abbreviations

BPM; bpm	beats per minute
BRP	bathroom privileges
BS	blood sugar; bowel sounds; breath sounds; barium swallow
BSA	body surface area
BUN	blood urea nitrogen
Bx	biopsy
C	Celsius, centigrade
Ca	cancer; calcium
CABG	coronary artery bypass graft
CAD	coronary artery disease
Cal	calorie
CAPD	chronic ambulatory peritoneal dialysis
cath	catheterize; catheterization
CC	chief complaint
cc	cubic centimeter
CBC	complete blood count
CCU	coronary care unit
CHF	congestive heart failure
cm	centimeter
CNS	central nervous system
COLD	chronic obstructive lung disease
COPD	chronic obstructive pulmonary disease
CPAP	continuous positive airway pressure
CPK	creatine kinase; creatine phosphokinase
CPR	cardiopulmonary resuscitation
CrCl	creatinine clearance
CRF	chronic renal failure; case report form
C & S	culture and sensitivity
CSF	cerebrospinal fluid
CT	computed tomography
CV	cardiovascular
CVA	cerebrovascular accident; costovertebral angle
CVP	central venous pressure
D & C	dilatation and curettage
d/c	discontinue
DIC	disseminated intra-vascular coagulation; drug information center
DKA	diabetic keotacidosis
DM	diabetes mellitus
DNR	do not resuscitate
DOA	dead on arrival
DOB	date of birth
Dx	disease; diagnosis
ECG	electrocardiogram
echo	echocardiogram
EEG	electroencephalogram
EENT	ear, eye, nose, and throat
EKG	electrocardiogram

Appendix A (continued): Common Medical Abbreviations

EPS	extrapyramidal symptoms
ERCP	endoscopic retrograde cholangio-pancreatography
ESR	erythrocyte sedimentation rate
ETOH	alcohol; ethyl alcohol; ethanol
FBG	fasting blood glucose
FBS	fasting blood sugar
FEF	forced expiratory flow
FEV_1	forced expiratory flow in one second
FH	family history
FMD	family medical doctor
FSH	follicle stimulating hormone
G^+	Gram-positive; guaiac positive
G^-	Gram-negative; guaiac negative
GERD	gastroesophageal reflux disease
GFR	glomerular filtration rate
GI	gastrointestinal
GTT	glucose tolerance test
GU	genitourinary
HA	headache
Hb	hemoglobin
Hct; hct; HCT	hematocrit
HEENT	head, eyes, ears, nose, and throat
Hgb; hgb	hemoglobin
H & H; H/H	hemoglobin and hematocrit
HIV	human immuno-deficiency virus
H/O	history of
H & P	history and physical
HPI	history of present illness
HR	heart rate
Hx	history
IBW	ideal body weight
ICU	intensive care unit
IDDM	insulin dependent diabetes mellitus
IPPB	intermittent positive pressure breathing
I & O	intake and output
ITP	idiopathic thrombocytopenic purpura
IU; I.U.	international unit
IUD	intrauterine device
IVDA	intravenous drug abuser
IVP	intravenous pyelogram
JVD	jugular venous distention
KO	keep open
KUB	kidneys, ureter, and bladder
KVO	keep vein open
LBBB	left bundle branch block
LBW	lean body weight; low birth weight

Appendix A (continued): Common Medical Abbreviations

L & D	labor and delivery
LD	lactic dehydrogenase
LDH	lactic dehydrogenase
LH	luteinizing hormone
LHRH	luteinizing hormone releasing hormone
LLQ	left lower quadrant
LMP	last menstrual period
LOC	loss of consciousness
LUQ	left upper quadrant
LTC	long term care
LVEDP	left ventricular end diastolic pressure
LVEDV	left ventricular end diastolic volume
LVEF	left ventricular ejection fraction
MAP	mean arterial pressure; mean airway pressure
MI	myocardial infarction
MIC	minimal inhibitory concentration
MICU	medical intensive care unit
MMR	measles, mumps, and rubella
MRI	magnetic resonance imaging
MVO_2	myocardial oxygen consumption; myocardial oxygen demand
NAD	no acute distress; no apparent distress
NCD	normal childhood diseases
neg	negative
NG	nasogastric
NKA	no known allergies
NKDA	no known drug allergies
NPO	nothing by mouth
N & V	nausea and vomiting
NVD	nausea, vomiting, and diarrhea
OBS	organic brain syndrome
OOB	out of bed
O & P	ova and parasites
OR	operating room
P & A	percussion and auscultation
Pa_{CO2}	partial pressure of carbon dioxide
Pa_{O2}	partial pressure of oxygen
PAT	paroxysmal atrial tachycardia
PCA	patient controlled analgesia
PCTA	percutaneous transluminal angioplasty
PCWP	pulmonary capillary wedge pressure
PE	physical examination; pulmonary embolism
PEFR	peak expiratory flow rate
PEEP	positive end expiratory pressure
PERL	pupils equal, reactive to light
PERRLA	pupils equal, round, react to light and accommodation
PET	positron emission tomography
PID	pelvic inflammatory disease

Appendix A (continued): Common Medical Abbreviations

PMD	private medical doctor
PMH	past medical history
PMS	premenstrual syndrome
PND	paroxysmal nocturnal dyspnea
P & O	parasites and ova
postop	postoperatively
PP	postprandial
PPD	packs per day, purified protein derivative
preop	preoperatively
Pro-time	prothrombin time
PSA	prostate specific antigen
PT	prothrombin time
PTA	percutaneous transluminal angioplasty
PTT	partial thromboplastin time
PUD	peptic ulcer disease
PVC	premature ventricular contraction; pulmonary venous congestion
PVD	peripheral vascular disease
RBBB	right bundle branch block
RBC	red blood cell
RIA	radioimmunoassay
RLQ	right lower quadrant
R/O	rule out
ROM	range of motion
RUQ	right upper quadrant
S_1	first heart sound
S_2	second heart sound
S_3	third heart sound
S_4	fourth heart sound
SH	social history
SICU	surgical intensive care unit
SIDS	sudden infant death syndrome
SLE	systemic lupus erythematosus
SOAP	subjective, objective, assessment, and plan
SOB	shortness of breath
S/P	status post
stat	immediately
T	temperature
TB	tuberculosis
temp	temperature
TLC	tender loving care; total lymphocyte count
TO	telephone order
TPN	total parenteral nutrition
TPR	temperature, pulse, and respiration; total peripheral resistance
TSH	thyroid stimulating hormone
TT	thrombin time
TURP	transurethral resection of prostate
U	unit

Appendix A (continued): Common Medical Abbreviations

UA	urinalysis
UTI	urinary tract infection
VO	verbal order
VS	vital signs
v. tach	ventricular tachycardia
WBC	white blood cell
WD	well developed
wk	week
WN	well nourished
WNL	within normal limits
wt	weight
W/U	work-up
yr	Year
@	at
~	about; approximately
>	greater than
<	less than
=	equal
↑	above; alive; greater than
↓	dead; down; less than

Appendix B: Common Pharmaceutical Abbreviations

aa	of each
ac	before meals
AD	right ear
ad lib	as much as desired
ADME	absorption, distribution, metabolism, excretion
AL	left ear
amp	ampule; ampul
agit	agitate (shake)
aq	water
ANDA	abbreviated new drug application
ATC	around the clock
AU	both ears
AUC	area under the curve
BID; bid	twice daily; two times a day
c	with
cap	capsule
cc	cubic centimeter
CCB	calcium channel blocker
collyr	eye wash
DAW	dispense as written
dL	deciliter
DTD; dtd	give/make such doses
D_5W	dextrose 5% in water
EC	enteric coated
FDA	Food and Drug Administration
G; g	gram
gal	gallon
gr	grain
gtt	drop
gtts	drops
H; h	hour
hr	hour
HS; hs	at bedtime
IM	intramuscular
inj	injection
IV	intravenous
IVP	intravenous push; intravenous pyelogram
IVPB	intravenous piggyback
kg; kG	kilogram
L	liter
LA	long acting
lb	pound
LTCF	long-term care facility
LVP	large volume parenteral
M	meter
MAR	medication administration record
MDI	metered dose inhaler

Appendix B (continued): Common Pharmaceutical Abbreviations

mEq	Milliequivalent
mg	milligram
mcg	microgram
min	minute
mL; ml	milliliter
mm	millimeter
mmol	millimole
mOsm	milliosmole
NDA	new drug application
ng	nanogram
noct	at night
NS	normal saline
OD	right eye
OS	left eye
os	by mouth
OTC	over the counter
OU	each eye; both eyes
oz	ounce
PC; pc	after meals
per diem	per day
PI	package insert, prescribing information, product information
PO	by mouth
PR	by rectum
PRN; prn	as needed
pt	pint
Q; q	every
QD; qd	every day
QH; qh	every hour
QID; qid	four times a day
QOD; qod	every other day
qs	quantity sufficient
qt	quart
Q2h	every 2 hrs
Q4h	every 4 hrs
Q6h	every 6 hrs
Q8h	every 8 hrs
Q12h	every 12 hrs
Rx	take though
s	without
SC;sc	subcutaneous
sig	let it be written (directions)
SL; sl	sublingual
sos	if needed
SQ	subcutaneous
SR	sustained release
ss	one-half
STAT; stat	immediately

Appendix B (continued): Common Pharmaceutical Abbreviations

supp	suppository
T½	half life
tab	tablet
tbsp	tablespoon
TID; tid	three times a day
troch	lozenge
tsp	teaspoon
ungt	ointment
ut dict	as directed
Vd	volume of distribution
wt	weight

Appendix C: Common Drug Name/Category
Abbreviations and Acronyms

Note: The use of abbreviations for drug names or drug categories is a potentially *dangerous* practice. Nevertheless, the abbreviations listed below are used. In order to prevent medication errors, health care professionals are strongly urged to check with the prescriber whenever an abbreviation is used.

ABCD	amphotericin B cholesteryl sulfate complex
ABLC	amphotericin B lipid complex
5-AC	azacitidine
ACEI; ACE-I	angiotensin converting enzyme inhibitor
Ach; ACH	acetylcholine
Act-D; ACT-D	dactinomycin
ACV	acyclovir
ADRIA	doxorubicin (Adriamycin)
APAP	acetaminophen
AMPT	metyrosine
Ara-A; ara-A	vidarabine
Ara-AC; ara-AC	fazarabine
Ara-C; ara-C	cytarabine
ASA	aspirin (acetylsalicylic acid)
4-ASA	aminosalicylic acid
5-ASA	mesalamine (5-aminosalicylic acid)
ATSO4	atropine sulfate
AZA	azathioprine
AZA-CR	azacitidine
5-AZC	azacitidine
AZT	zidovudine (azidothymidine); aztreonam (dangerous abbreviation as it is used for two drugs)
B_1	thiamine
B_2	riboflavin
B_3	nicotinic acid
B_6	pyridoxine
B_7	biotin
B_{12}	cyanocobalamin
BB	beta blocker
BCG	bacillus Calmette-Guérin (vaccine)
BCNU	carmustine
BCP	birth control pills
Bicarb	bicarbonate (HCO_3^-)
BiCNU	carmustine
Bleo	bleomycin
BSF	busulfan
BSP	Bromsulphalein
B & W	black and white (milk of magnesia and cascara fluidextract)
BZD; BZDZ	benzodiazepine
CBZ	carbamazepine
CCB	calcium channel blocker

Appendix C (continued): Common Drug Name/Category Abbreviations and Acronyms

CCNU	lomustine
CDDP	cisplatin
CeeNU	lomustine
CG	chorionic gonadotropin
CPM	chlorpheniramine maleate
CPZ	chlorpromazine; Compazine (dangerous abbreviation as it is used for two drugs)
CTM	Chlor-Trimeton
CTX	cyclophosphamide
CTZ	chlorothiazide
DA	dopamine
DCNU	chlorozotocin
DDAVP	desmopressin acetate
DDC; ddc	zalcitabine (dideoxycytidine)
DDI; ddi	didanosine (dideoxyinosine)
DDP	cisplatin
Dig	digoxin
D_5LR	dextrose 5% in lactated Ringer's
D_5NS	dextrose 5% in normal saline
D_5RL	dextrose 5% in Ringer's lactate
D_5W	dextrose 5% in water
$D_{50}W$	dextrose 50% in water
DM	dextromethorphan
DMSO	dimethyl sulfoxide
DOCA	desoxycorticosterone pivalate
DOSS	docusate sodium
Dox; DOX	doxorubicin
DPH	phenytoin (diphenylhydantoin); diphenhydramine (dangerous abbreviation as it is used for two drugs)
DPT	diphtheria and tetanus toxoids and pertussis vaccine adsorbed
DT	diphtheria and tetanus toxoids adsorbed
d4T	stavudine
DTIC	dacarbazine
ECASA	enteric coated aspirin
EES	erythromycin ethylsuccinate
EPI; Epi	epinephrine
EPO	erythropoietin
ETOH	alcohol; ethyl alcohol; ethanol
5-FC	flucytosine
5-FU	fluorouracil
FA	folic acid
FK506	tacrolimus
FSH/LH	follicle stimulating hormone/luteinizing hormone
FUDR	floxuridine
G-CSF	filgastrim (granulocyte colony stimulating factor)

Appendix C (continued): Common Drug Name/Category Abbreviations and Acronyms

GM-CSF	sargramostim (granulocyte-macrophage colony stimulating factor)
GnRH	gonadorelin acetate (gonadotropin-releasing hormone)
HC	hydrocortisone
hCG	human chorionic gonadotropin
HCT	hydrocortisone
HCTZ	hydrochlorothiazide
HMG-CoA	3-hydroxy-3-methyl-glutaryl-coenzyme A reductase
H_2RA	histamine$_2$-receptor antagonist
IDU	idoxuridine
IFN	interferon
INH	isoniazid
ISDN	isosorbide dinitrate
ISMO	isosorbide mononitrate
ISO	isoproterenol
K	potassium
K_1	phytonadione
LAAM	levomethadyl acetate HCl (levo-alpha-acetymethadol HCl)
L-ASP	asparaginase
l-dopa	levodopa
Li	lithium
L-PAM	melphalan
LR	lactated Ringers
MAOI	monoamine oxidase inhibitor
MCT	medium chain triglycerides
MITO-C	mitomycin
MOM	milk of magnesia
MMR	measles, mumps, and rubella
6-MP	6-mercaptopurine
MS	morphine sulfate
MTX	methotrexate
MTZ	mitoxantrone
NE	norepinephrine
NPH	isophane insulin
NS	normal saline solution
NSAID	nonsteroidal antiinflammatory drug
NTG	nitroglycerin
NTX	naltrexone
PAS	aminosalicylic acid
PB; Pb	phenobarbital
Pb	lead
PBZ	phenoxybenzamine; phenylbutazone; pyribenzamine (dangerous abbreviation as it is used for three drugs)
PCN	penicillin
PCP	phencyclidine; prochlorperazine (dangerous abbreviation as it is used for two drugs)

Appendix C (continued): Common Drug Name/Category Abbreviations and Acronyms

PNC	penicillin
PPA	phenylpropanolamine
PTZ	phenothiazine
PZA	pyrazinamide
PZI	protamine zinc insulin
RIG	rabies immune globulin
RL	Ringer's lactate
RTCA	ribavirin
t-RA	tretinoin (trans-retinoic acid)
r-tPA	alteplase (recombinant tissue plasminogen activator)
SMX/TMP; SMZ/TMP	sulfamethoxazole/trimethoprim (co-trimoxazole)
SSKI	saturated solution of potassium iodide
SSRIs	selective serotonin reuptake inhibitors
T_3	triiodothyronine; thyronine; liothyronine
T_4	levothyroxine; thyroxine
3TC	lamivudine
TCA	tricyclic antidepressant
TCN	tetracycline
THC	tetrahydrocannabinol
t-PA	alteplase (tissue plasminogen activator)
6-TG	thioguanine
TMP/SMX; TMP/SMZ	trimethoprim/sulfamethoxazole (co-trimoxazole)
VP-16	etoposide
VZIG	varicella-zoster immune globulin
ZDV	zidovudine

Appendix D: Key Laboratory Tests and Reference Intervals

Note: The reference intervals or "normal" values listed below are typical ones, but may not be in accordance with values established by individual laboratories. As a result, the values written below should be used as a *general guide only*. Note as well that laboratories may report test results using different units than those indicated here.

Complete Blood Count (CBC) and Differential	
Red blood cells	Male = 4.5–6 × 10^6/microliter
	Female = 4.2–5.5 × 10^6/microliter
Hemoglobin	Male = 13–18 g/dL
	Female = 12–16 g/dL
Hematocrit	Male = 40%–54%
	Female = 38%–47%
Mean corpuscular volume	80–100 µm^3
Mean corpuscular hemoglobin	26–32 pg
Mean corpuscular hemoglobin concentration	32%–36%
Platelets	140,000–400,000/mm^3
White blood cells	5–10,000/mm^3
White blood cell differential	
Neutrophils	55%–70%
Monocytes	2%–8%
Lymphocytes	20%–40%
Basophils	0.5%–1%
Eosinophils	1%–4%
Serum Electrolytes	
Bicarbonate	22–26 mEq/L or 22–26 mmol/L
Calcium, total	8.5–10.5 mg/dL
Chloride	90–110 mEq/L
Magnesium	1.5–2.4 mEq/L
Phosphate	2.5–4.5 mg/dL
Potassium	3.5–5 mEq/L
Sodium	135–145 mEq/L
Serum Enzyme Tests	
Acid phosphatase	1–10 U/L
Alanine aminotransferase (ALT)	5–40 U/L
Alkaline phosphatase	30–90 U/L
Aspartate aminotransferase (AST)	5–30 U/L
Creatine kinase (CK)	<200 U/L
Creatine kinase, MB isoenzyme	<6% of total CK

Appendix D (continued): Key Laboratory Tests and Reference Intervals

Serum Enzyme Tests (continued)	
Gama-glutamyl transferase (GGT)	Males = 6–45 U/L
	Females = 5–30 U/L
Lactate dehydrogenase (LD, LDH)	80–280 U/L
5'-Nucleotidase	10–18 U/L
Other Serum/Blood/Plasma Tests	
Activated partial thromboplastin time (APTT)	25–40 seconds
Albumin	3.5–5.5 g/dL
Bilirubin, total	0.3–1 mg/dL or 5–17 μmol/L
Bilirubin, direct	<0.4 mg/dL or <7 μmol/L
Blood urea nitrogen (BUN)	5–20 mg/dL
Cholesterol	
Total	<200 mg/dL
Low density lipoprotein	60–180 mg/dL
High density lipoprotein	Males = >45 mg/dL
	Females = >55 mg/dL
Creatinine	0.5–1.5 mg/dL
Glucose, fasting	70–110 mg/dL
Protein, total	6–8.5 g/dL
Prothrombin time	10–13 seconds
Thyroid function	
Total T_4	4–13 mcg/dL
T_3U	25%–35%
T_3U ratio	0.8–1.35
FT_4I	4.5–12
FT_4	1.2–2.5 mcg/dL
TSH	0.5–5 μU/mL or 1–10 μU/mL depending on assay
TT_3	6–220 ng/mL
FT_3I	85–205 ng/dL
FT_3	0.2–0.4 ng/dL
Uric acid	3–8 mg/dL
Urinalysis	
Bilirubin, glucose, ketones	none
pH	4.5–8
Protein	<150 mg/24 hrs
Red blood cells	≤2/high powered field
Specific gravity	1.005–1.030
White blood cells	≤1/high powered field

Appendix D (continued): Key Laboratory Tests and Reference Intervals

Reference Intervals for Some Common Non-antiinfective Medications	
Amitriptyline and nortriptyline	75–225 ng/mL
Nortriptyline (only)	50–150 ng/mL
Carbamazepine	2–10 mcg/mL
Cyclosporine	100–300 mg/mL
Digoxin	0.5–2 ng/mL
Digitoxin	20–35 ng/mL
Disopyramide	2–4.5 mcg/mL
Ethosuximide	40–75 mcg/mL
Felbamate	20–100 mcg/mL
Gabapentin	1–2 mcg/mL
Lamotrigine	2–4 mcg/mL
Imipramine and desipramine	125–225 ng/mL
Desipramine (only)	75–225 ng/mL
Lidocaine	2–5 mcg/mL
Lithium	0.8–1.2 mEq/L
Phenobarbital (adult)	20–40 mcg/mL
Phenytoin (total)	10–20 mcg/mL
Phenytoin (free)	1–2 mcg/mL
Procainamide	4–8 mcg/mL
N-acetylprocainamide (NAPA)	$\leq$30 mcg/mL
Procainamide and NAPA	<46 mcg/mL
Quinidine	2–5 mcg/mL
Salicylates (adults)	2–20 mg/dL
Theophylline (adults)	10–20 mcg/mL
Tocainide	5–12 mcg/mL
Valproic acid	100 mcg/mL (peak)
	40 mcg/mL (trough)
Reference Intervals for Some Common Antiinfectives	
Amikacin	20–25 mcg/mL (peak)
	5–10 mcg/mL (trough)
5-Flucytosine	100 mcg/mL (peak)
	50 mcg/mL (trough)
Gentamicin	4–8 mcg/mL (peak)
	1–2 mcg/mL (trough)
Netilmicin	4–8 mcg/mL (peak)
	1–2 mcg/mL (trough)

Appendix D (continued): Key Laboratory Tests and Reference Intervals

Reference Intervals for Some Common Antiinfectives (continued)	
Streptomycin	5–20 mcg/mL (peak)
	<5 mcg/mL (trough)
Tobramycin	4–8 mcg/mL (peak)
	1–2 mcg/mL (trough)
Vancomycin	20–40 mcg/mL (peak)
	5–10 mcg/mL (trough)

Appendix E: FDA Pregnancy Categories

Category A: No demonstrated risk to fetus.

Category B: Studies have shown no risk to the fetus. Either animal findings have shown risk but human findings have not, or animal findings have shown no risk and no adequate human studies have been performed.

Category C: Risk to the fetus cannot be ruled out. No adequate and well-controlled studies have been conducted.

Category D: May cause fetal harm if administered to a pregnant woman.

Category X: Contraindicated during pregnancy. Fetal risk clearly outweighs any possible benefit to the patient.

Appendix F: Selected Nonprescription (OTC) Agents Frequently Found in Combination Products*

Generic Name and Selected Trade Names	Normal Adult Dosage	Major Adverse Effects/Cautions	Key Counseling Points	Miscellaneous Issues
Acetaminophen	Individualize dosage. For analgesia and antipyresis, 325 to 500 mg Q3H or 325 to 650 mg Q4H or 650 mg to 1 G Q6H as needed. Frequently found in combination with prescription medications for treatment of pain, allergies, and insomnia — SEE Prescribing Information (PI) of prescription product	Considerations: Not recommended to be taken for more than 10 days for pain or 3 days for fever unless directed by the physician; use with caution in patients with liver or kidney disease and in patients consuming 3 or more alcohol-containing beverages per day. Most common AEs although rare include renal toxicity, allergic dermatitis, hepatotoxicity. Pregnancy category: Not specified	Considerations and adverse effects of the nonprescription agent should be taken into account when counseling a patient receiving a combination prescription product	If an overdose of acetaminophen is suspected the patient should seek emergency medical assistance immediately

Generic Name and Selected Trade Names	Normal Adult Dosage	Major Adverse Effects/Cautions	Key Counseling Points	Miscellaneous Issues
Aspirin	Individualize dosage For analgesia and antipyresis: 325 to 500 mg Q3H or 325 to 650 mg Q4H or 650 mg to 1 G Q6H as needed For antiinflammatory effect: Usually, 3.6 to 5.4 G/day in divided doses For MI prophylaxis: Usually, 80 to 325 mg/day	Contraindications: Children and teenagers with chicken pox or flu symptoms unless a physician is consulted about Reye's syndrome; patients with ulcers or stomach/other GI problems that persist or recur with administration of this agent; patients with bleeding disorders Considerations: Not recommended to be taken for more than 10 days for pain or 3 days for fever unless directed by the physician; use with caution in patients with liver or kidney disease; generally not recommended for use during pregnancy, especially during the last 3 months of pregnancy Most common AEs include stomach pain, heartburn, nausea/vomiting, bleeding Pregnancy category: Not specified, but not recommended	SEE acetaminophen	Numerous drug interactions (eg, with anticoagulants, antidiabetic agents, and antiarthritic agents) are possible — SEE Prescribing Information (PI)

Generic Name and Selected Trade Names	Normal Adult Dosage	Major Adverse Effects/Cautions	Key Counseling Points	Miscellaneous Issues
Aspirin (continued)	For reducing the risk of recurrent transient ischemic attacks or strokes in men: Usually, 650 mg BID or 325 mg QID Frequently found in combination with prescription medications for treatment of pain, allergies, and insomnia — SEE Prescribing Information (PI) of prescription product			

Generic Name and Selected Trade Names	Normal Adult Dosage	Major Adverse Effects/Cautions	Key Counseling Points	Miscellaneous Issues
Dextromethorphan	Individualize dosage For cough, 10 to 20 mg Q4H as needed; up to a maximum of 120 mg/day Frequently found in combination with prescription medications for treatment of cough and cold — SEE Prescribing Information (PI) of prescription product	<u>Considerations</u>: Not recommended for persistent or chronic cough such as with smoking, asthma, chronic bronchitis or emphysema, or if cough is accompanied by excess phlegm; do not take with or within 2 weeks of taking an MAO inhibitor (eg, phenelzine sulfate, tranyl-cypromine sulfate, selegiline) <u>Most common AEs</u> include mild dizziness or drowsiness, nausea/vomiting, stomach pain <u>Pregnancy category</u>: Not specified	SEE acetaminophen	Many preparations contain guaifenesin, an expectorant

Generic Name and Selected Trade Names	Normal Adult Dosage	Major Adverse Effects/Cautions	Key Counselling Points	Miscellaneous Issues
Phenylpropanolamine Bitartrate OR Phenylpropanolamine HCl	Individualize dosage For appetite suppression: Administer 25 mg TID; maximum of 75 mg/24 hrs For decongestion: Usually 25 mg Q4H as needed; maximum of 150 mg/24 hrs Frequently found in combination with prescription medications for treatment of cough, cold, and allergy symptoms — SEE Prescribing Information (PI) of prescription product	Considerations: Not recommended for use in patients with severe coronary artery disease or hypertension; use with caution in patients with cardiovascular disorders, diabetes mellitus, narrow-angle glaucoma, hyperthyroidism, prostatic hypertrophy, or psychiatric disorders Most common AEs include dizziness, dryness of nose or mouth, false sense of well-being, headache, insomnia, nausea, nervousness, restlessness Pregnancy category: Not specified	SEE acetaminophen	Numerous drug interactions are possible — SEE Prescribing Information (PI)

Generic Name and Selected Trade Names	Normal Adult Dosage	Major Adverse Effects/Cautions	Key Counseling Points	Miscellaneous Issues
Pseudo-ephedrine	Individualize dosage For decongestion, 60 mg Q 4–6H as needed; maximum of 240 mg/24 hrs Frequently found in combination with prescription medications for treatment of cough, cold, and allergy symptoms — SEE Prescribing Information (PI) of prescription product	Considerations and most common AEs: SEE phenylpropanolamine Pregnancy category: B	SEE acetaminophen	SEE phenylpropanol-amine

*As a rule, a medication should not be administered to a patient with a known hypersensitivity to it or a similar agent.

Appendix G: An English-Spanish Guide for Pharmacists

Table 1: Numbers

English	Spanish
One-half (1/2)	Medio/Media
One (1)	Uno
Two (2)	Dos
Three (3)	Tres
Four (4)	Cuatro
Five (5)	Cinco
Six (6)	Seis
Seven (7)	Siete
Eight (8)	Ocho
Nine (9)	Nueve
Ten (10)	Diez
Eleven (11)	Once
Twelve (12)	Doce
Thirteen (13)	Trece
Fourteen (14)	Catorce
Fifteen (15)	Quince
Sixteen (16)	Dieciséis
Seventeen (17)	Diecisiete
Eighteen (18)	Dieciocho
Nineteen (19)	Diecinueve
Twenty (20)	Veinte
Thirty (30)	Treinta
Forty (40)	Cuarenta
Fifty (50)	Cinquenta
Sixty (60)	Sesenta
Seventy (70)	Setenta
Eighty (80)	Ochenta
Ninety (90)	Noventa
One hundred (100)	Cien

Table 2: Colors

English	Spanish
White	Blanco/Blanca
Black	Negro/Negra
Blue	Azul
Brown	Café
Green	Verde
Orange	Naranja
Purple	Violeta/Púrpura
Red	Rojo/Roja
Yellow	Amarillo/Amarilla
Clear	Transparente

Table 3: Days of the Week and Terms Relating to Calendar

English	Spanish
Monday	Lunes
Tuesday	Martes
Wednesday	Miércoles
Thursday	Jueves
Friday	Viernes
Saturday	Sábado
Sunday	Domingo
Day	Día
Daily	Diariamente
Week	Semana
Weekly	Semanalmente
Month	Mes
Year	Año

Table 4: Dosage Forms

English	Spanish
Tablet	Tableta
Suppository	Supositorio
Liquid	Líquido
Suspension	Suspensión
Injection	Inyección
Subcutaneous	Subcutaneo
Intramuscular	Intramuscular
Capsule	Cápsula
Intravenous	Intravenoso
Inhaler	Inhalador
Intraocular (in the eye)	Intraocular (en el ojo)
Intranasal (in the nose)	Intranasal (en la nariz)
Intravaginal (in the vagina)	Intravaginal (en la vagina)
Sublingual (under the tongue)	Sublingual (bajo la lengua)
Eye drop	Gota para los ojos
Eye ointment	Ungüento para los ojos
Ointment	Ungüento
Cream	Crema
Patch	Parche
Enema	Enema

Table 5: Parts of the Body

English	Spanish
Abdomen	Abdómen
Arm	Brazo
Back	Espalda
Blood	Sangre
Bone	Hueso
Brain	Cerebro
Buttocks	Gluteos
Chest	Pecho
Ear	Oido
Eye	Ojo
Eyelid	Párpado
Face	Cara
Finger	Dedo
Foot	Pie
Hair	Pelo
Hand	Mano
Head	Cabeza
Heart	Corazón
Kidney	Riñón
Knee	Rodilla
Liver	Hígado
Lung	Pulmón
Muscle	Músculo
Mouth	Boca
Nose	Nariz
Rectum	Recto
Skin	Piel
Stomach	Estómago
Throat	Garganta
Tongue	Lengua
Vagina	Vagina

Table 6: Common Expressions

English	Spanish
May I help you?	Necesita ayuda usted?
What is the patient's name?	Cuál es el nombre del paciente?
How old is the patient?	Qué edad tiene el paciente?
Do you understand?	Me entiende usted?
Do you have any questions?	Tiene usted alguna pregunta?
Do you have insurance?	Tiene seguro médico?
Thank you	Gracias
You are welcome	De nada
Good-bye	Hasta luego/adiós
Please come back in ____ minutes	Por favor vuelva en ____ minutos
Please come back in ____ days	Por favor vuelva en ____ dias
Please come back in ____ weeks	Por favor vuelva en ____ semanas
Take one tablet/capsule every ___ hours	Tomar una tableta/capsula cada ___ horas
Take one tablet/capsule ___ times per day	Tomar una tableta/capsula ___ veces al día
Take ___ teaspoonful every ___ hours	Tomar ___ cucharadita cada ___ horas
Take ___ tablespoon every ___ hours	Tomar ___ cucharada cada ___ horas
Insert one suppository every ___ hours	Introduzca un supositorio cada ___ horas
Insert one suppository ___ times per day	Introduzca un supositorio ___ veces al día
Instill ___ drop into each/left/right eye	Aplique ___ gota en cada/izquierdo/derecho ojo
Instill ___ drop into each/left/right ear	Aplique ___ gota en cada/izquierdo/derecho oido
Apply under the eyelid	Aplique adentro del párpado
Apply the patch on the skin	Aplique el parche sobre la piel
Place under the tongue until it dissolves	Ponga debajo de la lengua hasta que se disuelva completamente
Use the inhaler this way	Use el inhalador de esta manera
Take as needed	Tomar cuando sea necesario
Use as directed	Uselo según las instrucciones
Take before meals	Tomar antes de las comidas
Take with meals	Tomar con las comidas
Take after meals	Tomar después de las comidas
Take at bedtime	Tomar antes de acostarse
Do not exceed recommended dosage	No tomar más de la dosis recomendada
Keep in the refrigerator	Mantenga en el refrigerador
Shake well before using	Agite bien antes de usar
Apply on the skin	Aplique en la piel
This prescription may be refilled ___ times	Esta receta se puede volver a llenar ___ veces
Keep this away from children	Guarde este medicamento lejos del alcance de los niños

Appendix H: Metered Dose Inhalers

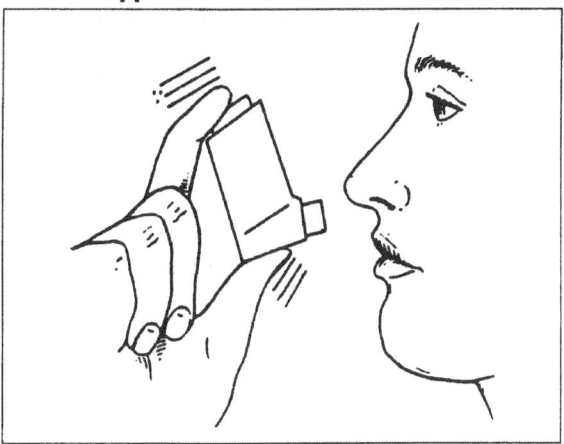

How to Use Your MDI

1. Remove the cap from the mouthpiece; shake the canister or inhaler with canister in place for 5–10 seconds.
2. Breathe out to the end of a normal breath.
3. Position the mouthpiece either:
   a. 2 to 3 finger widths from your mouth; open your mouth widely; or
   b. Close your lips around the mouthpiece.

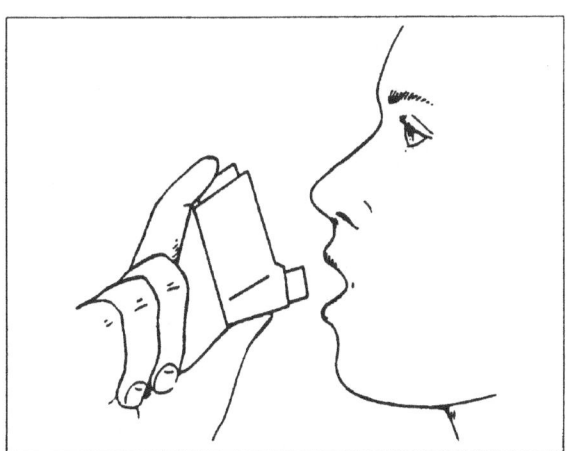

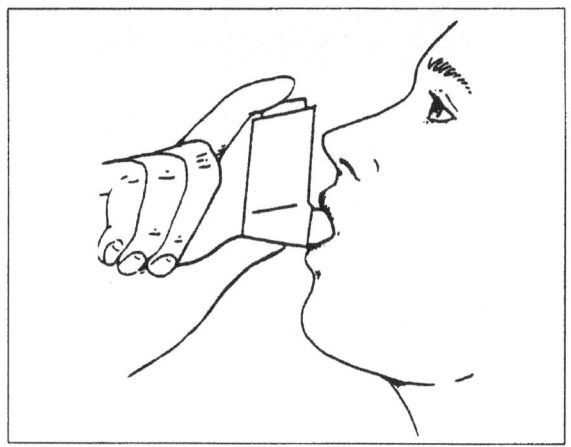

4. Tilt your head back slightly and begin a slow inhalation lasting 3–5 seconds, then depress the container once. Continue breathing slowly until the lungs are full.
5. Hold your breath for 10 seconds (or as long as you can) to allow medicine to reach deeply into the lungs.
6. Exhale SLOWLY through pursed lips.
7. If you need a second dose, wait one minute and repeat steps 1–6.
8. Rinse your mouth with water after each dose.

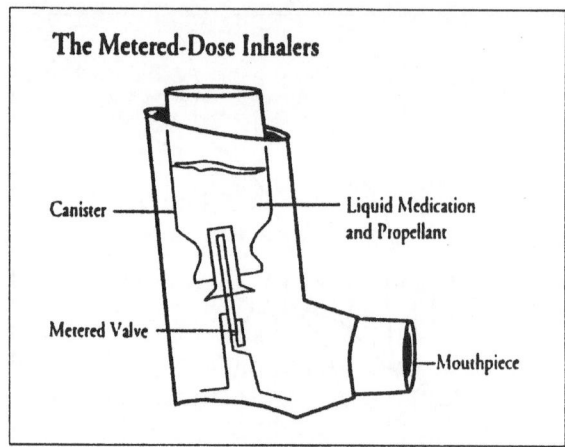

The Metered-Dose Inhalers

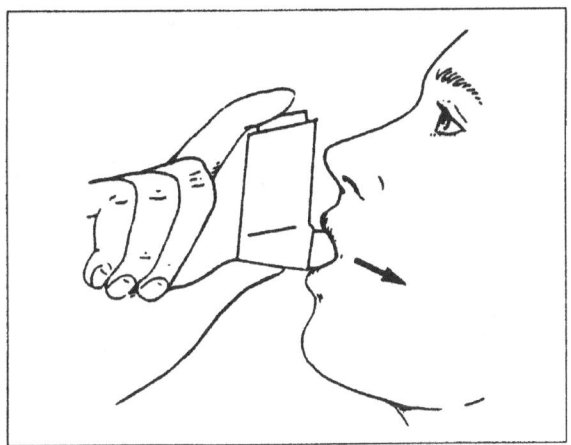

Storage and Maintenance: Store the canister at room temperature. It will not work well if stored in a cool place. The inhaler will work well again when the temperature rises.

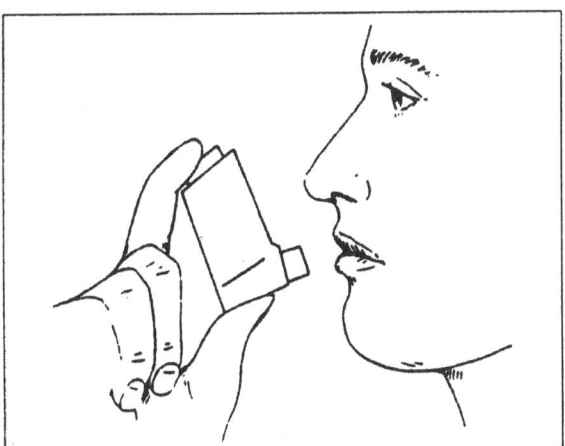

Originally published in American Pharmaceutical Association Special Report, "Asthma: The Pharmacist's Role in Optimizing Drug Delivery and Patient Compliance." Washington, DC: APhA, 1997. Reprinted with permission.

Appendix I: Spacers/Holding Chambers

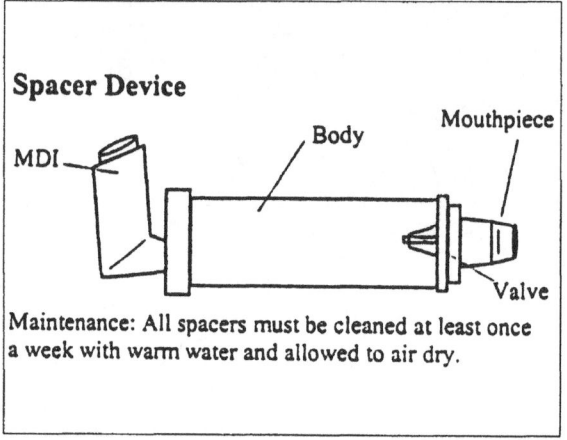

Maintenance: All spacers must be cleaned at least once a week with warm water and allowed to air dry.

How to Use Your Spacer

1. Remove the cap from the mouthpiece, shake the canister or inhaler with canister in place, and insert the inhaler into the device.
2. Place the mouthpiece in your mouth.
3. Press the canister once to release a dose of the drug.
4. Take a deep, slow breath. Hold the breath for about 10 seconds. Then breathe out SLOWLY through pursed lips.
5. Some spacer devices allow you to breathe again without re-pressing the canister, some do not. Please consult your health care provider for advice.

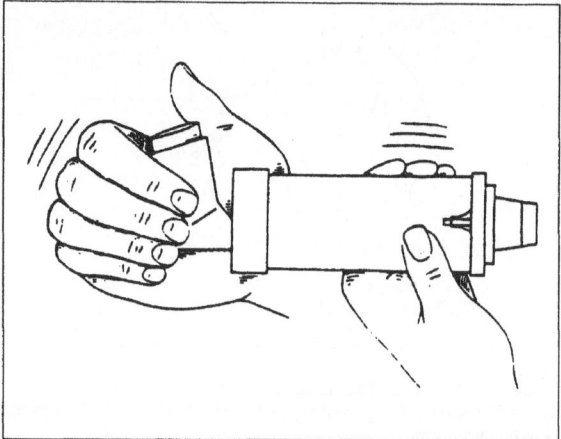

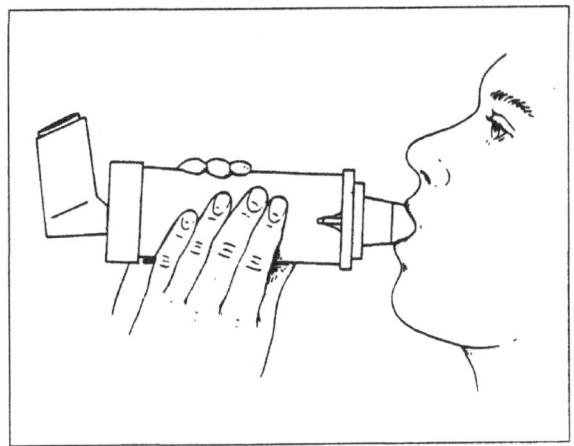

6. Remove the device from your mouth.
7. If you need a second dose. wait one minute and repeat steps 1–6.

Maintenance: All spacers must be cleaned at least once a week with warm water and allowed to dry.

Originally published in American Pharmaceutical Association Special Report, "Asthma: The Pharmacist's Role in Optimizing Drug Delivery and with Patient Compliance." Washington, DC: APhA, 1997. Reprinted with permission.

Appendix J: Nose Drops

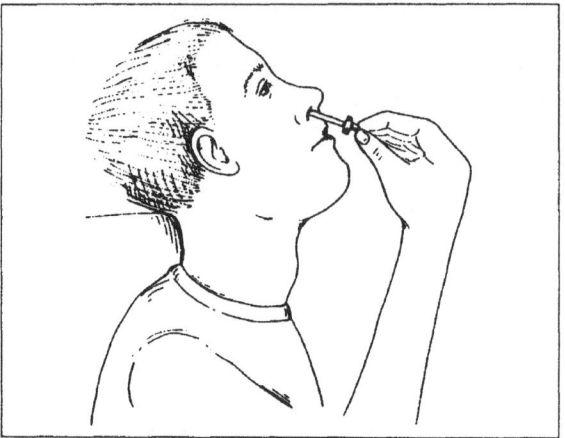

How to Use Nose Drops

Note: Giving nose drops to yourself can be difficult. If possible, have someone else administer the drops.

1. Have the patient blow his or her nose gently to clear the nostrils. Use a bulb syringe to gently clear the nostrils of an infant.
2. Clean the outer portion of the nose with a damp tissue.
3. Wash your hands with soap and warm water and dry them.
4. Lie down (or have the patient lie on his or her back) on a bed with the head tilted back and the neck supported (allow the head to hang over the edge of the bed or place a small pillow under the neck and shoulders). Cradle an infant in your arms with the head tilted back.
5. Shake the nose drops container.
6. Insert the dropper tip into the nostril about 1/3 inch, and place the prescribed dose or number of drops in the nostril. Try not to touch the nose with the dropper tip.
7. Stay (or have the patient stay) in the same position for at least five minutes.
8. Unless otherwise directed, repeat these steps for the other nostril.

9. Rinse the dropper tip with hot water and replace the cap on the container.
10. Wash your hands.

Originally published in American Pharmaceutical Association Special Report, "Achieving Optimal Outcomes from Nonprescription Drug Therapy for Allergic Rhinitis." Washington, DC: APhA, 1997. Reprinted with permission.

Appendix K: Nasal Sprays, Pumps, and Inhalers

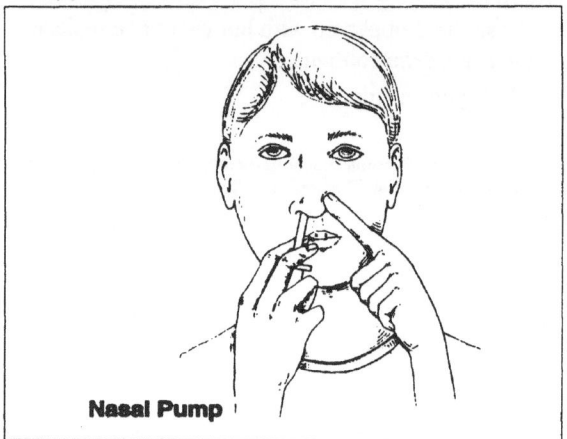
Nasal Pump

How to Use Nasal Sprays, Pumps, or Inhalers

1. Blow your nose gently to clear your nostrils.
2. Clean the outer portion of your nose with a damp tissue.
3. Wash your hands with soap and warm water and dry them.
4. Shake the medication container. If you think a nasal inhaler might be empty, test it by removing the metal canister and placing it in a container of water. If the canister floats, it is empty. Call your pharmacist to get a refill. Reassemble the inhaler if the canister sinks; it is not empty.

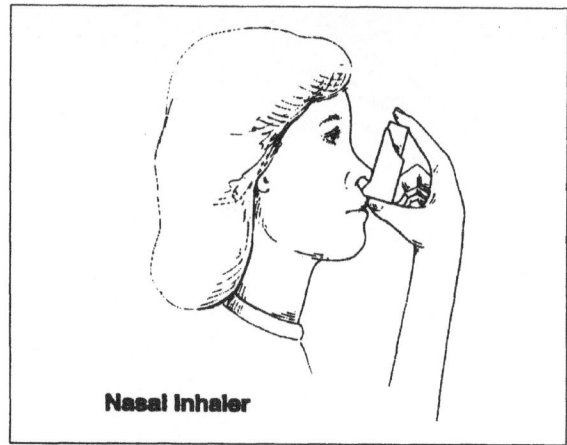
Nasal Inhaler

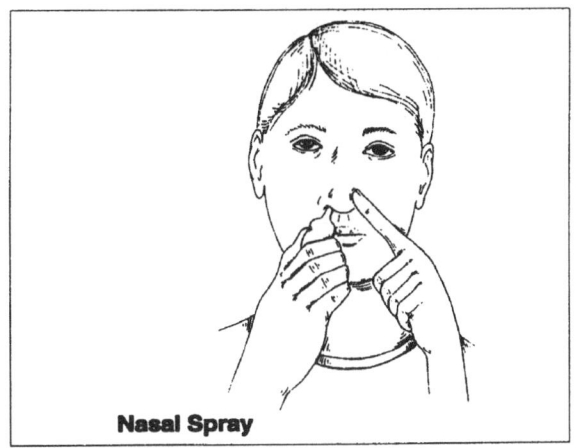
Nasal Spray

5. Keep your head upright. Press a finger against the side of your nose to close one nostril. With your mouth closed, insert the tip of the pump, spray, or inhaler into the open nostril. Sniff in through the nostril while quickly and firmly squeezing the spray container or activating the pump or inhaler.
6. Hold your breath for a few seconds and then breathe out through your mouth.
7. Repeat this procedure for the other nostril only if directed to do so.
8. Rinse the spray, pump, or inhaler tip with hot water and replace the cap on the container.
9. Wash your hands.

Originally published in American Pharmaceutical Association Special Report, "Achieving Optimal Outcomes from Nonprescription Drug Therapy for Allergic Rhinitis." Washington, DC: APhA, 1997. Reprinted with permission.

Appendix L: Eye Drops

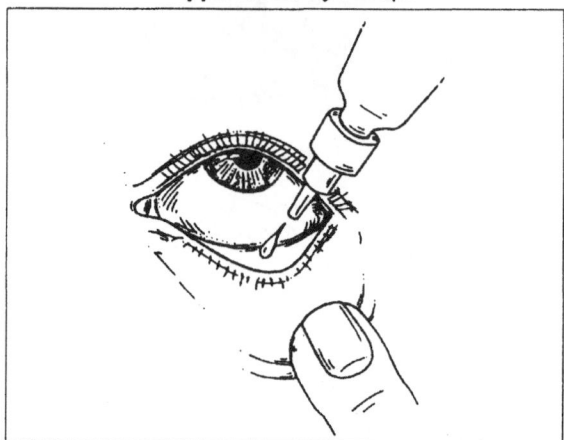

How to Use Eye Drops

1. Wash your hands with soap and warm water and dry them.
2. Shake the eye drops container.
3. Remove the cap. Do not touch the dropper tip. Eye drops must be kept clean.
4. Tilt the head back slightly.
5. Pull the lower eyelid down and away from the eyeball to form a pocket, as shown in the picture.
6. Hold the dropper tip directly over the eye, but do not allow it to touch the eye or eyelid. If self-administering the drops, you may want to brace your hand against your face to keep it steady.
7. Look up, or tell the patient to look up. Place one drop in the pocket and continue to hold the eyelid for a moment while the medication runs in. If you are self-administering the drops, look directly at the dropper tip when positioning it in front of your eye. To keep from blinking, look away from the dropper tip just before you release a drop.
8. Release the eyelid, close the eye for one or two minutes, and, unless you or the patient recently had eye surgery, press a finger against the inner corner of the eye. Do not squeeze the eye shut or rub it. The drops may sting or burn, but this feeling should go away quickly.

9. Wait at least five minutes before applying any more drops or another eye medication.
10. Replace the cap on the container.
11. Wash your hands.

Originally published in American Pharmaceutical Association Special Report, "Medication Administration Problem Solving in Ambulatory Care." Washington, DC: APhA, 1994. Reprinted with permission.

Appendix M: Eye Ointments and Gels

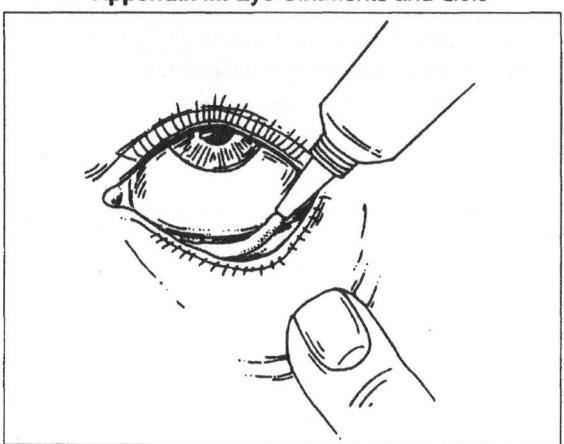

How to Use Eye Ointments and Gels

1. Wash your hands with soap and warm water and dry them.
2. Remove the cap from the medication tube. Do not touch the tip of the tube. Eye ointments and gels must be kept clean.
3. Tilt the head back slightly.
4. Pull the lower eyelid down and away from the eyeball to form a pocket, as shown in the picture. If self-administering eye ointment, you may wish to sit or stand in front of a mirror and brace your hand against your face to keep it steady.
5. Squeeze the tube and apply the prescribed amount of ointment or gel (usually a 1/4- to 1/2-inch ribbon) to the inner surface of the lower eyelid. Do not touch the tip of the medication tube to the eye or eyelid. When self administering eye ointment, look directly at the tip of the tube when positioning it in front of your eye. To keep from blinking, look up (away from the tube) just before you apply the ointment.
6. Release the eyelid, gently close the eye, and keep it closed for one or two minutes. While the eyelid is closed, rotate the eye to distribute the medication. Do not rub the eye.
7. Replace the cap on the medication tube.

8. Wipe off any excess ointment or gel with a clean tissue.
9. Wash your hands.
10. Eye ointments and gels can temporarily blur the vision. Avoid activities requiring good vision until your vision clears.

Originally published in American Pharmaceutical Association Special Report, "Medication Administration Problem Solving in Ambulatory Care." Washington, DC: APhA, 1994. Reprinted with permission.

Appendix N: Ear Drops

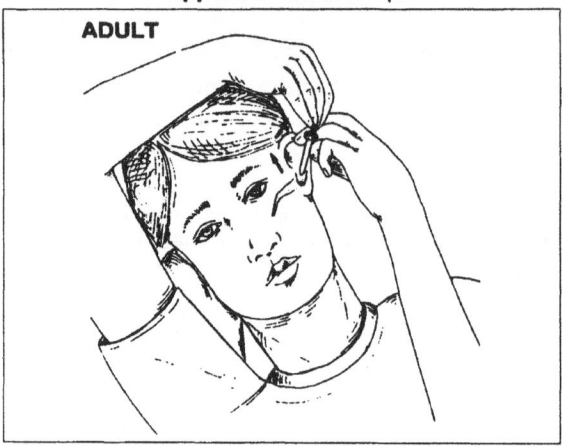

How to Use Ear Drops

Note: Self-administering ear drops can be difficult. If possible, have someone else administer the drops.

1. Wash your hands with soap and warm water and dry them thoroughly.
2. Carefully wash and dry the outside of the ear, taking care not to get any water in the ear canal.
3. Warm the ear drops to body temperature by holding the container in the palms of your hands for a few minutes. Do *not* warm the container in hot water. Hot ear drops can cause pain, nausea, and dizziness.

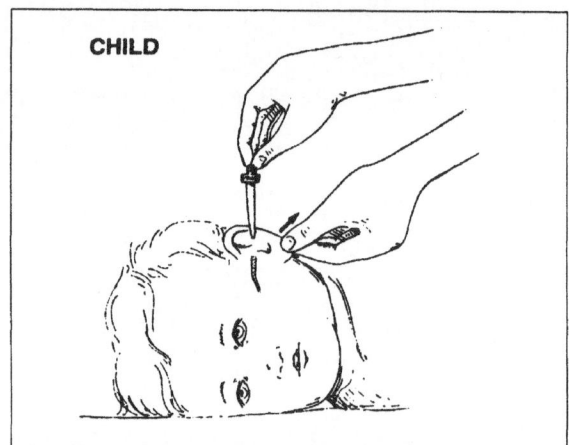

4. Shake the container.
5. Tilt your head (or have the patient tilt his or her head) to the side or lie down with the affected ear up. Use gentle restraint, if necessary, for an infant or a young child.
6. Open the container carefully. Position the dropper tip near, but not inside, the ear canal opening. Do not allow the dropper to touch the ear, because it could become contaminated or injure the ear. Ear drops must be kept clean.
7. Pull your ear (or the patient's ear) backward and upward to open the ear canal, as shown in the picture above. If the patient is a child younger than three years old, pull the ear backward and downward, as shown in the picture below.
8. Place the proper dose or number of drops into the ear canal. Replace the cap on the container.
9. Gently press the small, flat skin flap over the ear canal opening to force out air bubbles and push the drops down the ear canal.
10. Stay (or keep patient) in the same position for at least five minutes. If the patient is a child who cannot stay still, the doctor may tell you to place a clean piece of cotton gently into the child's ear, to prevent the medication from draining out.
11. Repeat the procedure for the other ear, if directed to do so.
12. Gently wipe any excess medication off the outside of the ear, using caution to avoid getting moisture in the ear canal. Wash your hands.

Originally published in American Pharmaceutical Association Special Report, "Medication Administration Problem Solving in Ambulatory Care." Washington, DC: APhA, 1994. Reprinted with permission.

Appendix O: Guidelines for Administering Subcutaneous Injections

1. Wash your hands
2. If the product was in the refrigerator, allow it to warm to room temperature by itself or roll it between the palms of your hands to aid the warming process
3. If the product is a suspension (it will be cloudy), gently mix the vial ("bottle") by rolling it between the palms of your hands; do not shake the medication
4. If it is a new vial remove the cap, do not remove the rubber stopper
5. Visually inspect the product to ensure that the color is uniform and no unwanted particles are in the solution/suspension
6. Take a needle/syringe out of any outer packaging
7. Wipe the rubber stopper of the vial with a new alcohol swab
8. Draw air into the syringe equal to the dose you will be administering
9. Push the needle through rubber stopper and inject air into vial by pushing down the plunger
10. Turn the vial and syringe upside down, draw up the indicated volume
11. Look at the syringe to make sure there are no air bubbles present in the syringe and check to make sure you have the correct volume/dose
12. Remove the needle from the vial, if you need to lay the syringe down place the cover on the needle
13. Cleanse the skin at the desired injection site with alcohol
14. Pinch a large area of skin and insert the needle into the skin at a 90° angle
15. Push the plunger in as far as it will go
16. Pull the needle out and apply gentle pressure over the injection site for a few seconds, do not rub the area
17. The next injection should be given in a different site

Appendix P: Nomograms to Determine Body Surface Area of Adults, Children, and Infants

Directions: To determine or calculate body surface area using the following nomograms, lay a straightedge on the corresponding height and weight (mass) points and read the intersecting point on the surface area scale.

Nomogram for Adults

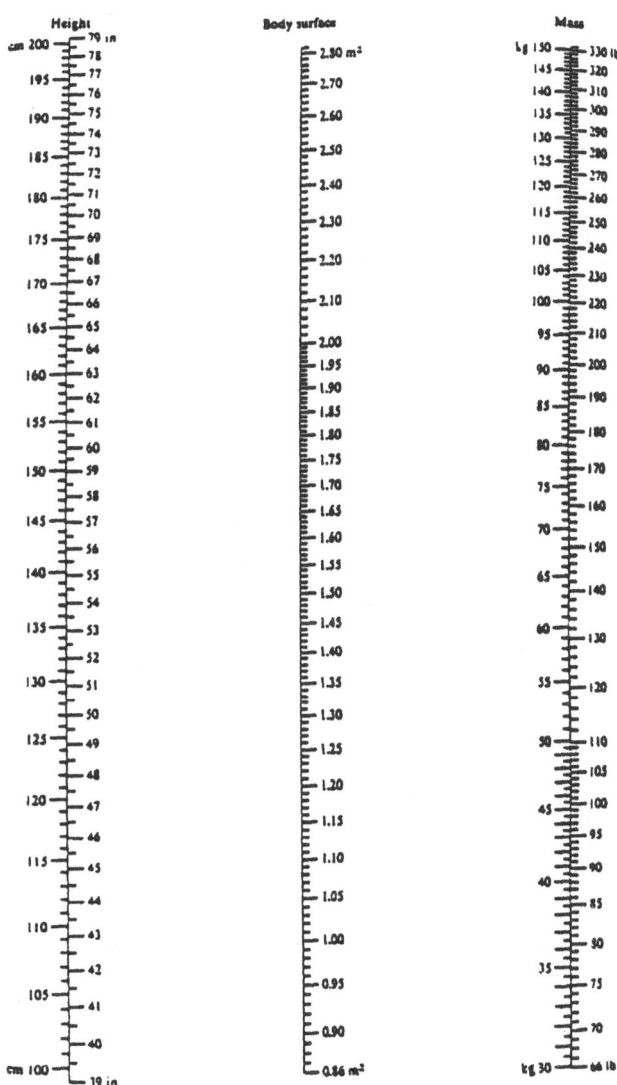

Reprinted from *Pharmaceutical and Clinical Calculations* by Mansoor A. Khan and Indra K. Reddy, Technomic Publishing Co., Inc., 1996, p. 256.

Nomogram for Children

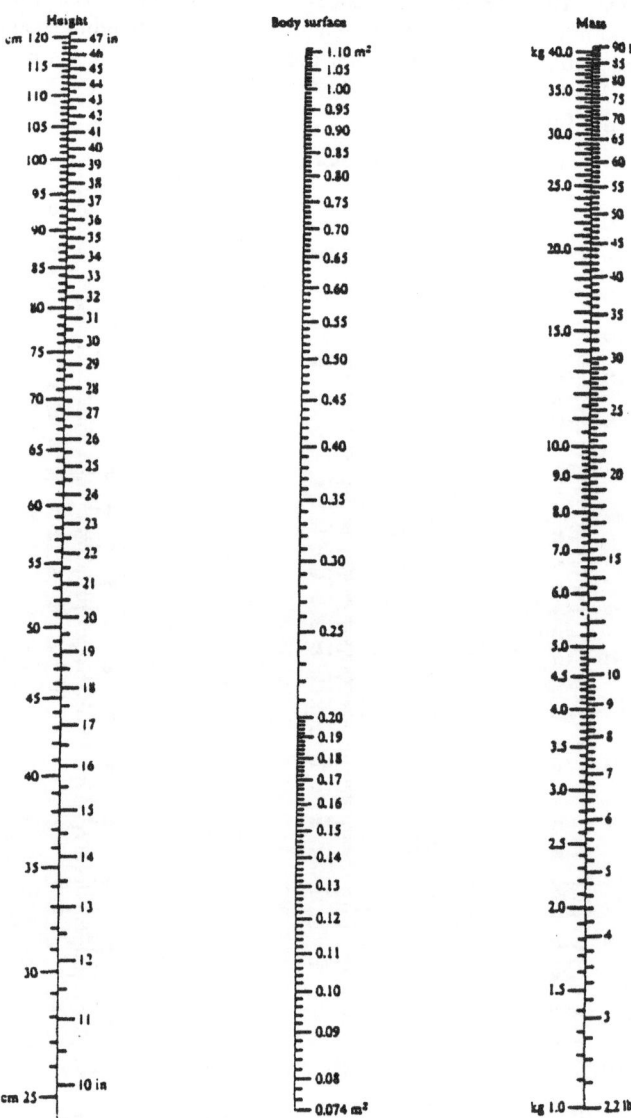

Reprinted from *Pharmaceutical and Clinical Calculations* by Mansoor A. Khan and Indra K. Reddy, Technomic Publishing Co., Inc., 1996, p. 255.

Nomogram for Infants

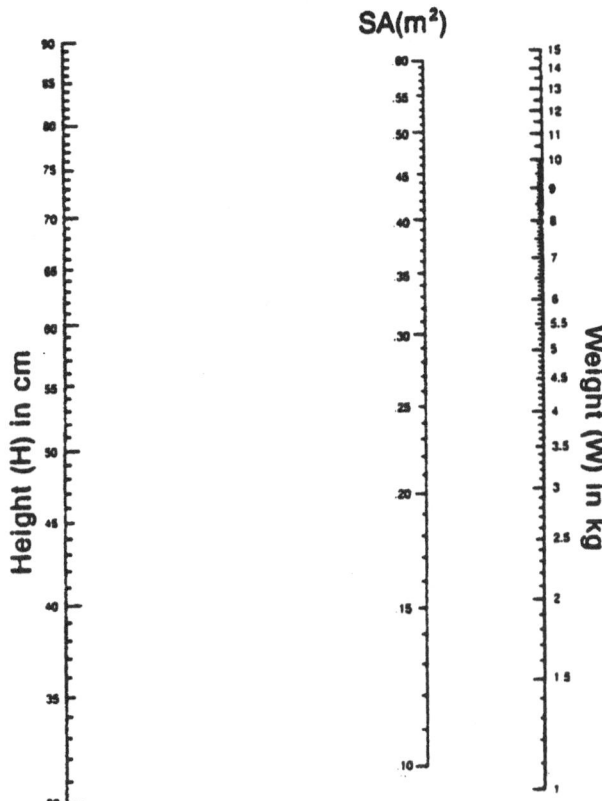

Reprinted from *Procter & Gamble Pharmacist's Handbook* by Dennis B. Worthen, Technomic Publishing Co., Inc., 1998, p. 317.

Appendix Q: Conversions Among Systems Used in Pharmaceutical Calculations

Metric Weight Equivalents

1 kilogram (kg) = 1000 grams
1 gram (g) = 1000 milligrams
1 milligram (mg) = 0.001 gram
1 microgram (mcg, µg) = 0.001 milligram
1 nanogram (ng) = 0.001 microgram
1 picogram (pg) = 0.001 nanogram
1 femtogram (fg) = 0.001 picogram

Metric Volume Equivalents

1 liter (L) = 1000 milliliters
1 deciliter (dL) = 100 milliliters
1 milliliter (mL) = 0.001 liter
1 microliter (µL) = 0.001 milliliter
1 nanoliter (nL) = 0.001 microliter
1 picoliter (pL) = 0.001 nanoliter
1 femtoliter (fL) = 0.001 picoliter

Apothecary Weight Equivalents

1 scruple (℈) = 20 grains (gr)
60 grains (gr) = 1 dram (ʒ)
8 drams (ʒ) = 1 ounce (℥)
1 ounce (℥) = 480 grains
12 ounces (℥) = 1 pound (lb)

Apothecary Volume Equivalents

60 minims (m) = 1 fluidram (flʒ)
8 fluidrams (flʒ) = 1 fluid ounce (fl℥)
1 fluid ounce (fl℥) = 480 minims
16 fluid ounces (fl℥) = 1 pint (pt)

Avoirdupois Equivalents

1 ounce (oz) = 437.5 grains
16 ounces (oz) = 1 pound (lb)

Weight/Volume Equivalents

1 mg/dL = 10 µg/mL
1 mg/dL = 1 mg%
1 ppm = 1 mg/L

Reprinted from *Procter & Gamble Pharmacist's Handbook* by Dennis B. Worthen, Technomic Publishing Co., Inc., 1998, pp. 311, 312.

Appendix Q (continued): Conversions Among Systems Used in Pharmaceutical Calculations

Conversion Equivalents	
1 gram (g)	= 15.43 grains
1 grain (gr)	= 64.8 milligrams
1 ounce (℥)	= 31.1 grams
1 ounce (oz)	= 28.35 grams
1 pound (lb)	= 453.6 grams
1 kilogram (kg)	= 2.2 pounds
1 milliliter (mL)	= 16.23 minims
1 minim (m)	= 0.06 milliliter
1 fluid ounce (fl oz)	= 29.57 mL
1 pint (pt)	= 473.2 mL
0.1 mg	= 1/600 gr
0.12 mg	= 1/500 gr
0.15 mg	= 1/400 gr
0.2 mg	= 1/300 gr
0.3 mg	= 1/200 gr
0.4 mg	= 1/150 gr
0.5 mg	= 1/120 gr
0.6 mg	= 1/100 gr
0.8 mg	= 1/80 gr
1.0 mg	= 1/65 gr

Appendix R: Calculating Milliequivalents

Milliequivalents

A milliequivalent is the gram weight of a substance that will combine with or replace one milligram (one millimole) of hydrogen. A milliequivalent is 1/1000 of an equivalent weight.

Milliequivalent per Liter (mEq/L)

$$mEq/L = \frac{\text{Weight of salt} \times \text{Valence of ion} \times 1000}{\text{Molecular weight of salt}}$$

$$\text{Weight of salt (g)} = \frac{mEq/L \times \text{Molecular Weight of salt}}{\text{Valence of ion} \times 1000}$$

Valences and Atomic Weights of Selected Ions.

Substance	Electrolyte	Valence	Molecular Weight
Calcium	Ca^{2+}	2	40
Chloride	Cl^-	1	35.5
Magnesium	Mg^{2+}	2	24
Phosphate	HPO_4^{2-} (80%)	1.8	96
(ph = 7.4)	$H_2PO_4^-$ (20%)	1.8	96
Potassium	K^+	1	39
Sodium	Na^+	1	23
Sulfate	SO_4^{2-}	2	96

Approximate Milliequivalents and Weights of Selected Ions.

Salt	mEq/g Salt	Mg Salt/mEq
Calcium Carbonate [$CaCO_3$]	20	50
Calcium Chloride [$CaCl_2$-$2H_2O$]	14	73
Calcium Gluconate (Ca gluconate$_2$-$1H_2O$)	4	224
Calcium Lactate [Ca lactate-$5H_2O$]	6	154
Magnesium sulfate ($MgSO_4$)	16	60
Magnesium sulfate ($MgSO_4$-$7H_2O$)	8	123
Potassium acetate (K acetate)	10	98
Potassium chloride (KCl)	13	75
Potassium citrate K_3 citrate-$1H_2O$)	9	108
Potassium iodide (KI)	6	166
Sodium bicarbonate ($NaHCO_3$)	12	84
Sodium chloride (NaCl)	17	58
Sodium citrate (Na_3 citrate-$2H_2O$)	10	98
Sodium iodide (NaI)	7	150
Sodium lactate (Na lactate)	9	112

Reprinted from *Procter & Gamble Pharmacist's Handbook* by Dennis B. Worthen, Technomic Publishing Co., Inc., 1998, pp. 313, 314.

Appendix S: Temperature Conversions

The Fahrenheit (F) scale establishes the freezing point of pure water at 32°F and the boiling point of pure water at 212°F. The Celsius (C) scale establishes the freezing point of pure water at 0°C and the boiling point at 100°C. The difference between boiling and freezing points in the Fahrenheit scale is 180 and in the Celsius scale it is 100. Thus, each degree Celsius equals 180/100 or 1.8 degrees Fahrenheit. A comparison of the Fahrenheit and Celsius scale is shown in the accompanying figure.

To convert the temperature from degrees Fahrenheit to degrees Celsius, any of the following three formulas may be used:

$$°C = \frac{°F - 32}{1.8}$$

$$°C = (°F - 32) \times 5/9$$

$$(9)°C = (5)°F - 160$$

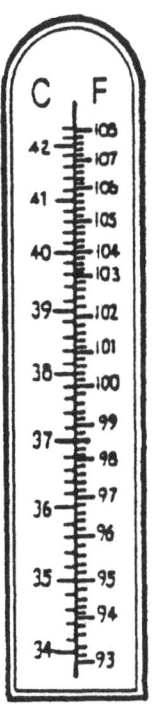

Comparison of Celsius and Fahrenheit temperatures.

Reprinted from *Pharmaceutical and Clinical Calculations* by Mansoor A. Khan and Indra K. Reddy, Technomic Publishing Co., Inc., 1996, p. 349.

Index

Acarbose, 605
Accolate (*see also* zafirlukast), 177–178
Accupril (*see also* quinapril HCl), 49–50
Acebutolol, 88, 89
Acebutolol HCl, 55–56
Aceon (*see also* perindopril erbumine), 48
Acetaminophen, 727
Acetazolamide, 693–694
Acetyl sulfisoxazole, 245–246
N-Acetylprocainamide, 724
Achromycin V (*see also* tetracycline HCl), 217
Aclometasone dipropionate, 683
Aclovate (*see also* aclometasone dipropionate), 683
Adalat (*see also* nifedipine), 11–12
Adalat CC (*see also* nifedipine), 11–12
Adriamycin PFS (*see also* doxorubicin HCl), 335–336
Adriamycin RDF (*see also* doxorubicin HCl), 335–336
Aerobid (*see also* flunisolide), 172
Aerolate (*see also* theophylline), 191–192
Airet (*see also* albuterol sulfate), 180–181
Akineton (*see also* biperiden HCl), 497
Albuterol, 180–181
Albuterol sulfate, 180–181
Aldactone (*see also* spironolactone), 131–132

Aldomet (*see also* methyldopa), 23–24
Alendronate sodium, 597–598
Alkeran (*see also* melphalan), 346–347
Allegra (*see also* fexofenadine HCl), 204
Allopurinol, 371–372
Alora (*see also* estradiol transdermal system), 559–560
Alphatrex (*see also* betamethasone dipropionate), 681
Alprazolam, 417–418, 454
Altace (*see also* ramipril), 51–52
Altretamine, 321–322
Alupent (*see also* metaproterenol sulfate), 186–187
Amantadine HCl, 493–494
Amaryl (*see also* glimepiride), 608
Ambien (*see also* zolpidem tartrate), 489–490
Amcinonide, 679
Amerge (*see also* naritriptan HCl), 536–537
Amikacin, 724
Amikacin sulfate, 256–257
Amikin (*see also* amikacin sulfate), 256–257
Amiloride, 129–130
Amiloride HCl, 88
Amiodarone HCl, 89–90
Amitriptyline and nortriptyline, 724
Amitriptyline HCl, 428–429
Amlodipine besylate, 3, 88
Amoxicillin, 225–226
Amoxicillin/clavulanate potassium, 227

Amoxil (*see also* amoxicillin), 225–226
Ampicillin, 228
Anafranil (*see also* clomipramine HCl), 432
Anaprox (*see also* naproxen sodium), 410–411
Anaprox DS (*see also* naproxen sodium), 410–411
Anastrozole, 323
Ancobon (*see also* flucytosine), 279–280
Androderm (*see also* testosterone, topical system), 553
Android (*see also* methyltestosterone), 548–549
Antivert (*see also* meclizine HCl), 642
A.P.L. (*see also* gonadotropin, human chorionic), 590
Apresoline (*see also* hydralazine HCl), 35
Aquatensen (*see also* methyclothiazide), 118
Aralen (*see also* chloroquine phosphate), 301–302
Ardeparin sodium, 151–152
Aricept (*see also* donepezil HCl), 687
Arimidex (*see also* anastrozole), 323
Aristocort (*see also* triamcinolone; triamcinolone acetonide), 575, 680, 682
Artane (*see also* trihexyphenidyl HCl), 507
Aspirin, 728–729
Astemizole, 195–196
Atacand (*see also* candesartan cilexetil), 25
Atamet (*see also* carbidopa and levodopa), 499–500
Atapryl (*see also* selegiline HCl), 505
Atarax (*see also* hydroxyzine HCl), 204, 425, 642
Atenolol, 57–58, 88, 90
Ativan (*see also* lorazepam), 426, 482

Atorvastatin calcium, 137–138
Atovaquone, 310
Atropine sulfate and difenoxin HCl, 629–630
Atropine sulfate and diphenoxylate HCl, 631–632
Atrovent (*see also* ipratropium bromide), 183
Augmentin (*see also* amoxicillin/clavulanate potassium), 227
Auranofin, 359–360
Aurothioglucose, 361–362
Avapro (*see also* irbesartan), 26
Axanil (*see also* hydroxyzine HCl), 425
Axid (*see also* nizatidine), 669
Azatadine maleate, 197
Azathioprine, 363–364
Azithromycin dihydrate, 218
Azmacort (*see also* triamcinolone acetonide), 176
Azulfidine En-Tabs (*see also* sulfasalazine), 248

Bacampicillin HCl, 228
Bactrim (*see also* trimethoprim and sulfamethoxazole), 249–250
Bactrim DS (*see also* trimethoprim and sulfamethoxazole), 249–250
Baycol (*see also* cerivastatin sodium), 139
Beclomethasone dipropionate, 165
Beclovent (*see also* beclomethasone dipropionate), 165–166
Beepen-VK (*see also* penicillin V potassium), 229
Belladonna alkloids, 652–653
Benadryl (*see also* diphenhydramine; diphenhydramine HCl), 203, 639
Benadryl Allergy (*see also* diphenhydramine), 203
Benadryl Kapseals (*see also* diphenhydramine), 203
Benazepril, 38–39

Benazepril HCl, 88
Bendroflumethiazide, 88, 111–112
Benemid (*see also* probenecid), 375–376
Bentyl (*see also* dicyclomine HCl), 655–656
Benzthiazide, 88, 113
Benztropine mesylate, 495–496
Bepridil HCl, 4
Betamethasone, 569–570
Betamethasone acetate, 569–570
Betamethasone benzoate, 681
Betamethasone dipropionate, 681
Betamethasone dipropionate, augmented, 677–678, 679
Betamethasone sodium phosphate, 569–570
Betamethasone valerate, 679, 681
Betapace (*see also* sotalol HCl), 74–75
Betapen-VK (*see also* penicillin V potassium), 229
Betatrex (*see also* betamethasone valerate), 679, 681
Beta-Val (*see also* betamethasone valerate), 679, 681
Betaxolol, 88
Betaxolol HCl, 59, 695
Betoptic (*see also* betaxolol HCl), 695
Betoptic S (*see also* betaxolol HCl), 695
Biaxin (*see also* clarithromycin), 219–220
BiCNU (*see also* carmustine), 328
Biperiden HCl, 497
Biphasic contraceptive products, 554
Bisoprolol, 88
Bisoprolol fumarate, 60
Bitolterol mesylate, 182
Blocadren (*see also* timolol maleate), 76–77, 543
Brethine (*see also* terbutaline sulfate), 190
Brevicon (*see also* monophasic contraceptive products), 562

Bricanyl (*see also* terbutaline sulfate), 190
Bromfenac sodium, 394–395
Bromocriptine mesylate, 498, 585–586
Bromphen (*see also* brompheniramine maleate), 198
Brompheniramine maleate, 198
Bronkometer (*see also* isoetharine), 184
Bronkosol (*see also* isoetharine), 184
Budesonide, 167–168
Bumetanide, 88, 122–123
Bumex (*see also* bumetanide), 122–123
Buprenex (*see also* buprenorphine), 379–380
Buprenorphine, 379–380
Bupropion HCl, 430–431
Buspar (*see also* buspirone HCl), 419–420
Buspirone HCl, 419–420
Busulfan, 324–325
Butorphanol tartrate, 381

Cafergot (*see also* ergotamine tartrate and caffeine), 534
Caffeine, ergotamine tartrate with, 534
Calan (*see also* verapamil HCl), 14–15
Calan SR (*see also* verapamil HCl), 14–15
Calcimar (*see also* calcitonin salmon), 599–600
Calcitonin salmon, 599–600
Candesartan cilexetil, 25, 88
Capoten (*see also* captopril), 40–41
Captopril, 40–41, 88
Carafate (*see also* sucralfate), 674
Carbachol, 696
Carbamazepine, 511–512, 724
Carbenicillin indanyl sodium, 228
Carbidopa and levodopa, 499–500
Carboplatin, 326–327

Cardene (*see also* nicardipine HCl), 9–10
Cardene SR (*see also* nicardipine HCl), 9–10
Cardioquin (*see also* quinidine polygalacturonate), 103
Cardizem (*see also* diltiazem HCl), 5–6
Cardizem CD (*see also* diltiazem HCl), 5–6
Cardizem SR (*see also* diltiazem HCl), 5–6
Cardura (*see also* doxazosin), 16
Carmustine, 328
Carteolol, 88
Carteolol HCl, 61
Cartrol (*see also* carteolol HCl), 61
Carvedilol, 62–63, 88
Cataflam (*see also* diclofenac potassium), 397
Catapres (*see also* clonidine), 21–22
Catapres-TTS (*see also* clonidine), 21–22
Ceclor (*see also* cefaclor), 230–231
Ceclor CD (*see also* cefaclor), 230–231
Cedax (*see also* ceftibuten), 234
CeeNU (*see also* lomustine), 345
Cefaclor, 230–231
Cefadroxil monohydrate, 232
Cefixime, 232
Cefpodoxime proxetil, 233
Cefprozil, 233
Ceftibuten, 234
Ceftin (*see also* cefuroxime axetil), 234
Cefuroxime axetil, 234
Cefzil (*see also* cefprozil), 233
Celestone (*see also* betamethasone), 569–570
Cephalexin, 235
Cephalexin HCl, 235
Cerivastatin sodium, 139
Cetirizine HCl, 199
Chlorambucil, 329

Chlordiazepoxide HCl, 421
Chlordiazepoxide HCl and clidinium bromide, 654
Chloroquine phosphate, 301–302
Chlorothiazide, 88, 114
Chlorpheniramine maleate, 199
Chlorpromazine, 460–462, 639
Chlorpropamide, 606–607
Chlorspan-12 (*see also* chlorpheniramine maleate), 199
Chlortab-4 (*see also* chlorpheniramine maleate), 199
Chlorthalidone, 88, 115
Chlor-Trimeton (*see also* chlorpheniramine maleate), 199
Cholestyramine, 140–141
Choline salicylate and magnesium salicylate, 396
Chorionic gonadotropin, human, 590
Ciloxan (*see also* ciprofloxacin HCl ophthalmic solution), 237–238
Cimetidine, 661–662
Cimetidine HCl, 661–662
Cipro (*see also* ciprofloxacin HCl), 237–238
Ciprofloxacin HCl, 237–238
Ciprofloxacin HCl ophthalmic solution, 237–238
Cisapride, 663
Cisplatin, 330–331
Clarithromycin, 219–220
Claritin (*see also* loratadine), 205
Claritin Reditabs (*see also* loratadine), 205
Clemastine fumarate, 200
Cleocin (*see also* clindamycin HCl), 311–312
Cleocin HCl (*see also* clindamycin HCl), 311–312
Cleocin T (*see also* clindamycin HCl), 311–312
C-Lexin (*see also* cephalexin), 235
Clidinium bromide and chlordiazepoxide HCl, 654

Climara (*see also* estradiol transdermal system), 559–560
Clindamycin HCl, 311–312
Clindex (*see also* clidinium bromide and chlordiazepoxide HCl), 654
Clinoril (*see also* sulindac), 413
Clobetasol propionate, 677–678
Clocortolone pivalate, 681
Cloderm (*see also* clocortolone pivalate), 681
Clomid (*see also* clomiphene citrate), 587–588
Clomiphene citrate, 587–588
Clomipramine HCl, 432
Clonazepam, 455–456, 518
Clonidine, 21–22, 88
Clopidogrel bisulfate, 159–160
Clorazepate dipotassium, 422–423
Clozapine, 463–464
Clozaril (*see also* clozapine), 463–464
Codeine phosphate, 382
Codeine sulfate, 382
Cogentin (*see also* benztropine mesylate), 495–496
Cognex (*see also* tacrine HCl), 688–689
Colchicine, 373–374
Colestid (*see also* colestipol), 142
Colestipol, 142
Compazine (*see also* prochlorperazine), 473–474, 647
Conjugated estrogens, 554–555, 601
Conjugated estrogens plus medroxyprogesterone, 556–557, 601
Cordarone (*see also* amiodarone HCl), 89–90
Cordran (*see also* flurandrenolide), 682
Coreg (*see also* carvedilol), 62–63
Corgard (*see also* nadolol), 69
Cormax (*see also* clobetasol propionate), 677–678
Cortef (*see also* hydrocortisone), 572
Cortisone acetate, 571

Cortone (*see also* cortisone acetate), 571
Coumadin (*see also* warfarin sodium), 157–158
Covera-HS (*see also* verapamil HCl), 14–15
Cozaar (*see also* losartan potassium), 27
Crinone 4% gel (*see also* progesterone gel), 593–594
Crinone 8% gel (*see also* progesterone gel), 593–594
Crixivan (*see also* indinavir sulfate), 291–292
Cromolyn sodium, 169–170
Crystodigin (*see also* digitoxin), 107–108
Cuprimine (*see also* penicillamine), 369–370
Cutivate (*see also* fluticasone propionate), 682
Cyclocort (*see also* amcinonide), 679
Cyclophosphamide, 332
Cycloserine, 261–262
Cyclosporine, 365–366, 724
Cyclothiazide, 88
Cyproheptadine, 200
Cytomel (*see also* liothyronine sodium), 567–568
Cytospaz (*see also* hyoscyamine sulfate), 659
Cytotec (*see also* misoprostol), 668
Cytoxan (*see also* cyclophosphamide), 332

Dalmane (*see also* flurazepam HCl), 481
Dalteparin sodium, 153
Danaparoid sodium, 154
Danazol, 576–577
Danocrine (*see also* danazol), 576–577
Dapsone, 313–314
Daranide (*see also* dichlorphenamide), 698

Daraprim (*see also* pyrimethamine), 306–307
Darvon (*see also* propoxyphene HCl), 393
Darvon-N (*see also* propoxyphene napsylate), 392–393
Daypro (*see also* oxaprozin), 412
Dazamide (*see also* acetazolamide), 693–694
DDAVP (*see also* desmopressin), 578–579
Decadron (*see also* dexamethasone), 571
Declomycin (*see also* demeclocycline HCl), 213–214
Delavirdine mesylate, 288
Delta-Cortef (*see also* prednisolone), 574
Deltasone (*see also* prednisone), 574
Demadex (*see also* torsemide), 127–128
Demecarium bromide, 697
Demeclocycline HCl, 213–214
Demerol (*see also* meperidine HCl), 388
Demulen (*see also* monophasic contraceptive products), 562
Depakene (*see also* valproic acid), 528
Depakote (*see also* divalproex sodium), 454, 513–514, 531
Depakote Sprinkle (*see also* divalproex sodium), 513–514
Depen (*see also* penicillamine), 369–370
Deponit (*see also* nitroglycerin, transdermal), 86
Desipramine, 724
Desipramine and imipramine, 724
Desipramine HCl, 433
Desmopressin, 578–579
Desogen (*see also* monophasic contraceptive products), 562
Desonide, 683
DesOwen (*see also* desonide), 683
Desoximetasone, 679, 682

Desyrel (*see also* trazodone HCl), 449–450
Dexacort (*see also* dexamethasone sodium phosphate), 171
Dexamethasone, 571, 683
Dexamethasone phosphate, 571
Dexamethasone sodium phosphate, 171, 683
Dexchlor (*see also* dexchlorpheniramine maleate), 201
Dexchlorpheniramine maleate, 201
Dextromethorphan, 730
D.H.E. 45 (*see also* dihydroergotamine mesylate injection), 535
Diabeta (*see also* glyburide), 611–612
Diabinese (*see also* chlorpropamide), 606–607
Diamine TD (*see also* brompheniramine maleate), 198
Diamox (*see also* acetazolamide), 693–694
Diamox Sequels (*see also* acetazolamide), 693–694
Diazepam, 424–425
Dichlorphenamide, 698
Diclofenac potassium, 397
Diclofenac sodium, 398
Dicyclomine HCl, 655–656
Didanosine, 289–290
Difenoxin HCl and atropine sulfate, 629–630
Diflorasone diacetate, 677–678, 679
Diflucan (*see also* fluconazole), 277–278
Diflunisal, 399
Digitoxin, 107–108, 724
Digoxin, 109–110, 724
Dihydroergotamine mesylate injection, 535
Dilacor XR (*see also* diltiazem HCl), 5–6
Dilantin (*see also* phenytoin; phenytoin sodium), 98, 523–524

Dilantin-125 (*see also* phenytoin), 523–524
Dilantin Infatabs (*see also* phenytoin), 523–524
Dilantin Kapseals (*see also* phenytoin), 523–524
Dilatrate-SR (*see also* isosorbide dinitrate), 78–79
Dilaudid (*see also* hydromorphone HCl), 385–386
Diltiazem, 88, 90
Diltiazem HCl, 5–6
Dimenhydrinate, 202
Dimetabs (*see also* dimenhydrinate), 202
Dimetapp Allergy (*see also* brompheniramine maleate), 198
Dimetapp Extentabs (*see also* brompheniramine maleate), 198
Diovan (*see also* valsartan), 28
Diphenhydramine, 203
Diphenhydramine HCl, 639
Diphenoxylate HCl and atropine sulfate, 631–632
Diphenylan (*see also* phenytoin), 523–524
Diprolene (*see also* betamethasone dipropionate, augmented), 677–678
Diprolene AF (*see also* betamethasone dipropionate, augmented), 679
Diprosone (*see also* betamethasone dipropionate), 681
Disalcid (*see also* salsalate), 413
Disopyramide, 724
Disopyramide phosphate, 91–92
Diucardin (*see also* hydroflumethiazide), 117
Diurese (*see also* trichlormethiazide), 121
Diurigen (*see also* chlorothiazide), 114
Diuril (*see also* chlorothiazide), 114
Divalproex sodium, 454, 513–514, 531
Docetaxel, 333–334

Dolobid (*see also* diflunisal), 399
Dolophine (*see also* methadone HCl), 389
Donepezil HCl, 687
Donnatal (*see also* belladonna alkloids), 652–653
Dopar (*see also* levodopa), 501
Doral (*see also* quazepam), 485
Doryx (*see also* doxycycline hyclate), 215
Dorzolamide HCl, 699
Doxazosin, 16, 88
Doxepin HCl, 433
Doxorubicin HCl, 335–336
Doxycycline calcium, 215
Doxycycline hyclate, 215
Doxycycline monohydrate, 216
Dramamine (*see also* dimenhydrinate), 202
Dramamine Liquid (*see also* dimenhydrinate), 202
Dronabinol, 640
Duract (*see also* bromfenac sodium), 394–395
Duragesic (*see also* fentanyl transdermal system), 383–384
Duricef (*see also* cefadroxil monohydrate), 232
Dynacin (*see also* minocycline HCl), 216
DynaCirc (*see also* isradipine), 8
DynaCirc CR (*see also* isradipine), 8
Dyrenium (*see also* triamterene), 133

EC-Naprosyn (*see also* naproxen), 410–411
Edecrin (*see also* ethacrynic acid), 124
EES (*see also* erythromycin ethylsuccinate), 223
Effexor (*see also* venlafaxine HCl), 452–453
Efudex (*see also* fluorouracil), 338–339

Elavil (*see also* amitriptyline HCl), 428–429
Eldepryl (*see also* selegiline HCl), 505
Elixophyllin (*see also* theophylline), 191–192
Elocon (*see also* mometasone furoate), 682
Eltroxin (*see also* levothyroxine sodium), 565–566
E-Mycin (*see also* erythromycin tablets, delayed-release), 221–222
Enalapril maleate, 42–43, 88
Enduron (*see also* methyclothiazide), 118
Enoxacin, 239
Enoxaparin sodium, 155
Epifrin (*see also* epinephrine), 700
Epinephrine, 700
Epivir (*see also* lamivudine), 293
Ergomar (*see also* ergotamine tartrate), 532–533
Ergostat (*see also* ergotamine tartrate), 532–533
Ergotamine tartrate, 532–533
Ergotamine tartrate and caffeine, 534
ERYC (*see also* erythromycin capsules, delayed-release), 221–222
Ery-Ped (*see also* erythromycin ethylsuccinate), 223
Ery-Tab (*see also* erythromycin tablets, delayed-release), 221–222
Erythrocin (*see also* erythromycin stearate), 224
Erythromycin, 221–222
Erythromycin Base, 221–222
Erythromycin capsules, delayed-release, 221–222
Erythromycin estolate, 223
Erythromycin ethylsuccinate, 223
Erythromycin ophthalmic ointment, 221–222
Erythromycin stearate, 224

Erythromycin tablets, delayed-release, 221–222
Esidrix (*see also* hydrochlorothiazide), 116
Eskalith (*see also* lithium carbonate), 457–458
Eskalith CR (*see also* lithium carbonate), 457–458
Estazolam, 480–481
Esterified estrogens, 558
Estraderm (*see also* estradiol transdermal system), 559–560
Estradiol transdermal system, 559–560
Estratab (*see also* estrogens, esterified), 558
Estrogens, conjugated, 554–555, 601
Estrogens, conjugated, plus medroxyprogesterone, 556–557, 601
Estrogens, esterified, 558
Estropipate, 561, 601
Ethacrynic acid, 88, 124
Ethambutol HCl, 263–264
Ethionamide, 265–266
Ethmozine (*see also* moricizine HCl), 97
Ethosuximide, 515–516, 724
Etodolac, 400
Etoposide, 337
Eulexin (*see also* flutamide), 340
Exna (*see also* benzthiazide), 113
Ezide (*see also* hydrochlorothiazide), 116

Famotidine, 664–665
Felbamate, 724
Feldene (*see also* piroxicam), 412
Felodipine, 7, 88
FemPatch (*see also* estradiol transdermal system), 559–560
Fenoprofen calcium, 401
Fentanyl transdermal system, 383–384
Fexofenadine HCl, 204

Flagyl (*see also* metronidazole), 315–316
Flavored Colestid (*see also* colestipol), 142
Flecainide acetate, 93–94
Flomax (*see also* tamsulosin HCl), 18
Florinef (*see also* fludrocortisone acetate), 580
Florone (*see also* diflorasone diacetate), 677–678, 679
Flovent 44 mcg (*see also* fluticasone propionate), 173
Flovent 110 mcg (*see also* fluticasone propionate), 173
Flovent 220 mcg (*see also* fluticasone propionate), 173
Floxin (*see also* ofloxacin), 243
Fluconazole, 277–278
Flucytosine, 279–280
5-Flucytosine, 724
Fludrocortisone acetate, 580
Flunisolide, 172
Fluocinolone acetonide, 680, 682
Fluocinonide, 680
Fluonex (*see also* fluocinonide), 680
Fluoroplex (*see also* fluorouracil), 338–339
Fluorouracil, 338–339
Fluoxetine HCl, 434–435
Fluoxymesterone, 547
Flurandrenolide, 682
Flurazepam HCl, 481
Flutamide, 340
Flutex (*see also* triamcinolone acetonide), 680, 682
Fluticasone propionate, 173, 682
Fluvastatin sodium, 142
Fluvoxamine maleate, 436
Follicle-stimulating hormone, 591–592
Fosamax (*see also* alendronate sodium), 597–598
Fosfomycin tromethamine, 251
Fosinopril, 44

Fosinopril sodium, 88
Fragmin (*see also* dalteparin sodium), 153
Fulvicin P/G (*see also* griseofulvin), 281–282
Furadantin (*see also* nitrofurantoin), 254–255
Furazolidone, 633
Furosemide, 88, 125–126
Furoxone (*see also* furazolidone), 633

Gabapentin, 517–518, 724
Gantanol (*see also* sulfamethoxazole), 247
Gantrisin (*see also* acetyl sulfisoxazole), 245–246
Garamycin (*see also* gentamicin sulfate), 258–259
Gemfibrozil, 143–144
Genahist (*see also* diphenhydramine), 203
Genora (*see also* monophasic contraceptive products), 562
Gentamicin, 724
Gentamicin sulfate, 258–259
Geocillin (*see also* carbenicillin indanyl sodium), 228
Glaucon (*see also* epinephrine), 700
Glimepiride, 608
Glipizide, 609–610
Glucophage (*see also* metformin HCl), 613–614
Glucotrol (*see also* glipizide), 609–610
Glucotrol XL (*see also* glipizide), 609–610
Glyburide, 611–612
Glycopyrrolate, 657–658
Glynase Pres Tab (*see also* glyburide), 611–612
Gold sodium thiomalate, 367–368
Gonadorelin acetate, 589
Gonadotropin, human chorionic, 590

Gonadotropin-releasing hormone, synthetic, 589
Granisetron HCl, 641
Grifulvin V (*see also* griseofulvin), 281–282
Griseofulvin, 281–282
Gris-PEG (*see also* griseofulvin), 281–282
Growth hormone, 582
Guanabenz acetate, 29, 88
Guanadrel, 30–31
Guanethidine, 32–33
Guanethidine monosulfate, 88
Guanfacine HCl, 34, 88

Halcinonide, 680
Halcion (*see also* triazolam), 488
Haldol (*see also* haloperidol), 465
Halobetasol propionate, 677–678
Halog (*see also* halcinonide), 680
Haloperidol, 465
Halotestin (*see also* fluoxymesterone), 547
Heparin sodium, 156
Hexalen (*see also* altretamine), 321–322
Hismanal (*see also* astemizole), 195–196
Hivid (*see also* zalcitabine), 298
Humalog (*see also* insulin lispro), 624–625
Humatrope (*see also* somatropin), 582
Humegon (*see also* menotropins), 591–592
Humorsol (*see also* demecarium bromide), 697
Humulin L (*see also* insulin, Lente human, intermediate acting), 622
Humulin N (*see also* insulin, NPH human, intermediate acting), 621
Humulin R (*see also* insulin, regular human, rapid acting), 618–619
Humulin U (*see also* insulin, Ultralente human, slow acting), 623

Hydeltrasol (*see also* prednisolone), 574
Hydeltra-T.B.A. (*see also* prednisolone), 574
Hydralazine HCl, 35, 88
Hydrea (*see also* hydroxyurea), 341
Hydrochlorothiazide, 88, 116
Hydrocodone bitartrate, 384
Hydrocortisone, 572, 683
Hydrocortisone acetate, 572, 683
Hydrocortisone butyrate, 682
Hydrocortisone cypionate, 572
Hydrocortisone sodium phosphate, 572
Hydrocortisone sodium succinate, 572
Hydrocortisone valerate, 682
Hydrocortone (*see also* hydrocortisone), 572
HydroDiuril (*see also* hydrochlorothiazide), 116
Hydroflumethiazide, 88, 117
Hydromorphone HCl, 385–386
Hydromox (*see also* quinethazone), 121
Hydro-Par (*see also* hydrochlorothiazide), 116
Hydroxychloroquine sulfate, 303–304
Hydroxyurea, 341
Hydroxyzine HCl, 204, 425, 642
Hydroxyzine pamoate, 204, 425, 642
Hygroton (*see also* chlorthalidone), 115
Hylorel (*see also* guanadrel), 30–31
Hyoscyamine sulfate, 659
Hytrin (*see also* terazosin HCl), 19–20

Ibuprofen, 402
Ilosone (*see also* erythromycin estolate), 223
Ilotycin (*see also* erythromycin ophthalmic ointment), 221–222
Imdur (*see also* isosorbide mononitrate), 80
Imipramine and desipramine, 724

Imipramine HCl, 437
Imipramine pamoate, 438
Imitrex (*see also* sumatriptan succinate), 541–542
Immodium capsules (*see also* loperamide HCl), 634
Immunex (*see also* methotrexate sodium), 349–350
Imuran (*see also* azathioprine), 363–364
Indapamide, 88, 117
Inderal (*see also* propranolol HCl), 72–73, 538
Inderal LA (*see also* propranolol HCl), 72–73, 538
Indinavir sulfate, 291–292
Indocin (*see also* indomethacin), 403–404
Indocin SR (*see also* indomethacin), 403–404
Indomethacin, 403–404
Insulin, Lente human, intermediate acting (recombinant DNA origin), 622
Insulin Lispro, 624–625
Insulin, NPH human, intermediate acting (recombinant DNA origin), 621
Insulin, regular human, rapid acting (recombinant DNA origin), 618–619
Insulin, Semilente human, rapid acting (recombinant DNA origin), 620
Insulin, Ultralente human, slow acting (recombinant DNA origin), 623
Intal (*see also* cromolyn sodium), 169–170
Intal Nebulizer Solution (*see also* cromolyn sodium), 169–170
Interferon alfa-2a, 344
Interferon alfa-2b, 342–343
Intron A (*see also* interferon alfa-2b), 342–343
Invirase (*see also* saquinavir mesylate), 296

Ipratropium bromide, 183
Irbesartan, 26, 88
Ismelin (*see also* guanethidine), 32–33
ISMO (*see also* isosorbide mononitrate), 81
Isoetharine, 184
Isoniazid, 267–268
Isoproterenol HCl, 185
Isoptin (*see also* verapamil HCl), 14–15
Isoptin SR (*see also* verapamil HCl), 14–15
Isopto Carbachol (*see also* carbachol), 696
Isopto Carpine (*see also* pilocarpine), 701
Isordil (*see also* isosorbide dinitrate), 78–79
Isordil Sub-lingual (*see also* isosorbide dinitrate), 78–79
Isordil Tembids (*see also* isosorbide dinitrate), 78–79
Isordil Titradose (*see also* isosorbide dinitrate), 78–79
Isosorbide dinitrate, 78–79
Isosorbide mononitrate, 80–82
Isradipine, 8, 88
Isuprel (*see also* isoproterenol HCl), 185
Itraconazole, 283–284

Jenest-28 (*see also* biphasic contraceptive products), 554

Kadian (SR) (*see also* morphine sulfate), 390
Keflex (*see also* cephalexin), 235
Keftab (*see also* cephalexin HCl), 235
Kemadrin (*see also* procyclidine HCl), 504
Kenacort (*see also* triamcinolone), 575
Kenalog (*see also* triamcinolone acetonide), 680, 682

Kenalog-40 (*see also* triamcinolone), 575
Kerlone (*see also* betaxolol HCl), 59
Ketoconazole, 285
Ketoprofen, 405
Ketorolac tromethamine, 406–407
Klonopin (*see also* clonazepam), 455–456, 518
Kytril (*see also* granisetron HCl), 641

Labetalol HCl, 64, 88
Lamictal (*see also* lamotrigine), 519–520
Lamisil (*see also* terbinafine HCl), 286–287
Lamivudine, 293
Lamotrigine, 519–520, 724
Laniazid (*see also* isoniazid), 267–268
Lanoxicaps (*see also* digoxin), 109–110
Lanoxin (*see also* digoxin), 109–110
Lanoxin Elixir (*see also* digoxin), 109–110
Lansoprazole, 666–667
Lariam (*see also* mefloquine HCl), 305
Larodopa (*see also* levodopa), 501
Lasix (*see also* furosemide), 125–126
Ledercillin-VK (*see also* penicillin V potassium), 229
Lescol (*see also* fluvastatin sodium), 142
Leukeran (*see also* chlorambucil), 329
Leuprolide acetate, 581
Levaquin (*see also* levofloxacin), 240
Levatol (*see also* penbutolol sulfate), 70
Levbid (*see also* hyoscyamine sulfate), 659
Levlen (*see also* monophasic contraceptive products), 562
Levodopa, 501
Levodopa and carbidopa, 499–500
Levo-Dromoran (*see also* levorphanol tartrate), 388
Levofloxacin, 240

Levomethadyl acetate HCl, 387
Levorphanol tartrate, 388
Levo-T (*see also* levothyroxine sodium), 565–566
Levothroid (*see also* levothyroxine sodium), 565–566
Levothyroxine sodium (T_4), 565–566
Levoxyl (*see also* levothyroxine sodium), 565–566
Levsin (*see also* hyoscyamine sulfate), 659
Levsinex (*see also* hyoscyamine sulfate), 659
Librax (*see also* clidinium bromide and chlordiazepoxide HCl), 654
Librium (*see also* chlordiazepoxide HCl), 421
Lidex (*see also* fluocinonide), 680
Lidocaine, 724
Lidocaine HCl, 95
Liothyronine sodium (T_3), 567–568
Lipitor (*see also* atorvastatin calcium), 137–138
Lisinopril, 45–46, 88
Lithium, 724
Lithium carbonate, 457–458
Lithobid (*see also* lithium carbonate), 457–458
Lithonate (*see also* lithium carbonate), 457–458
Lithotabs (*see also* lithium carbonate), 457–458
LoCholest Light Powder (*see also* cholestyramine), 140–141
LoCholest Powder (*see also* cholestyramine), 140–141
Locoid (*see also* hydrocortisone butyrate), 682
Lodine (*see also* etodolac), 400
Lodine XL (*see also* etodolac), 400
Loestrin 21 (*see also* monophasic contraceptive products), 562
Loestrin Fe (*see also* monophasic contraceptive products), 562

Lomefloxacin HCl, 241
Lomotil (*see also* diphenoxylate HCl and atropine sulfate), 631–632
Lomustine, 345
Loniten (*see also* minoxidil), 36
Lo/Ovral (*see also* monophasic contraceptive products), 563
Loperamide HCl, 634
Lopid (*see also* gemfibrozil), 143–144
Lopressor (*see also* metoprolol tartrate), 67–68
Lorabid (*see also* loracarbef), 236
Loracarbef, 236
Loratadine, 205
Lorazepam, 426, 482
Losartan potassium, 27, 88
Lotensin (*see also* benazepril), 38–39
Lovastatin, 145
Lovenox (*see also* enoxaparin sodium), 155
Lozol (*see also* indapamide), 117
Lupron (*see also* leuprolide acetate), 581
Lupron Depot (*see also* leuprolide acetate), 581
Luteinizing hormone, 591–592
Lutrepulse (*see also* gonadorelin acetate), 589
Luvox (*see also* fluvoxamine maleate), 436
Lysodren (*see also* mitotane), 351

Macrobid (*see also* nitrofurantoin), 254–255
Macrodantin (*see also* nitrofurantoin), 254–255
Magnesium salicylate and choline salicylate, 396
Marinol (*see also* dronabinol), 640
Mavik (*see also* trandolapril), 53–54
Maxair (*see also* pirbuterol acetate), 188
Maxalt (*see also* rizatriptan benzoate), 539–540

Maxalt-MLT (*see also* rizatriptan benzoate), 539–540
Maxaquin (*see also* lomefloxacin HCl), 241
Maxiflor (*see also* diflorasone diacetate), 677–678, 679
Maxivate (*see also* betamethasone dipropionate), 681
Meclizine HCl, 642
Medihaler Ergotamine (*see also* ergotamine tartrate), 532–533
Medihaler-Iso (*see also* isoproterenol HCl), 185
Medrol (*see also* methylprednisolone), 573
Medroxyprogesterone, conjugated estrogens with, 556–557, 601
Mefenamic acid, 408
Mefloquine HCl, 305
Melphalan, 346–347
Menest (*see also* estrogens, esterified), 558
Menotropins, 591–592
Meperidine HCl, 388
Mepron (*see also* atovaquone), 310
Mercaptopurine, 348
Mesoridazine besylate, 466–467
Metahydrin (*see also* trichlormethiazide), 121
Metaprel (*see also* metaproterenol sulfate), 186–187
Metaproterenol sulfate, 186–187
Metformin HCl, 613–614
Methadone HCl, 389
Methadose (*see also* methadone HCl), 389
Methotrexate sodium, 349–350
Methyclothiazide, 88, 118
Methyldopa, 23–24, 88
Methylprednisolone, 573
Methylprednisolone sodiuim succinate, 573
Methyltestosterone, 548–549
Meticorten (*see also* prednisone), 574

Metoclopramide, 643–644
Metolazone, 88, 119–120
Metoprolol, 95
Metoprolol succinate, 65–66, 88
Metoprolol tartrate, 67–68, 88
Metronidazole, 315–316
Mevacor (*see also* lovastatin), 145
Mexiletine HCl, 96
Mexitil (*see also* mexiletine HCl), 96
Miacalcin (*see also* calcitonin salmon), 599–600
Micronase (*see also* glyburide), 611–612
Midamor (*see also* amiloride), 129–130
Minipress (*see also* prazosin HCl), 17
Minitran (*see also* nitroglycerin, transdermal), 86
Minocin (*see also* minocycline HCl), 216
Minocycline HCl, 216
Minoxidil, 36, 88
Mirtazapine, 439–440
Misoprostol, 668
Mistometer (*see also* isoproterenol HCl), 185
Mitotane, 351
Modicon (*see also* monophasic contraceptive products), 563
Moexipril HCl, 47, 88
Mometasone furoate, 682
Monodox (*see also* doxycycline monohydrate), 216
Mono-gesic (*see also* salsalate), 413
Monoket (*see also* isosorbide mononitrate), 82
Monophasic contraceptive products, 562–563
Monopril (*see also* fosinopril), 44
Monurol (*see also* fosfomycin tromethamine), 251
Moricizine HCl, 97
Morphine sulfate, 390
Motofen (*see also* difenoxin HCl and atropine sulfate), 629–630

Motrin (*see also* ibuprofen), 402
MS Contin (*see also* morphine sulfate), 390
MSIR (*see also* morphine sulfate), 390
Myambutol (*see also* ethambutol HCl), 263–264
Mycobutin (*see also* rifabutin), 271–272
Myidil (*see also* triprolidine HCl), 209
Mykrox (*see also* metolazone), 119–120
Myleran (*see also* busulfan), 324–325
Myochrysine (*see also* gold sodium thiomalate), 367–368
Mysoline (*see also* primidone), 525–526

Nabumetone, 409
Nadolol, 69, 88, 97
Nalfon (*see also* fenoprofen calcium), 401
Nalfon 200 (*see also* fenoprofen calcium), 401
Nalidixic acid, 252–253
Naloxone HCl and pentazocine HCl, 391
Naprosyn (*see also* naproxen), 410–411
Naprosyn Suspension (*see also* naproxen), 410–411
Naproxen, 410–411
Naproxen sodium, 410–411
Naqua (*see also* trichlormethiazide), 121
Nardil (*see also* phenelzine sulfate), 445–446
Naritriptan HCl, 536–537
Naturetin (*see also* bendroflumethiazide), 111–112
Navane (*see also* thiothixene), 477–478
Nebcin (*see also* tobramycin sulfate), 260
Nedocromil sodium, 174–175

Nefazodone HCl, 441
NegGram (*see also* nalidixic acid), 252–253
Nelfinavir mesylate, 294
Nelova (*see also* monophasic contraceptive products), 563
Nelova 10/11 (*see also* biphasic contraceptive products), 554
Neoral (*see also* cyclosporine), 365–366
Netilmicin, 724
Neurontin (*see also* gabapentin), 517–518
Nevirapine, 295
Nicardipine HCl, 9–10, 88
Nico-Vert (*see also* dimenhydrinate), 202
Nifedipine, 11–12, 88
Nimodipine, 13
Nimotop (*see also* nimodipine), 13
Nisaval (*see also* pyrilamine maleate), 207
Nitro-Bid (*see also* nitroglycerin, topical), 87
Nitro-Derm (*see also* nitroglycerin, transdermal), 86
Nitrodisc (*see also* nitroglycerin, transdermal), 86
Nitro-Dur (*see also* nitroglycerin, transdermal), 86
Nitrofurantoin, 254–255
Nitroglycerin, 83–87, 88
Nitroglycerin, sublingual, 83–84
Nitroglycerin, topical, 87
Nitroglycerin, transdermal, 86
Nitroglycerin, translingual, 85
Nitrol (*see also* nitroglycerin, topical), 87
Nitrolingual Spray (*see also* nitroglycerin, translingual), 85
Nitrostat (*see also* nitroglycerin, sublingual), 83–84
Nizatidine, 669
Nizoral (*see also* ketoconazole), 285

Nolvadex (*see also* tamoxifen citrate), 353–354
Nordette (*see also* monophasic contraceptive products), 563
Norditropin (*see also* somatropin), 582
Norethin 1/35E (*see also* monophasic contraceptive products), 563
Norethin 1/50M (*see also* monophasic contraceptive products), 563
Norfloxacin, 242
Norinyl 1 + 35 (*see also* monophasic contraceptive products), 563
Norinyl 1 + 50 (*see also* monophasic contraceptive products), 563
Normiflo (*see also* ardeparin sodium), 151–152
Normodyne (*see also* labetalol HCl), 64
Noroxin (*see also* norfloxacin), 242
Norpace (*see also* disopyramide phosphate), 91–92
Norpace CR (*see also* disopyramide phosphate), 91–92
Norpramin (*see also* desipramine HCl), 433
Nortriptyline, 724
Nortriptyline and amitriptyline, 724
Nortriptyline HCl, 442
Norvasc (*see also* amlodipine besylate), 3
Norvir (*see also* ritonavir), 296
Novo-Lexin (*see also* cephalexin), 235
Novolin L (*see also* insulin, Lente human, intermediate acting), 622
Novolin N (*see also* insulin, NPH human, intermediate acting), 621
Novolin R (*see also* insulin, regular human, rapid acting), 618–619
Nu-Cephalex (*see also* cephalexin), 235
Numorphan (*see also* oxymorphone HCl), 391
Nutropin (*see also* somatropin), 582

Octreotide acetate, 635–636
Ocusert Pilo-20 (*see also* pilocarpine), 701
Ocusert Pilo-40 (*see also* pilocarpine), 701
Ofloxacin, 243
Ogen (*see also* estropipate), 561
Olanzapine, 468–469
Omeprazole, 670–671
Omnipen (*see also* ampicillin), 228
Oncovin (*see also* vincristine sulfate), 355–356
Ondansetron, 645–646
Opium tincture, camphorated, 638
Opium tincture, deodorized, 637
Optimine (*see also* azatadine maleate), 197
OraMorph SR (*see also* morphine sulfate), 390
Orap (*see also* pimozide), 471–472
Orasone (*see also* prednisone), 574
Oretic (*see also* hydrochlorothiazide), 116
Oreton Methyl (*see also* methyltestosterone), 548–549
Orgaran (*see also* danaparoid sodium), 154
Orinase (*see also* tolbutamide), 616
Orlaam (*see also* levomethadyl acetate HCl), 387
Ortho-Cyclen (*see also* monophasic contraceptive products), 563
Ortho-est (*see also* estropipate), 561, 601
Ortho-Novum (*see also* monophasic contraceptive products), 563
Ortho-Novum 7/7/7 (*see also* triphasic contraceptive products), 554
Ortho-Novum 10/11 (*see also* biphasic contraceptive products), 554
Ortho Tri-Cyclen (*see also* triphasic contraceptive products), 554
Orudis (*see also* ketoprofen), 405
Oruvail (*see also* ketoprofen), 405

Ovcon-50 (*see also* monophasic contraceptive products), 563
Ovral (*see also* monophasic contraceptive products), 563
Oxaprozin, 412
Oxazepam, 427
Oxycodone HCl, 390
OxyContin (*see also* oxycodone HCl), 390
Oxymorphone HCl, 391
Oxytetracycline, 217

Paclitaxel, 352
Pamelor (*see also* nortriptyline HCl), 442
Paraplatin (*see also* carboplatin), 326–327
Paregoric, 638
Parlodel (*see also* bromocriptine mesylate), 498, 585–586
Parlodel Snap Tabs (*see also* bromocriptine mesylate), 498, 585–586
Parnate (*see also* tranylcypromine sulfate), 448
Paroxetine HCl, 443–444, 459
Paxil (*see also* paroxetine HCl), 443–444, 459
PBZ (*see also* tripelennamine HCl), 209
PBZ-SR (*see also* tripelennamine HCl), 209
PCE (*see also* erythromycin tablets, delayed-release), 221–222
Pediapred (*see also* prednisolone), 574
Penbutolol sulfate, 70, 88
Penetrex (*see also* enoxacin), 239
Penicillamine, 369–370
Penicillin V potassium, 229
Pentazocine HCl and naloxone HCl, 391
PenVee K (*see also* penicillin V potassium), 229
Pepcid (*see also* famotidine), 664–665

Pergolide mesylate, 502–503
Pergonal (*see also* menotropins), 591–592
Periactin (*see also* cyproheptadine), 200
Perindopril erbumine, 48
Permax (*see also* pergolide mesylate), 502–503
Perphenazine, 470, 647
Phenelzine sulfate, 445–446
Phenergan (*see also* promethazine HCl), 206–207, 483–484, 647
Phenetron Lanacaps (*see also* chlorpheniramine maleate), 199
Phenetron Syrup (*see also* chlorpheniramine maleate), 199
Phenobarbital, 482, 521–522, 724
Phenylpropanolamine bitartrate, 731
Phenylpropanolamine HCl, 731
Phenytoin, 523–524, 724
Phenytoin sodium, 98
Pilocar (*see also* pilocarpine), 701
Pilocarpine, 701
Pimozide, 471–472
Pindolol, 71, 88
Pirbuterol acetate, 188
Piroxicam, 412
Plaquenil (*see also* hydroxychloroquine sulfate), 303–304
Platinol (*see also* cisplatin), 330–331
Platinol-AQ (*see also* cisplatin), 330–331
Plavix (*see also* clopidogrel bisulfate), 159–160
Plendil (*see also* felodipine), 7
Poladex T.D. (*see also* dexchlorpheniramine maleate), 201
Polaramine (*see also* dexchlorpheniramine maleate), 201
Polaramine Repetabs (*see also* dexchlorpheniramine maleate), 201
Polythiazide, 88, 121
Ponstel (*see also* mefenamic acid), 408

Pravachol (*see also* pravastatin sodium), 146
Pravastatin sodium, 146
Prazosin HCl, 17, 88
Precose (*see also* acarbose), 605
Prednisolone, 574
Prednisolone sodium phosphate, 574
Prednisolone terbutate, 574
Prednisone, 574
Pregnyl (*see also* gonadotropin, human chorionic), 590
Prelone (*see also* prednisolone), 574
Premarin (*see also* estrogens, conjugated), 554–555, 601
Premphase (*see also* estrogens, conjugated, plus medroxyprogesterone), 556–557, 601
Prempro (*see also* estrogens, conjugated, plus medroxyprogesterone), 556–557, 601
Prevacid (*see also* lansoprazole), 666–667
Prilosec (*see also* omeprazole), 670–671
Primidone, 525–526
Prinivil (*see also* lisinopril), 45–46
Pro-Banthine (*see also* propantheline bromide), 660
Probenecid, 375–376
Procainamide, 724
Procainamide and NAPA, 724
Procainamide HCl, 98–99
Procan SR (*see also* procainamide HCl), 98–99
Procanbid-extended release (*see also* procainamide HCl), 98–99
Procardia (*see also* nifedipine), 11–12
Procardia XL (*see also* nifedipine), 11–12
Prochlorperazine, 473–474, 647
Procyclidine HCl, 504
Profasi (*see also* gonadotropin, human chorionic), 590

Progesterone gel, 593–594
Promethazine HCl, 206–207, 483–484, 647
Pronestyl (*see also* procainamide HCl), 98–99
Pronestyl-SR (*see also* procainamide HCl), 98–99
Propafenone HCl, 100
Propantheline bromide, 660
Propoxyphene HCl, 393
Propoxyphene napsylate, 392–393
Propranolol HCl, 72–73, 88, 101, 538
Propulsid (*see also* cisapride), 663
Prosom (*see also* estazolam), 480–481
Protriptyline HCl, 447
Protropin (*see also* somatropin), 582
Proventil (*see also* albuterol sulfate), 180–181
Proventil Repetabs (*see also* albuterol sulfate), 180–181
Prozac (*see also* fluoxetine HCl), 434–435
Pseudoephedrine, 732
Pulmicort Turbuhaler (*see also* budesonide), 167–168
Purinethol (*see also* mercaptopurine), 348
Pyrazinamide, 269–270
Pyrilamine maleate, 207
Pyrimethamine, 306–307

Quazepam, 485
Questran Light (*see also* cholestyramine), 140–141
Questran Powder (*see also* cholestyramine), 140–141
Quinaglute Dura-Tabs (*see also* quinidine gluconate), 101–102
Quinapril, 88
Quinapril HCl, 49–50
Quinethazone, 121
Quinidex Extentabs (*see also* quinidine sulfate), 104
Quinidine, 724

Quinidine gluconate, 101–102
Quinidine polygalacturonate, 103
Quinidine sulfate, 104
Quinine sulfate, 308–309
Quinora (*see also* quinidine sulfate), 104

Ramipril, 51–52, 88
Rantidine HCl, 672–673
Reglan (*see also* metoclopramide), 643–644
Relafen (*see also* nabumetone), 409
Remeron (*see also* mirtazapine), 439–440
Renese (*see also* polythiazide), 121
Repronex (*see also* menotropins), 591–592
Rescriptor (*see also* delavirdine mesylate), 288
Reserpine, 37, 88
Respbid (*see also* theophylline), 191–192
Restoril (*see also* temazepam), 487
Retrovir (*see also* zidovudine), 299–300
Rezulin (*see also* troglitazone), 617
Rheumatrex (*see also* methotrexate sodium), 349–350
Ridaura (*see also* auranofin), 359–360
Rifabutin, 271–272
Rifadin (*see also* rifampin), 273–274
Rifampin, 273–274
Rimactane (*see also* rifampin), 273–274
Risperdal (*see also* risperidone), 475–476
Risperidone, 475–476
Ritonavir, 296
Rizatriptan benzoate, 539–540
Robinul (*see also* glycopyrrolate), 657–658
Robinul Forte (*see also* glycopyrrolate), 657–658

Roferon-A (*see also* interferon alfa-2a), 344
Roxanol (*see also* morphine sulfate), 390
Roxanol-T (*see also* morphine sulfate), 390
Rufen (*see also* ibuprofen), 402
Rythmol (*see also* propafenone HCl), 100

Saleto (*see also* ibuprofen), 402
Salflex (*see also* salsalate), 413
Salicylates, 724
Salmeterol xinafoate, 189
Salsalate, 413
Saluron (*see also* hydroflumethiazide), 117
Sandimmune (*see also* cyclosporine), 365–366
Sandostatin (*see also* octreotide acetate), 635–636
Saquinavir mesylate, 296
Scopolamine, 648–649
Secobarbital sodium, 486
Seconal (*see also* secobarbital sodium), 486
Sectral (*see also* acebutolol HCl), 55–56
Seldane (*see also* terfenadine), 208
Selegiline HCl, 505
Septra (*see also* trimethoprim and sulfamethoxazole), 249–250
Septra DS (*see also* trimethoprim and sulfamethoxazole), 249–250
Serax (*see also* oxazepam), 427
Serentil (*see also* mesoridazine besylate), 466–467
Serevent (*see also* salmeterol xinafoate), 189
Seromycin (*see also* cycloserine), 261–262
Serophene (*see also* clomiphene citrate), 587–588
Sertraline, 447, 459

Serzone (*see also* nefazodone HCl), 441
Sildenafil citrate, 705–706
Simvastatin, 147
Sinemet (*see also* carbidopa and levodopa), 499–500
Sinemet CR (*see also* carbidopa and levodopa), 499–500
Sinequan (*see also* doxepin HCl), 433
Slo-Bid (*see also* theophylline), 191–192
Slo-Phyllin (*see also* theophylline), 191–192
Solganal (*see also* aurothioglucose), 361–362
Solu-Cortef (*see also* hydrocortisone), 572
Solu-Medrol (*see also* methylprednisolone), 573
Somatropin, 582
Sorbitrate (*see also* isosorbide dinitrate), 78–79
Sorbitrate Chewable (*see also* isosorbide dinitrate), 78–79
Sorbitrate Oral Tablets (*see also* isosorbide dinitrate), 78–79
Sorbitrate Sub-lingual (*see also* isosorbide dinitrate), 78–79
Sotalol HCl, 74–75, 88, 104
Sparfloxacin, 244
Spectrobid (*see also* bacampicillin HCl), 228
Spironolactone, 88, 131–132
Sporanox (*see also* itraconazole), 283–284
Stadol (*see also* butorphanol tartrate), 381
Stadol NS (*see also* butorphanol tartrate), 381
Stavudine, 297
Stelazine (*see also* trifluoperazine HCl), 479
Streptomycin, 725
Streptomycin sulfate, 275–276

Sucralfate, 674
Sulfamethoxazole, 247
Sulfamethoxazole and trimethoprim, 249–250
Sulfasalazine, 248
Sulindac, 413
Sumatriptan succinate, 541–542
Suprax (*see also* cefixime), 232
Surmontil (*see also* trimipramine maleate), 451
Symadine (*see also* amantadine HCl), 493–494
Symmetrel (*see also* amantadine HCl), 493–494
Synalar (*see also* fluocinolone acetonide), 680, 682
Synemol (*see also* fluocinolone acetonide), 680, 682
Synthroid (*see also* levothyroxine sodium), 565–566

Tacrine HCl, 688–689
Tagamet (*see also* cimetidine), 661–662
Talwin Nx (*see also* pentazocine HCl and naloxone HCl), 391
Tambocor (*see also* flecainide acetate), 93–94
Tamoxifen citrate, 353–354
Tamsulosin HCl, 18
Tasmar (*see also* tolcapone), 506
Tavist (*see also* clemastine fumarate), 200
Taxol (*see also* paclitaxel), 352
Taxotere (*see also* docetaxel), 333–334
Tebamide (*see also* trimethobenzamide HCl), 651
Tegretol (*see also* carbamazepine), 511–512
Tegretol-XR (*see also* carbamazepine), 511–512
Telador (*see also* betamethasone dipropionate), 681

Temazepam, 487
Temovate (*see also* clobetasol propionate), 677–678
Tenex (*see also* guanfacine HCl), 34
Tenormin (*see also* atenolol), 57–58
Terazosin HCl, 19–20, 88
Terbinafine HCl, 286–287
Terbutaline sulfate, 190
Terfenadine, 208
Terramycin (*see also* oxytetracycline), 217
Testoderm (*see also* testosterone, scrotal system), 551–552
Testoderm with Adhesive (*see also* testosterone, scrotal system), 551–552
Testosterone, injectable, 550
Testosterone, scrotal system, 551–552
Testosterone, topical system, 553
Testred (*see also* methyltestosterone), 548–549
Tetracycline HCl, 217
T-Gen (*see also* trimethobenzamide HCl), 651
Thalitone (*see also* chlorthalidone), 115
Theo-24 Extended Release (*see also* theophylline), 191–192
Theobid (*see also* theophylline), 191–192
Theo-Dur (*see also* theophylline), 191–192
Theolair (*see also* theophylline), 191–192
Theophylline, 191–192, 724
Theo-X Extended Release (*see also* theophylline), 191–192
Thiethylperazine maleate, 650
Thiothixene, 477–478
Thorazine (*see also* chlorpromazine), 460–462, 639
Tiazac (*see also* diltiazem HCl), 5–6
Ticlid (*see also* ticlopidine HCl), 161–162

Ticlopidine HCl, 161–162
Tigan (see also trimethobenzamide HCl), 651
Tilade (see also nedocromil sodium), 174–175
Timolol, 104
Timolol maleate, 76–77, 88, 543, 702
Timoptic (see also timolol maleate), 702
Timoptic Ocudose (see also timolol maleate), 702
Timoptic-XE (see also timolol maleate), 702
Tobramycin, 725
Tobramycin sulfate, 260
Tocainide, 724
Tocainide HCl, 105
Tofranil (see also imipramine HCl), 437
Tofranil-PM (see also imipramine pamoate), 438
Tolazamide, 615
Tolbutamide, 616
Tolcapone, 506
Tolectin 200 (see also tolmetin sodium), 414
Tolectin 600 (see also tolmetin sodium), 414
Tolectin DS (see also tolmetin sodium), 414
Tolinase (see also tolazamide), 615
Tolmetin sodium, 414
Tonocard (see also tocainide HCl), 105
Topamax (see also topiramate), 527
Topicort (see also desoximetasone), 679
Topicort-LP (see also desoximetasone), 682
Topiramate, 527
Toprol-XL (see also metoprolol succinate), 65–66
Toradol (see also ketorolac tromethamine), 406–407

Torecan (see also thiethylperazine maleate), 650
Tornalate (see also bitolterol mesylate), 182
Torsemide, 88, 127–128
Trandate (see also labetalol HCl), 64
Trandolapril, 53–54, 88
Transderm-Nitro (see also nitroglycerin, transdermal), 86
Transderm-Scop (see also scopolamine), 648–649
Tranxene SD (see also clorazepate dipotassium), 422–423
Tranxene SD Half Strength (see also clorazepate dipotassium), 422–423
Tranxene T-Tab (see also clorazepate dipotassium), 422–423
Tranylcypromine sulfate, 448
Trazodone HCl, 449–450
Trecator-SC (see also ethionamide), 265–266
Triamcinolone, 575
Triamcinolone acetonide, 176, 575, 680, 682
Triamcinolone diacetate, 575
Triamolone 40 (see also triamcinolone), 575
Triamonide 40 (see also triamcinolone), 575
Triamterene, 88, 133
Triazolam, 488
Trichlormethiazide, 88, 121
Tridesilon (see also desonide), 683
Trifluoperazine HCl, 479
Trihexyphenidyl HCl, 507
Trilafon (see also perphenazine), 470, 647
Tri-Levlen (see also triphasic contraceptive products), 554
Trilisate (see also choline salicylate and magnesium salicylate), 396
Trilone (see also triamcinolone), 575
Trimazide (see also trimethobenzamide HCl), 651

Trimethobenzamide HCl, 651
Trimethoprim and sulfamethoxazole, 249–250
Trimipramine maleate, 451
Tri-Norinyl (*see also* triphasic contraceptive products), 554
Triostat (*see also* liothyronine sodium), 567–568
Tripelennamine HCl, 209
Triphasic contraceptive products, 554
Triphasil (*see also* triphasic contraceptive products), 554
Triprolidine HCl, 209
Troglitazone, 617
Trusopt (*see also* dorzolamide HCl), 699
Tusstat (*see also* diphenhydramine), 203

Ultracef (*see also* cefadroxil monohydrate), 232
Ultravate (*see also* halobetasol propionate), 677–678
Unicontin (*see also* theophylline), 191–192
Unicort (*see also* betamethasone benzoate), 681
Uni-Dur Extended-Release (*see also* theophylline), 191–192
Uniphyl (*see also* theophylline), 191–192
Univasc (*see also* moexipril HCl), 47

Valisone (*see also* betamethasone valerate), 679, 681
Valium (*see also* diazepam), 424–425
Valproic acid, 528, 724
Valsartan, 28, 88
Vanceril (*see also* beclomethasone dipropionate), 165–166
Vanceril Double Strength (*see also* beclomethasone dipropionate), 165–166
Vancocin HCl (*see also* vancomycin HCl), 317–318

Vancomycin, 725
Vancomycin HCl, 317–318
Vantin (*see also* cefpodoxime proxetil), 233
Vascor (*see also* bepridil HCl), 4
Vasopressin, 578–579
Vasotec (*see also* enalapril maleate), 42–43
Vectrin (*see also* minocycline HCl), 216
Veetids (*see also* penicillin V potassium), 229
Veltane (*see also* brompheniramine maleate), 198
Venlafaxine HCl, 452–453
Ventolin (*see also* albuterol; albuterol sulfate), 180–181
Ventolin Nebules (*see also* albuterol sulfate), 180–181
Ventolin Rotacaps (*see also* albuterol sulfate), 180–181
VePesid (*see also* etoposide), 337
Verapamil, 88, 106
Verapamil HCl, 14–15
Verelan (*see also* verapamil HCl), 14–15
Viagra (*see also* sildenafil citrate), 705–706
Vibramycin Calcium (*see also* doxycycline calcium), 215
Vibramycin Hyclate (*see also* doxycycline hyclate), 215
Vibramycin Monohydrate (*see also* doxycycline monohydrate), 216
Vibra-Tabs (*see also* doxycycline hyclate), 215
Videx (*see also* didanosine), 289–290
Vincristine sulfate, 355–356
Viracept (*see also* nelfinavir mesylate), 294
Viramune (*see also* nevirapine), 295
Visken (*see also* pindolol), 71
Vistaril (*see also* hydroxyzine pamoate), 204, 425, 642

Vivactil (*see also* protriptyline HCl), 447
Vivelle (*see also* estradiol transdermal system), 559–560
Voltaren (*see also* diclofenac sodium), 398
Voltaren-XR (*see also* diclofenac sodium), 398

Warfarin sodium, 157–158
Wellbutrin (*see also* bupropion HCl), 430–431
Wellbutrin SR (*see also* bupropion HCl), 430–431
Westcort (*see also* hydrocortisone valerate), 682
Wigraine (*see also* ergotamine tartrate and caffeine), 534
Wytensin (*see also* guanabenz acetate), 29

Xanax (*see also* alprazolam), 417–418, 454
Xylocaine (*see also* lidocaine HCl), 95

Zafirlukast, 177–178
Zagam (*see also* sparfloxacin), 244
Zalcitabine, 298
Zantac (*see also* rantidine HCl), 672–673
Zarontin (*see also* ethosuximide), 515–516
Zaroxolyn (*see also* metolazone), 119–120
Zebeta (*see also* bisoprolol fumarate), 60
Zerit (*see also* stavudine), 297
Zestril (*see also* lisinopril), 45–46
Zidovudine, 299–300
Zileuton, 179
Zithromax (*see also* azithromycin dihydrate), 218
Zocor (*see also* simvastatin), 147
Zofran (*see also* ondansetron), 645–646
Zolmitriptan, 543–544
Zoloft (*see also* sertraline), 447, 459
Zolpidem tartrate, 489–490
Zomig (*see also* zolmitriptan), 543–544
Zyban (*see also* bupropion HCl), 430–431
Zyflo (*see also* zileuton), 179
Zyloprim (*see also* allopurinol), 371–372
Zyprexa (*see also* olanzapine), 468–469
Zyrtec (*see also* cetirizine HCl), 199